Lecture Notes of the Institute for Computer Sciences, Social Informatics and Telecommunications Engineering 181

More information about this series at http://www.springer.com/series/8197

Kostas Giokas · Laszlo Bokor
Frank Hopfgartner (Eds.)

eHealth 360°

International Summit on eHealth
Budapest, Hungary, June 14–16, 2016
Revised Selected Papers

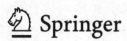 Springer

Editors
Kostas Giokas
Applied Informatics in mHealth
National Technical University of Athens
Zografou
Greece

Frank Hopfgartner
University of Glasgow
Glaswow
UK

Laszlo Bokor
Budapest University of Technology
Budapest
Hungary

ISSN 1867-8211 ISSN 1867-822X (electronic)
Lecture Notes of the Institute for Computer Sciences, Social Informatics
and Telecommunications Engineering
ISBN 978-3-319-49654-2 ISBN 978-3-319-49655-9 (eBook)
DOI 10.1007/978-3-319-49655-9

Library of Congress Control Number: 2016958513

Printed on acid-free paper

This Springer imprint is published by Springer Nature
The registered company is Springer International Publishing AG
The registered company address is: Gewerbestrasse 11, 6330 Cham, Switzerland

Preface

These proceedings represent the work presented by the researchers who participated in the eHealth360 International Summit, that took place during June 14–16 in Budapest, Hungary. This summit represented the latest work by researchers in the area of electronic health, especially in the way that technology empowers health care.

This particular summit was strengthened by the fact that six co-located conferences took place (Track on Games for Well-being, Track on Wearables in Healthcare, Track on Personal, Pervasive and Mobile Health, Track on IoT and Big Data Technologies for Health Care, Track on Mobile Medical Multimedia Technologies, Applications and Services and Track on Ambient-Assisted Living Technologies Based on Internet of Things), each one focusing in the specialized domain with the help of high-quality papers.

However, the main reason why eHealth360 was so successful, was the traction it generated among the top health care technology providers (such as LG) and representatives from the Hungarian government and the European Union. The pace of the conference was very fast with exciting speakers, lively presentations, and alternating discussion themes (round tables, birds of feather, technology forecasts, keynotes) and a setup that kept the audience very energized. With an excellent balance between the technology and the community track, the audience proved to be the most important challenge for the speakers. The audience posed very difficult questions on the societal challenges we are facing.

Although I am sure that you will enjoy the high-quality articles presented during the conference, you can never beat the vibe of real-life participation in such a wonderful event. Looking forward to next year's event and hope to see all of you there.

October 2016   Kostas Giokas

Organization

IoTCare 2016

Steering Committee

Imrich Chlamtac	Create-Net, EAI (Co-chair)
Abdur Rahim Biswas	CREATE-NET, Italy (Co-chair)
Timo Jamsa	University of Oulu, Finland

Organizing Committee

General Chairs

Timo Jamsa	University of Oulu, Finland
Abdur Rahim Biswas	CREATE-NET, Italy

Technical Program Committee Chair

Vera Stavroulaki	WINGS ICT Solutions, Greece

Technical Program Committee Co-chair

Kazuo Hashimoto	Center for Research Strategy, Waseda University, Japan

Publicity and Social Media Chair

Rango Rao Venkatesha Prasad	TU Deflt, The Netherlands

Publicity and Social Media Co-chair

Shinsaku Kiyomoto	Senior Manager, KDDI R&D Labs, Japan

Sponsorship and Exhibits Chair

Philippe Cousin	EGM, France

Publications Chairs

Stylianos Georgoulas	Research Fellow, ICS, University of Surrey, UK

Web Chair

Iqbal Hossain, Programmer	CSE, BUET, Bangladesh

GOWELL 2016

Steering Committee

Imrich Chlamtac	CREATE-NET, Italy (Chair)
Laura Anna Ripamonti	University of Milan, Italy
Dario Maggiorini	University of Milan, Italy

Organizing Committee

General Co-chairs

Laura Anna Ripamonti	University of Milan, Italy
Dario Maggiorini	University of Milan, Italy
Daniela Villani	Università Cattolica del S. Cuore, Italy

Technical Program Chair

Davide Gadia	University of Milan, Italy

Publicity and Social Media Chairs

Claudio Palazzi	University of Padova, Italy
Armir Bujari	University of Padova, Italy

Publications Chair

Davide Gadia	University of Milan, Italy

Web Chair

Dario Maggiorini	University of Milan, Italy

HealthWear 2016

Steering Committee

Imrich Chlamtac	CREATE-NET, Italy (Chair)
Frank Hopfgartner	University of Glasgow, UK

Organizing Committee

General Chair

Frank Hopfgartner	University of Glasgow, UK

Technical Program Chairs

Huiru (Jane) Zheng	Ulster University, UK
Jakob Eg Larsen	Technical University of Denmark, Denmark

Publicity and Social Media Chair

Federica Cena	Technical University of Turin, Italy

Publications Chairs

Thierry Urruty	University of Poitiers, France
Jochen Meyer	OFFIS, Germany

Panels Chairs

Cathal Gurrin	INSIGHT Centre, Ireland
Udo Kruschwitz	University of Essex, UK

Tutorials Chairs

Klaus Schöffmann	Klagenfurt University, Austria
Na Li	Dublin City University, Ireland

Web Chair

Till Plumbaum	Berlin Institute of Technology, Germany

PPmH 2016

Steering Committee

Imrich Chlamtac	CREATE-NET, Italy (Chair)
Emmanouil G. Spanakis	Foundation for Research and Technology — Hellas (FORTH), Greece

Organizing Committee

General Chair

Emmanouil G. Spanakis	Foundation for Research and Technology — Hellas (FORTH), Greece

General Co-chairs

Kostas Marias	Institute of Computer Science at FORTH (ICS-FORTH), Greece
Manolis Tsiknakis	Technological Educational Institute of Crete, Computational BioMedicine, Laboratory (CBML) FORTH-ICS, Greece

Vangelis Sakkalis   Institute of Computer Science at FORTH
                             (ICS-FORTH), Greece

Technical Program Chair

Emmanouil G. Spanakis   Foundation for Research and Technology — Hellas
                             (FORTH), Greece

Publicity and Social Media Chair

Matthew Pediaditis   Institute of Computer Science at FORTH
                             (ICS-FORTH), Greece

Workshops Chairs

Vangelis Sakkalis   Institute of Computer Science at FORTH
                             (ICS-FORTH), Greece
Kostas Marias   Institute of Computer Science at FORTH
                             (ICS-FORTH), Greece
Manolis Tsiknakis   Technological Educational Institute of Crete,
                             Computational BioMedicine Laboratory (CBML)
                             FORTH-ICS, Greece

Sponsorship and Exhibits Chair

Matthew Pediaditis   Institute of Computer Science at FORTH
                             (ICS-FORTH), Greece

Publications Chair

Emmanouil G. Spanakis   Foundation for Research and Technology — Hellas
                             (FORTH), Greece

Web Chair

Matthew Pediaditis   Institute of Computer Science at FORTH
                             (ICS-FORTH), Greece

M3Apps 2016

Steering Committee

Imrich Chlamtac   CREATE-NET, Italy (Chair)
Csaba A. Szabo   Budapest University of Technology and Economics,
                             Hungary (Co-chair)

Organizing Committee

General Chair

László Bokor   Budapest University of Technology and Economics
(BME), Hungary

Technical Program Chairs

Maria Martini   Kingston University London, UK
Levente Kovács   Óbuda University, Hungary
Lorenzo Iacobelli   Thales Communications and Security SAS, France

Publicity and Social Media Chairs

Adrian Pekar   Technical University of Kosice, Slovakia
Lukasz Budzisz   Technical University of Berlin, Germany
Matteo Mazzotti   University of Bologna, Italy

Publications Chair

Tiia Ojanperä   VTT Technical Research Centre of Finland Ltd.,
Finland

Web Chair

Norbert Varga   Budapest University of Technology and Economics,
Hungary

AALIoT 2016

Steering Committee

Imrich Chlamtac   CREATE-NET, Italy (Chair)
Dimitris Koutsouris   Biomedical Engineering Laboratory,
National Technical University of Athens, Greece
Kostas Giokas   Applied Informatics in mHealth, National Technical
University of Athens, Greece

Organizing Committee

General Chair

Dimitris Koutsouris   Biomedical Engineering Laboratory,
National Technical University of Athens, Greece

General Co-chair

Kostas Giokas   Applied Informatics in mHealth, National Technical
University of Athens, Greece

Technical Program Committee Chair

Ioannis Kouris   Applied Informatics in mHealth, National Technical
                                University of Athens, Greece

Publicity and Social Media Chair

Kostas Giokas   Applied Informatics in mHealth, National Technical
                                University of Athens, Greece

Workshops Chair

Athanasios Anastasiou   Applied Informatics in mHealth, National Technical
                                University of Athens, Greece

Sponsorship and Exhibits Chair

Kostas Giokas   Applied Informatics in mHealth, National Technical
                                University of Athens, Greece

Publications Chair

Vassileia Costarides   Applied Informatics in mHealth, National Technical
                                University of Athens, Greece

Web Chair

Panagiotis Katrakazas   Applied Informatics in mHealth, National Technical
                                University of Athens, Greece

Contents

GOWELL 2016

HealthWear 2016

PPmH 2016

M3Apps + AALIoT 2016

IoTCare 2016

Remote Assistance for Elderly to Find Hidden Objects in a Kitchen

Zeeshan Asghar[1,2(✉)], Goshiro Yamamoto[3], Takafumi Taketomi[2], Christian Sandor[2], Hirokazu Kato[2], and Petri Pulli[1]

[1] Department of Information Processing Science, University of Oulu, 90014 Oulu, Finland
{zeeshan.asghar,petri.pulli}@Oulu.fi
[2] Graduate School of Information Science, Nara Institute of Science and Technology,
Takayama, Ikoma, Nara 8916-5, Japan
{takafumi-t,sandor,kato}@is.naist.jp
[3] Kyoto University Hospital, Shogoin Kawahara-cho 54, Sakyo-ku, Kyoto, Japan
goshiro@is.naist.jp

Abstract. Remote assistive technologies are one of the most promising solutions for an aging society in the future. This paper describes a design of a remote assistive system to guide elderly to find and recognize hidden objects in a kitchen through ubiquitous technologies utilizing sensing and light projection. These intelligent technologies can play a vital role in taking care of the elderly with cognitive impairments when the caregiver's lives or work far away. The main goal of this research is to provide visual guidance to elderly to overcoming the deficits of initiation, planning, attention and memory deficits while performing kitchen-based activities of daily living such as locating and identifying items for cooking. In a standard kitchen where objects can be placed in open and closed spaces, it is difficult for elderly with cognitive impairment to find and locate objects that are invisible and sometimes hidden behind other objects. In this situation the RFID technology can directly provide the location of the items and projection technology can display the image of the object at the exact location. An initial prototype has been developed and a user study with twelve elderly people has been conducted. The initial results show that the visual guidance makes the task of finding and identifying objects easier and simpler. Additionally, results show promise for further development and system can be used for other kitchen activities.

Keywords: Remote assistance · Elderly · Caregiver · RFID · Projection

1 Introduction

The world population is aging and people aged over 65 are increasing faster in number than any other age group [1]. In general, people of this age group prefer to live at home independently as long as possible and able to age well [2]. In fact, more than 31% people older than 65 or above, live independently within the European Union (EU) [3]. As people grow older it is difficult for them to live independently without assistance because of different cognitive and physical impairments. Caregivers reported that people with Mild Cognitive Impairment (MCI) with decreased initiation were cooking, using the

© ICST Institute for Computer Sciences, Social Informatics and Telecommunications Engineering 2017
K. Giokas et al. (Eds.): eHealth 2016, LNICST 181, pp. 3–8, 2017.
DOI: 10.1007/978-3-319-49655-9_1

telephone, and taking medication [4]. The kitchen is the focus of this study where elderly spent most of the time doing different activities. These activities are key for their autonomy such as cooking, preparing food, storing provisions, etc. [12]. Generally, a kitchen task comprises of a set of step-by-step instructions and to complete each step requires a different kind of objects. An object can be found in an open and a closed place in a kitchen environment. Ikeda et al. [5] and Uranishi et al. [6] have developed a kitchen assistive system to support elderly by indicating with light projection visually. These systems support them to find and work with various cooking objects located in an open place such as a table top. In this work, we improve the efficiency of the elderly and caregivers to find and locate objects from not only an open place, but also hidden places such as cabinets or drawers in a kitchen. In remote assistance, it takes time to express positions and appearances of objects located in hidden places by verbal communication. In the case when a remote caregiver is guiding an elderly in an unfamiliar environment, explanations with only verbal communication take caregiver's time and increased burden.

In this paper, we present the design and initial prototype of a remote assistive system for elderly to find and recognize objects from hidden places required during a kitchen task. The system has two main features (1) find and locate the objects used during a task (2) display image of the object at the exact location of the kitchen cabinet. To achieve this goal, we utilized Radio Frequency Identification Technology (RFID) and projection technology. Our system can minimize the cognitive overhead of elderly while storing and retrieving objects from the cabinet and shelves during a task. That can also make the kitchen task more efficient and simple. Moreover, we can reduce the workload from the caretakers and by activating and encouraging the elderly in daily activities would promote independent living.

2   Related Work

There are several related works to keep track of human or objects locations. Active Bats [7] is a high accuracy ultrasound positioning system that uses ultrasonic tags on objects or person for tracking but as a disadvantage it requires a large number of ultrasound receivers around the ceiling. Another indoor location tracking system RADAR [8] use radiofrequency signals Received Signal Strength Information (RSSI). This system is easy to setup with existing Wi-Fi network with few base stations but RSSI approaches are less accurate for smaller spaces like kitchen environment.

RFID is a contact-less technology locating objects in an indoor environment and more accurate than ultrasound and infrared-based indoor tracking technologies. Moreover, battery-free passive RFID tags offer cheap tagging option with everyday objects such as cup, plates and salad bowl, etc. in a kitchen environment [9].

Moving form tracking technologies, we discuss research work developed kitchen assistive systems. Ficocelli et al. [10] developed an assistive kitchen with speech communication and automated cabinet system to help the users to storing and retrieving items, and obtaining recipes for meal preparation. But this system lacks the picture of available items and needs RFID tags to keep track the location of the required items.

Sato et al. [11] used a projector and a depth camera to designed Shadow Cooking system to guide users with step-by-step information projected on a kitchen counter. A Smart Kitchen [12] that provides ambient assisted living services, a smart environment that increases the autonomy of elderly and disabled people in their kitchen related activities. Bonani et al. [13] used augmented reality techniques in a conventional kitchen with the projection of information on objects and surfaces to help people cook more easily and safely. We combined the RFID and projection technology to help the elderly with cognitive impairment to carry out the regular kitchen activities independently such as finding and identifying objects. This system also has a remote application for the care-givers that can assist elderly remotely whenever needed.

3 Remote Assistive System

A remote assistive system has been designed using the projection technology that augments visual prompts in a kitchen environment. The design of the remote assistive system consists of two sites: a local site where the elderly is performing the task in a kitchen and a remote site where the remote caregiver is assisting. An overview of the whole system is illustrated in Fig. 1. The system starts working when an elderly in the kitchen environment is looking for an object needed in a kitchen task and the object is hidden in the cabinet. The caregiver at the remote site using an application simply selects the required object from a list of objects. The application retrieves stored objects from the database. At the local site projection system displays the image of the selected object at the exact location. Location of the object is obtained automatically. The elderly picks up the required object easily and he/she doesn't need to search out all the shelves of the cabinet.

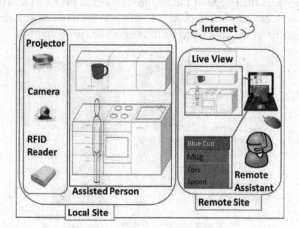

Fig. 1. Overview of the whole system: a local site where RFID and projection technology is installed to assist a person and a remote site where a caregiver using an application gives step-by-step instructions to that person via Internet.

The local site consists of a projector, camera, and an RFID system. All these tools are installed at the local site. The camera and projector attach to ceiling and pointing towards the kitchen cabinet. The projector displays the visual information on the cabinet surface and the camera only provides the live view to the remote caregiver. The live view helps the caregiver to see the real environment. Kitchen cabinet involves RFID readers in some specific shelves location. When objects with RFID tags put on these shelves, objects are detected with RFID readers. For example, if cup, glass, plates, etc. enters or leaves from the cabinet, RFID readers detects the objects. By this way, objects can be tracked on a kitchen cabinet. The remote site contains an interactive graphical interface that shows all required objects to the caregivers that assist them in any kitchen task. This application is connected via Internet to the remote site application. During a kitchen task, remote caregiver provides step-by-step instruction to the elderly using the audio connection. Remote caregiver selects the required object from the remote application and the projection system displays the image of the required object on the cabinet wall. Using this process, the elderly can easily find and locate the required object.

4   Implementation and User Study

Our prototype consists of a camera (Logitech C210 640 × 480 pixels), a projector (Epson H431B LCD 1280 × 768 pixels) and an RFID system (Takaya TR3-LN003FW4-16). We setup the proposed system in a laboratory environment. Figure 2(a) displays the camera and projector on a pole, while the RFID system is placed inside the cabinet. Figure 2(b) shows the scene from the local site with the projected image at the exact location of the cabinet. The cabinet with four shelves is shown in Fig. 2(c). The geometry between the camera, the projector, and the door surface must be calibrated in advance. The projector provides the image of the required object at the exact location and RFID reader updates the location of each object. Moreover, the camera was also intended to capture the live scene of the cabinet to facilitate remote caregiver.

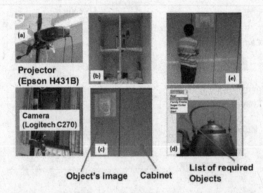

Fig. 2. (a) Our prototype system consists of a camera and a projector on the pole and RFID system placed inside the cabinet (b) the scene of the local site with the projected image (c) A cabinet with four shelves (c) Application interface used by the remote caregiver (e) live view of the local site.

The graphical user interface for remote caregiver was developed using OpenCV and MySQL database. The database is used to store the tag information attached to every kitchen object. This tag information will update the location of an object in the database automatically when an object leaves the cabinet and returns to the cabinet. The image of each object has been stored in the database along with an RFID tag. The graphical user interface lists all the stored objects used during a kitchen task. A remote caregiver using this interface selects the required object from the list and gives instruction via audio connection to the local user to pick an object from the required location. Figure 2(d) shows the interface used by the remote caregiver. After this instruction the system will show the required object at the exact location that makes the object retrieval process straightforward. Figure 2(e) shows the real scene where a person at the local site is picking an item from the cabinet. We conducted a user study with twelve elderly participants to assess the feasibility of the implemented system. All the participants performed a simple kitchen task in a laboratory environment. The task was to find and recognize objects from a kitchen cabinet. They received step-by-step instructions from the remote caregiver. Both the participants were not familiar with the kitchen environment. All the elderly participants completed the task easily and efficiently.

5   Discussion

The system is intended to help elderly living independently to locate and recognize objects from hidden places in a kitchen. The initial results show that by combining RFID technology along with the projection technology can increase the efficiency and decrease the burden of caregivers taking care of elderly people with different disabilities via Internet. Although the current prototype system uses only one projector that covers only a small area of kitchen, we can easily expand the projection area with multiple projectors. As a result of our observation, there are some limitations such as the registration of a new object when it arrives in the kitchen environment. Currently, we attached an RFID tag to each object and save it to the database before starting the actual system. To make the system more efficient in the future, the system needs to scan all the tags and register the new tag automatically. The camera can take pictures of new objects and the pictures along with the new tags can be saved to the database. In the future, we would like to compare the efficiency of our proposed system with central projection mode and with searchlight [14] system.

6   Conclusion

In this paper, we have proposed a remote assistive system that help elderly people to find objects in hidden places during a kitchen task. We implemented a prototype system with an RFID system to locate the objects from hidden places and a projector to display the image of the required object. Additionally, a user study has been conducted with twelve elderly participants in a laboratory environment to confirm feasibility of the proposed system. The initial results shows promise for the use of the system for other kitchen activities, although the user study were focusing on a small sample of older adults. Our future work will consist of adding more features to the prototype to conduct longer studies with the larger user groups.

Acknowledgements. This research work has been funded by the "Teleassistance for seniors with Dementia – A Novel Concept for Safety" project for the Japan-Finland Research Cooperative Program by Japan Science and Technology Agency.

References

1. World Population Ageing (2013). http://www.un.org/en/development/desa/. Accessed 15 May 2016
2. Marek, K., Rantz, M.: Aging in place: a new model for long-term care. Nurs. Adm. Q. **24**(3), 1–11 (2000)
3. Stula, S.: Living in Old Age in Europe-Current Developments and Challenges. German Association for Public and Private Welfare (DV), Berlin (2012)
4. Cook, C., Fay, S., Rockwood, K.: Decreased initiation of usual activities in people with mild-to-moderate alzheimer's disease: a descriptive analysis from the VISTA clinical trial. Int. Psychogeriatr. **20**(05), 952–963 (2008)
5. Ikeda, S., Asghar, Z., Hyry, J., Pulli, P., Pitkanen, A., Kato, H.: Remote assistance using visual prompts for demented elderly in cooking. In: Proceedings of the 4th International Symposium on Applied Sciences in Biomedical and Communication Technologies, pp. 1–5 (2011)
6. Uranishi, Y., Yamamoto, G., Asghar, Z., Pulli, P., Kato, H., Oshiro, O.: Work step indication with grid-pattern projection for demented senior people. In: Proceedings of 35th Annual International Conference of the IEEE Engineering in Medicine and Biology Society, pp. 4698–4701 (2013)
7. Hazas, M., Ward, A.: A novel broadband ultrasonic location system. In: Borriello, G., Holmquist, L.E. (eds.) UbiComp 2002. LNCS, vol. 2498, pp. 264–280. Springer, Heidelberg (2002). doi:10.1007/3-540-45809-3_21
8. Bahl, P., Padmanabhan, V.N.: RADAR: an in-building RF-based user location and tracking system. In: Nineteenth Annual Joint Conference of the IEEE Computer and Communications Societies. INFOCOM 2000, pp. 775–784. IEEE (2000)
9. Surie, D., Baydan, B., Lindgren, H.: proxemics awareness in kitchen As-A-Pal: tracking objects and human in perspective. In: Proceedings of the 9th International Conference on Intelligent Environments (IE), pp. 157–164. IEEE (2013)
10. Ficocelli, M., Nejat, G.: The design of an interactive assistive kitchen system. Assist. Technol. **24**(4), 246–258 (2012)
11. Sato, A., Watanabe, K., Rekimoto, J.: Shadow cooking: situated guidance for a fluid cooking experience. In: Stephanidis, C., Antona, M. (eds.) UAHCI 2014. LNCS, vol. 8515, pp. 558–566. Springer, Heidelberg (2014). doi:10.1007/978-3-319-07446-7_54
12. Blasco, R., Marco, Á., Casas, R., Cirujano, D., Picking, R.: A smart kitchen for ambient assisted living. Sensors **14**(1), 1629–1653 (2014)
13. Bonanni, L., Lee, C.H., Selker, T.: CounterIntelligence: augmented reality kitchen. In: Proceedings of CHI, vol. 2239, p. 44 (2005)
14. Butz, A., Schneider, M., Spassova, M.: Searchlight–a lightweight search function for pervasive environments. In: Ferscha, A., Mattern, F. (eds.) PERVASIVE 2004, pp. 351–356. Springer, Heidelberg (2004)

Tele-guidance Based Navigation System for the Visually Impaired and Blind Persons

Babar Chaudary[✉], Iikka Paajala, Eliud Keino, and Petri Pulli

Department of Information Processing Science (TOL),
University of Oulu, Oulu, Finland
{babar.chaudary,petri.pulli}@oulu.fi,
Iikkaa.paajala@gmail.com, eliud.keino@gmail.com

Abstract. The design and development of tele-assistance services have taken a great consideration in the domain of healthcare lately. With the growing proportion of dependent people (ageing, disabled users) in the society, tele-assistance and tele-monitoring platforms will play a significant role to provide an efficient and economical remote care. It will allow aged or disabled persons to maintain their independence and lessen the burden and cost of care by caregivers. The concept of proposed tele-guidance system is based on the idea that a blind pedestrian can be assisted by spoken instructions from a remote caregiver who receives a live video stream from a camera carried by the visually impaired persons (VIP). The ICT based assistive tools have acceptance issues by visually impaired persons. It is important while designing navigation tools for the VIP to keep in view the factors that restrain them from the adoption of assistive technology. This paper presents a tele-guidance based navigation assistance system for the VIP and blind persons and reports a qualitative study about attitude of VIP towards technological navigation assistance.

Keywords: Tele-assistance · Tele-presence · Real-time · Navigation · Remote care · Caregiver · Visually impaired · Blind · Acceptance · Qualitative · UTAUT

1 Introduction

Vision loss is a serious impairment that deprives a human of approx. 80–90% perceptual abilities and has a detrimental effect on professional, social and personal quality of life. WHO estimates the number of VIP to be 285 million, majority being over 50 years of age [1]. Even in modern societies, common understanding of blindness and the needs of the VIP are poorly identified. The white cane and more rarely a guide dog are the primary mobility aids that are mainly associated with this disability. In spite of recent remarkable advancements in information and communication technologies (ICT) and electronics, the devices that are termed as Electronic Travel Aids (ETA) are very slowly fighting their ways into the community of the VIP. In fact, no single ETA has been widely accepted by the VIP and blind as a useful aid [2].

© ICST Institute for Computer Sciences, Social Informatics and Telecommunications Engineering 2017
K. Giokas et al. (Eds.): eHealth 2016, LNICST 181, pp. 9–16, 2017.
DOI: 10.1007/978-3-319-49655-9_2

ETA is the general term encompassing a large class of assistive devices. The idea of sensory substitution, i.e. replacing lack of stimuli from one sense by appropriate stimuli for another sense is the operating principle of all ETAs [2].

Following is a functional, rather than technological classification of ETAs:

1. Obstacle Detectors
2. Environment Imagers
3. Orientation & Navigation Systems (ONSs)

The first two classes of ETAs are personal (wearable) devices that scan the environment in personal and near spaces. These devices have the task to assist VIP to intercept obstacles on their path. On the other hand, the third group is systems that offer sensing of far-spaces and can acquire data from larger scale distributed networks, e.g. GPS, GIS, Digital Maps, and through wide access to the Internet and wireless communication networks (e.g. RFID, Bluetooth, Wi-Fi, and GSM). An innovative class of ONSs is based on guiding the VIP by a remote human guide termed as Tele-assistance/Tele-guidance systems [3].

The first reported system for remote guidance of the blind was the system developed at the Brunel University, UK [4]. Three ICT technologies were combined to offer the Tele-assistance functionality; namely, GPS, GIS and video/voice transmission over the 3G mobile network. [5] was a Tele-assistance system developed using GPS, Digital maps, Bluetooth, and voice/video link was established over the GSM network within the High-Speed Downlink Packet Access (HSDPA). The system comprised of an ultra-mobile laptop computer worn in a shoulder bag, a digital webcam, and a GPS receiver attached to the shoulder strap, and a single-ear head-phone with a microphone and the assistant who remotely aided the VIP used any PC with a public IP address. In [6], the authors developed a remote guidance system where the VIP was equipped with a digital camera, a GPS receiver and a headset. Internet and GSM connections transmitted video/audio information and GPS data between the remote operator and the user. Similar tele-assistance systems were developed in [7–9].

These systems either used bulky back packs or special purpose mobile terminals to be carried by the VIP. This fact affected the acceptability of such systems by VIP at large. The advancement in computation capabilities of mobile devices and electronics miniaturization presented newer possibilities for developers to develop more user-friendly tele-guidance systems for the VIP. The proposed tele-guidance system enables remote caregiver to assist VIP through voice or vibration using live video feed of VIP's field of view and relative IoT data.

2 System Description

System comprises of two modules, VIP's terminal and remote caregiver's terminal.

2.1 VIP's Terminal

VIP's terminal comprises of four components:

(1) **Smart Phone:** It provides connectivity with the remote caregiver's terminal. The readily available sensors e.g. GPS, Gyroscope, Proximity sensor and network connectivity are used to provide remote caregiver with real time IoT data about VIP.

(2) **Bluetooth Webcam:** A Bluetooth webcam connected to the smart phone through Bluetooth connection is mounted on the chest of the VIP. It sends real time video of the field of view of the VIP to remote caregiver.

(3) **Bluetooth Headset (Earpiece, Speaker):** The Bluetooth head set is used for voice communication.

(4) **Smart Cane:** The Smart Cane contains tactile braille cell, directional vibrators, and Bluetooth interface. It is being developed as part of this project.

The VIP initiates a video call to pre-configured remote caregiver when in need of assistance. The VIP receives guidance either through voice commands using headset or smart cane's directional vibrators or tactile braille cell. During the tele-guidance session, VIP will be able to mute the voice of the remote caregiver anytime if she wants to make sense of the surroundings by listening proximity sounds. The remote caregiver will get a notification about voice muting. VIPs will be able to configure more than one person as caregiver. If either of those higher in priority is not available, the help call will be automatically handed over to the one available. The selection of caregiver and hand over can also be based on need based support (Fig. 1).

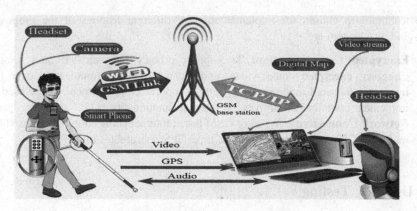

Fig. 1. Tele-guidance system concept

2.2 Remote Caregiver's Terminal

The remote caregiver can either use a workstation, tablet or phablet as terminal. It receives and initiates the VoIP video calls and renders VIP's real-time location coordinates. As VIP can configure many people as his caregiver, the system will help caregivers to mediate time and load of the assistance through availability status info. It will be studied if there is a need for the caregiver to override voice muting by VIP.

The Fig. 2 shows the system's communication and response schematic sequence.

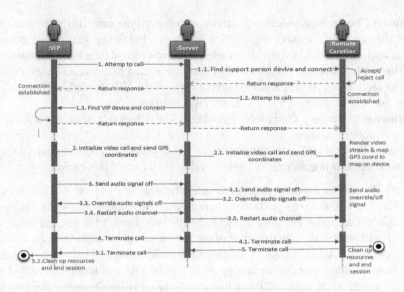

Fig. 2. The communication and response schematic

2.3   Technologies

The technologies chosen for implementation of different features of the proposed tele-guidance system are:

(1) **Encrypted Communication:** To support privacy between VIP and remote caregiver, encrypted voice, video, and location data communication over the internet is chosen. Linphone API [10] that supports ZRTP protocol will be used to implement communication over the internet functionality [11].

(2) **Network Connectivity:** Wi-Fi or GSM based internet connection will be used for making VOIP calls and sending real time GPS coordinates of VIP.

3   Usability Testing

The usability testing will be conducted with real blind and VIP in three countries i.e. Finland, Pakistan, and Sweden as part of the ongoing qualitative study by the project [12].

Usability testing by VIP:

- **1st phase:** VIP initiated tele-guidance session and followed voice commands remote caregiver to navigate.
- **2nd phase:** VIP followed tactile guidance by remote caregiver to navigate.
- **3rd phase:** User muted the voice.

Usability testing by remote caregiver:

- **1st phase:** The remote caregiver received a tele-guidance VoIP video call from the VIP and guided him through voice commands.

- **2nd phase:** The remote caregiver guided VIP through tactile commands to navigate.
- **3rd phase:** Remote caregiver gets indication voice about channel muting.
- **Test phase:** Remote caregiver overrides voice muting by VIP.

4 Study for Acceptance of Technological Navigation Assistance Aids by VIP

This study uses an extended version of Unified Theory of Acceptance and Use of Technology (UTAUT2). This model can be used by organizations to gain knowledge on improving the design and marketing of their consumer product [13]. UTAUT2 questionnaire was altered paying attention to the special needs of VIP [14] [Appendix A]. The UTAUT2 constructs are performance expectancy (PE), effort expectancy (EE), social influence (SI), facilitating conditions (FC), hedonic motivation (HM), price value (PV) and habit (HA). Questionnaire includes background questions (BG) and original UTAUT questions from constructs of anxiety (ANX) and attitude (ATT) [15]. Also few questions about special assistive technology themed (SPE) and user's previous experience (PEx) were included in the questionnaire. The questionnaire is intended for both general acceptance study about navigation assistance for VIP and for finding out acceptance issues affecting tele-guidance technologies. During analysis of collected data after earlier reported study [14], it was felt that questionnaires should be extended with users' previous experience specifically about general technological assistance, navigational technological assistance. The qualitative analysis was conducted paying attention on tele-guidance issues and user needs. Those figured out issues were sought by added question about special assistive technology (SPE), user's previous experience (PEx) and routines (RO).

4.1 Preliminary Results of Acceptance Study

19 VIP and blind are interviewed (10 female, 9 male, aged 21–82) in Oulu region in Finland. Our study supports earlier mentioned fact that no single ETA has been widely accepted by the VIP and blind people. None of the sample group used ETAs, and in fact had never even tried those apart from occasional GPS support. It seems that there may be too little information available on ETAs.

9 of the sample group didn't know enough on available tools, 9 perceived that they do have enough information on available tools. 10 participants did like the idea of sending their location information to person(s) close to them. 5 did object this matter. 12 wanted to select themselves the moments when they are being located. 1 participant would have given permission to location data when needed when support person would have been the spouse. If presented an option of new kind of assistance device, 14 of the participants were willing to alter their daily routines, and 13 were willing to use own money on those devices. Nearly all 19 participants were willing to try to learn to use new kind of assistance method.

An accompanying qualitative study addresses the caregivers' needs and acceptance of navigational caretaking tools and services [16].

5 Future Research

Future research will focus on experiments in different outdoor environments and development of efficient navigation training methods for VIP and remote caregivers. The focus will be on how to address and negotiate the situation if remote connection is lost, reduction mechanism of communication delay, and if some miscommunication or non-availability occurs between the VIP traveler and remote caregiver.

6 Conclusion

In this article, a tele-guidance navigation system for VIP in was presented. The approach of the system is based on the idea that a VIP/blind pedestrian can be assisted by spoken instructions from a remote caregiver who receives a video stream from a camera carried by the VIP. The scenarios for the usability testing of overall system for both VIP and remote caregiver to evaluate the usability were presented. A qualitative study to investigate attitude of VIP and blind persons towards navigation assistance tools was also presented.

Acknowledgement. This paper has been written as part of the ASTS (Assisted Living for Senior Citizens) Project funded by Academy of Finland and Japan Science technology Agency (JST).

Appendix: A

The Questionnaire with UTAUT Constructs		
Serial #	Construct	Questions
1	BG	Age
2	BG	Gender
3	BG	Did you acquire visual impairment with birth or did you lost vision? How long ago?
4	BG	What is your visual acuity?
5	SP	Do you have a support person(s) whom you can contact when you need help? Which hours available?
6	PEx, TA	Do you use smartphone or any other mobile device? What brand? Which apps?
7	PEx	Do you use white cane? When/why did you start using it?
8	PEx, TA	What other assistance tools do you use?
9	PEx, RO, IP	In what situations do you use navigation assistance?

(*continued*)

(continued)

Serial #	Construct	Questions
The Questionnaire with UTAUT Constructs		
10	PEx	Have you used navigation assistance tools previously? Why did you quit?
Statements		
11	HM	Navigation assistance makes going outdoors more pleasant
12	HM	I like using navigation assistance
13	PV	Navigation assistance tools are reasonably priced
14	HA	Using navigation assistance has become a habit to me
15	PE	I need navigation assistance every time I go outdoors
16	PE	In my opinion navigation assistance is useful when I am outdoors
17	PE	Navigation assistance increases the speed of doing chores
18	PE	If I use navigation assistance, I will increase my chances to get where I want
19	EE	I find navigation assistance tools easy to use
20	EE	Learning to use navigation assistance tools is easy for me
21	SI	People, who are important to me, think that I should use navigation assistance
22	IP	I find it annoying when surrounding people notice I am visually impaired
23	SI	The society has been supportive in the use of assistive
24	SI	Instructors or medical staff have been supportive in the use of assistive
25	FC	My knowledge of using navigation assistance is sufficient
26	FC	If I have problem navigation assistance, I know from who I ask help
27	ANX	I feel nervous using navigation assistance
28	ANX	Navigation assistance is somewhat intimidating
29	ATT	Using navigation assistance is a good idea
30	ATT	Navigation assistance makes me feel safe
31	PV	I am willing to spend money in order to buy new navigation assistance
32	PV, RO	I am willing to spend my time in order to learn to use new navigation assistance
33	RO	I am willing to change my daily routines, if I receive a new kind of navigation assistance
34	RO	I think that people close to me are willing to change their daily routines, if I receive a new kind of navigation assistance
35	IP, SPE	It is good that people close to me know my location
36	IP, SPE	I would like to select when people close to me know my location

References

1. Global data on visual impairments (2010). http://www.who.int/blindness/GLOBALDATAFINALforweb.pdf?ua=1
2. Bourbakis, N.: Sensing surrounding 3-D space for navigation of the blind. IEEE Eng. Med. Biol. Mag. **27**(1), 49–55 (2008)
3. Garaj, V., Hunaiti, Z., Balachandran, W.: Using remote vision: the effects of video image frame rate on visual object recognition performance. IEEE Trans. Syst. Man Cybern. Part A: Syst. Hum. **40**(4), 698–707 (2010)
4. Garaj, V., Jirawimut, R., Ptasinski, P., Cecelja, F., Balachandran, W.: A system for remote sighted guidance of visually impaired pedestrians. Br. J. Vis. Impair. **21**, 55–63 (2003)
5. Bujacz, M., Baranski, P., Moranski, M., Strumillo, P., Materka, A.: Remote mobility and navigation aid for the visually disabled. In: Sharkey, P.M., Lopesdos-Santos, P., Weiss, P.L., Brooks, A.L. (eds.) Proceedings of 7th International Conference on Disability, Virtual Reality and Associated Technologies with Art ArtAbilitation, pp. 263–270, September 2008
6. Baranski, P., Polanczyk, M., Strumillo, P.: A remote guidance system for the blind. In: Proceedings of IEEE International Conference on e-Health Networking Applications and Services, pp. 386–390 (2010)
7. Bujacz, M., Baranski, P., Moranski, M., Strumillo, P., Materka, A.: Remote guidance for the blind - a proposed teleassistance system and navigation trials. In: Proceedings of International Conference on Human System Interaction, pp. 888–892 (2008)
8. Koley, S., Mishra, R.: Voice operated outdoor navigation system for visually impaired person. Int. J. Eng. Trends Technol. **3**(2), 153–157 (2012)
9. Hunaiti, Z., Garaj, V., Balachandran, W.: A remote vision guidance system for visually impaired pedestrians. Int. J. Navig. **59**(3), 497–504 (2006)
10. http://www.linphone.org/
11. https://silentcircle.com/faq-zrtp
12. Chaudary, B., Pulli, P.: Smart cane outdoor navigation system for visually impaired and blind persons. J. Commun. Disord. Deaf Stud. Hear. Aids **2**, 125 (2014)
13. Venkatesh, V., Thong, J.Y.L., Xu, X.: Consumer acceptance and use of information technology: extending the unified theory of acceptance and use of technology. MIS Q. **36**(1), 157–178 (2012)
14. Paajala, I.J., Keränen, N.: Study for acceptance on new navigation assistance by visually impaired people. In: 2015 9th International Symposium on Medical Information and Communication Technology (ISMICT), pp. 64–67. IEEE, March 2015
15. Venkatesh, V., Morris, M.G., Davis, G.B., Davis, F.D.: User acceptance of information technology: toward a unified view. MIS Q. **27**(3), 425–478 (2003)
16. Hautala, M., Keränen, N.S., Leinonen, E., Kangas, M., Jämsä, T.: ICT use in family caregiving of elderly and disabled subjects. In: Giokas, K. (ed.) IoTCare 2016. LNCS, pp. 42–48. Springer, Heidelberg (2016)

Twinkle Megane: Near-Eye LED Indicators on Glasses for Simple and Smart Navigation in Daily Life

Aryan Firouzian[1]([✉]), Yukitoshi Kashimoto[2], Zeeshan Asghar[1,2],
Niina Keranen[1], Goshiro Yamamoto[2], and Petri Pulli[1]

[1] University of Oulu, Box 3000, 90014 Oulu, Finland
{aryan.firouzian,zeeshan.asghar,niina.s.keranen,petri.pulli}@oulu.fi
[2] Nara Institute of Science and Technology, 8916-5, Takayama, Ikoma, Nara, Japan
{kashimoto.yukitoshi.km3,goshiro}@is.naist.jp

Abstract. We present an eyeglass-type wearable device that has light emitting diode (LED) indicators on the frame of it. The device produces lighting patterns of 14 RGB LEDs near user's eyes as guiding information. Since installed LEDs on the frame of glasses are light and saving power, it is feasible to develop it for daily use. On the other hand, it cannot provide rich information such as text or images. In this study, we aim to realize a remote assistive system that provides assistive commands by lighting patterns of the eyeglass-type device from remote sites. Especially, we consider elderlies who are suffering from mild cognitive impairment as users. They would be one of potential user groups since the device does not block their sights by text or images and it can be worn in daily life without the additional sense of restraint. This paper explains our conceptual assistive system structure, a prototype eyeglass-type device with near-eye LED indicators and usability experimentation in simple navigational tasks.

Keywords: Eyeglass-type wearable device · LED indicators · Assistive system · Elderly · Mild cognitive impairment

1 Introduction

Aged society is one of the common crucial issues in the world. In this study, we mainly focus on elderly-user-friendly interface in a telepresence caretaking system. Bharucha et al. [1] estimated 28 million people suffered from dementia in 2009, and it costs 156 billion dollars annually for caretaking them directly. The analysis of the elderly adults demographic suffering from memory loss has drawn attention to the use of technologies, to involve less human and financial resources in the caretaking process. Symptoms of memory problems are categorized into several stages. In most of cases, elderly in an early stage is shifted to a severe stage because of an aggravation of their condition. Considering the increasing population of elderly suffering from memory problems, this study aims to restrain

© ICST Institute for Computer Sciences, Social Informatics and Telecommunications Engineering 2017
K. Giokas et al. (Eds.): eHealth 2016, LNICST 181, pp. 17–22, 2017.
DOI: 10.1007/978-3-319-49655-9_3

the aggravation by supporting elderly in an early stage of memory problem such as mild cognitive impairment.

In the last decades, wearable technologies have been developed to support human activities. Recently, wearable devices can have cameras, display, and some of the sensors on itself. One of the most significant aspects of development is light weight design since it needs to be comfortable for wearing in daily life. In this paper, we show near-eye LED indicators on the frame of glasses as a light-weight wearable device for an assistive interface. Although most of the elderlies suffering mild cognitive impairment can live by themselves, it is necessary to support them in different cases to avoid the aggravation of their condition due to anxiety, etc.

2   Related Work

One of the assistive applications for a daily tasks is navigation. In wearable computing research field, navigation has been studied as a major topic. Thomas et al. have developed a hands-free navigational aid by implementing head-mounted display system for outdoor guiding and they believe wearable technology has the potential for wayfinding application [9]. In recent, there are many advanced head-mounted displays such as Google Glass or Epson Moverio BT-200 and so forth. In the future, it is expected that light wearable displays provide high-quality images in front of the user. Poppinga et al. used off-the-shelf ambiglasses to provide users with notification with LED indicators and intuitive navigation instruction. Our near-eye LED indicator prototype is similar to ambiglasses and it can be customized and combined with advanced head-mounted and give simple navigational instruction. In addition, LED indicators do not disturb a user to see objects located at the center of the user's sight [8].

3   Design of Assistive System with Eyeglass-Type Device

We have developed the prototype of the indicator-based smart glasses to provide users with the visual cues, which do not interfere with their vision on the physical environment. Android applications are developed to form messages and send them as binary data to the prototypes. The application has been improved iteratively. The communication protocol between the application and device is promoted to Bluetooth low energy to provide faster communication and consume less power. The first prototype includes 12 LED indicators, while the second prototype has 14 indicators to widen different form of blinking patterns and more meaningful messages. After conducting experimentation phase, test subjects complain about physical design and weight of the device, and it derived us to design more fashionable and light-weight prototype. Figure 1(b) shows the first prototype. Figure 1(a) shows the second prototype, and the position of indicators. We followed similar approach to Poppinga et al. to form four main navigation commands. However, since our prototype cover more parts of the frame,

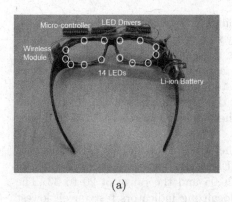
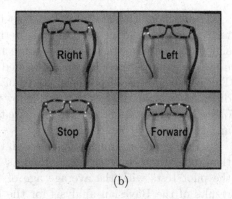

(a)   (b)

Fig. 1. (a): Second constructed prototype; white circles depict the position of LED indicators implanted on the frame of the eyeglasses. (b): Lightweight and user friendly design of the prototype

we achieved different results. In addition to LED indicators, the conceptual prototype includes the mounted camera, global positioning system, gyroscope, and step detector sensors. The abovementioned sensors and cameras help the remote caretaker to localize the senior citizens in home and city environment, while the glasses provide the visual cues to guide the users [2].

4   Experimentation of of Near-Eye LED Indicators

The design science research method is used in the study, and the experiment phase evaluates the usability of the device for further improvement [4]. We designed experiments with different user groups. The Wizard of Oz method with unstructured interviews, living lab approach, and video recording are used to collect and interpret the data [6].

We previously published a paper to explain settings, protocols and different steps of experimentation with near eye indicator display. The first step is to measure visibility of visual indicators; then forming meaningful notifications with different combination of indicators, and finally evaluate the efficiency of the notification in real life tasks. We conducted controlled experiments to measure satisfactory LED frequencies, brightnesses [7].

In the first experiment, Bayesian analysis indicates what indicators on the frame might be missed when they are blinking, and what indicators might be mistakenly chosen as blinking. In addition, the results clarify the satisfactory blinking pattern for blinking indicators including optimized brightness and frequency. In the second experiment, different sets of LED indicators' combinations blink simultaneously, and users choose interpreted navigational command such as left, right, stop and so on. We found optimized frequency, optimized brightness, and most distinguishable indicators on the frame. We formed most meaningful indicators configurations to convey navigational commands. Figure 1(b) shows the four most simple and intuitive navigational commands.

The last experiment evaluates the usability of the visual cues in a navigational task, which is a real life problem for elderly suffering from dementia. We simulate simple navigational tasks for the subjects in an open indoor environment. The users are supposed to walk on predefined map while the visual cues guide them. The map contains a specific number of stops and turning left and right with different rotation degrees. Figure 3 shows the predefined map. One of the main objectives of experiment was to evaluate the simple guidance system in 90-degree and 180-degree turning point.

Two main user groups participate in the experiments and Fig. 2 demonstrate the order of the conducted experiments. Eleven student subjects participate in the pilot tests with the average age of 26.05 and the range of 20 to 33. The results of the Bayesian analysis for the localizing indicators test unveil lowest sensitivity and specificity for nasal indicators (indicators close to the nose). In other word, the nasal LED indicators can be missed while blinking, and they can be mistakenly considered as blinking while they are not. In the next experiment, four out of 48 combinations are chosen as the navigational commands based on the users' preferences. In the last experiment, the student users accomplish their task by following the navigation guidance to walk the predefined route.

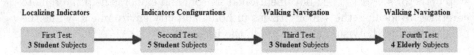

Fig. 2. It shows the sequence of the experiments and the number and type of subjects in the experiments.

Eight elderly subjects participate in the usability experiments. Four subjects suffered from severe dementia and four subjects suffered from mild dementia [3]. The severity of dementia deteriorates following track of topic and concentrating conditions [5]. These difficulties prevent severe demented elderly subjects to accomplish their tasks in experiments. Before conducting walking test, we request all the subjects to identify individual blinking indicators and confirm the meaning of navigational cues. The subjects with severe dementia fail in preliminary test and withdraw the experiment.

All the subjects suffering from mild dementia accomplish their tasks by following the visual cues and walking on the predefined route. Table 1 shows the most important collected data in the experiment. The subjects react more accurately to the visual cues at the end part of the walking task. It shows high adaptability to the system in performing the tasks. Figure 3 depicts the map of the navigation area in an open indoor environment. Considering turn-by-turn navigation, the result of the experiment proves that conveying different degree angles rotation with simple navigation instruction is the most challenging part. In turning points, subjects can detect the direction that the glasses indicate while the amount of rotation confuse them. The perception of turning commands differ in the subjects, and it means that some subjects always consider

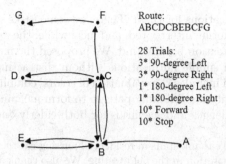

Route:
ABCDCBEBCFG

28 Trials:
3* 90-degree Left
3* 90-degree Right
1* 180-degree Left
1* 180-degree Right
10* Forward
10* Stop

Fig. 3. The predefined map contains number of rotations to the left and right in an open area.

Table 1. The relevant descriptive statistics and factors are measured for four elderly subjects suffering from mild dementia in walking experiment.

Variable	Subject A	Subject B	Subject C	Subject D
Age	81	80	83	74
Gender	Male	Male	Female	Male
Using eyeglasses	No	Yes	Yes	Yes
Mistakes by subjects	8	7	7	5
Correction via device	6	0	3	4
Correction via human assistant	2	7	4	1
Accomplishment time	220 s	390 s	286 s	136 s
Average speed	0.068 m/s	0.038 m/s	0.052 m/s	0.110 m/s
Path length	15 m	15 m	15 m	15 m

turning command as a 90-degree turn and some subjects turn continuously until the stop command is triggered. The indicators blink with the frequency of 1 Hz, 1, 5 Hz, and 2 Hz in the pilot and usability experiments. The subjects achieve the best results while indicators blink with the frequency of 1 Hz. Nevertheless, the unstructured interviews uncover that the elderly adults would rather the frequency less than 1 Hz. The test subjects also highly emphasize on the common-shape design of the glasses and they prefer the visual cues not to be seen by outsider to preserve their dignity in real life.

5   Conclusions

We have implemented an interface as eyeglasses which are common among senior citizens. The device has the potential to be used in diverse scenarios by different target user groups. Most of the users suffering from cognitive decline fail to interact with advanced user interfaces, while our prototype can be used to generate simple notifications for them. There are some tasks such as driving and biking which should not be interrupted, and meanwhile, the user needs to receive information in the attention background. We proposed the mentioned prototype to provide users with simple notifications without distracting them from main tasks. Our future plan includes the evaluation of colors' combinations, indicators' positions, light intensity and blinking pattern to form meaningful notification in different real life challenges and scenarios for both elderly and young users.

Acknowledgment. We thank staffs in residential nursing care centers of Karpalokoti and ODL for the collaboration in the field testing. We also thank Jarmo Lehtonen and the design team from the University of Lapland for designing conceptual models.

References

1. Bharucha, A.J., Anand, V., Forlizzi, J., Dew, M.A., Reynolds, C.F., Stevens, S., Wactlar, H.: Intelligent assistive technology applications to dementia care: current capabilities, limitations, and future challenges. Am. J. Geriatr. Psychiatry **17**(2), 88–104 (2009)
2. Firouzian, A., Asghar, Z., Tervonen, J., Pulli, P., Yamamoto, G.: Conceptual design, implementation of indicator-based smart glasses: a navigational device for remote assistance of senior citizens suffering from memory loss. In: 2015 9th International Symposium on Medical Information and Communication Technology (ISMICT), pp. 153–156. IEEE (2015)
3. Folstein, M.F., Folstein, S.E., McHugh, P.R.: Mini-mental state: a practical method for grading the cognitive state of patients for the clinician. J. Psychiatr. Res. **12**(3), 189–198 (1975)
4. Hevner, A., Chatterjee, S.: Design Research in Information Systems: Theory And Practice, vol. 22. Springer Science & Business Media, Heidelberg (2010)
5. Hubbard, G., Downs, M.G., Tester, S.: Including older people with dementia in research: challenges and strategies. Aging Ment. Health **7**(5), 351–362 (2003)
6. Lääkkö, M., Firouzian, A., Tervonen, J., Yamamoto, G., Pulli, P.: Attention control and eyesight focus for senior citizens. In: Shumaker, R., Lackey, S. (eds.) VAMR 2014. LNCS, vol. 8526, pp. 309–315. Springer, Heidelberg (2014). doi:10.1007/978-3-319-07464-1_29
7. Manel, S., Williams, H.C., Ormerod, S.J.: Evaluating presenceabsence models in ecology: the need to account for prevalence. J. Appl. Ecol. **38**(5), 921–931 (2001)
8. Poppinga, B., Henze, N., Fortmann, J., Heuten, W., Boll, S.: Ambiglasses-information in the periphery of the visual field. In: Mensch & Computer, pp. 153–162 (2012)
9. Thomas, B., Demczuk, V., Piekarski, W., Hepworth, D., Gunther, B.: A wearable computer system with augmented reality to support terrestrial navigation. In: Second International Symposium on Wearable Computers, 1998. Digest of Papers, pp. 168–171. IEEE (1998)

Proposal of a New Privacy Protection Scheme for the Data Subject on the International Cooperation Information Sharing Platform

Naonori Kato$^{(\boxtimes)}$, Haruo Takasaki, and Yosuke Murakami

KDDI Research Institute Ltd., Tokyo, Japan
{xan-katou,ha-takasaki,yk-murakami}@kddi.com

Abstract. A novel project called iKaaS (intelligent Knowledge-as-a-Service) was adapted as a Strategic Information and Communications R&D Promotion Programme (SCOPE), one of the projects funded by Ministry of Internal Affairs and Communications. This project aims an advanced knowledge-intensive platform that enables to provide and distribute the relevant information under strict consideration of privacy. This information distribution includes a cross-border one between EU and Japan, where privacy protection of the data subject is a major issue. To settle the privacy issues inside the project, DPEC (Data Protection and Ethical Community) was established as a governing organization for privacy. In this paper, we consider issues on the cross-border data distribution from the viewpoint of the legal system comparison between EU and Japan. As a result of the consideration, we introduce the governance framework of DPEC. Moreover, we clarify the issues to be discussed in the future cross-border data distribution and propose a privacy enhanced data protection scheme.

Keywords: Act on the protection of personal information · KaaS · Privacy · Cross-border data distribution · Big Data · Data protection

1 Introduction

Recently, "Big Data" or "IoT (Internet of Things)" have increasingly emerged as buzzwords in the field of network technology. This phenomenon means that any type of data has practical potential to be used in any field. A variety of approaches to data utilization have been tried both in research and in business. During this turmoil on the data processing, misuses of personal data have appeared as a serious social problem.

The experiment which National Institute of Information and Communications Technology (NICT) in Japan planned provoked an issue of an appropriate use of surveillance cameras[1]. In this case, the surveillance cameras collected the movies of

---

[1] See. Investigative report which was written by a third-party committee (Only in Japanese), http://www.nict.go.jp/nrh/iinkai/report.pdf. That concluded the experiment was no illegal, but needs explicit notices. NICT planned to use surveillance cameras to control streams of people in the station.

© ICST Institute for Computer Sciences, Social Informatics and Telecommunications Engineering 2017
K. Giokas et al. (Eds.): eHealth 2016, LNICST 181, pp. 23–28, 2017.
DOI: 10.1007/978-3-319-49655-9_4

pedestrians at the station without any consents or notices. That is similar with Google street view case. The public announcement from NICT on the experiment provoked a social argument. This situation compelled NICT to establish a third-party committee and to publish its report. This report concluded the experiment was not illegal, but needed explicit notices, although NICT had planned to use surveillance cameras for control of people streams in the station.

In other case, the personal data disclosure which Japan Railway East (JR East) planned to the business partner induced an issue on the definition of "personal information"[2]. JR East sold the passengers' records to the third party without any consent from each passengers. JR East's public announcement to start this disclosure to the third party inflamed a social argument. This situation also imposed JR East to publish a report on the disclosure of passengers' records outside JR East. In this report, JR East didn't mention illegality of the disclosure. JR East planned to disclose chronical passenger boarding data after only removing names of the passengers, and leaving all other data as they were. This procedure faced severe social criticism because a passenger can be estimated by the disclosed chronical data.

Meanwhile, EU has shown constant concerns on data protection, and has recognized the data protection as a hot issue. In October 2015, the European Court of Justice declared invalidity of the Safe Harbour Decision. Under the promoting pressures for data utilization, we acknowledge the urgent clarifying the proper and legitimate sharing of the personal data.

The one hand "Big Data" is considered as "new oil", the situation to utilize data in the society is becoming complex more and more. The In this paper, we analyse.

2   Issues on the Information Sharing in the Society

On the information sharing platforms, a wide variety of data are exchanged and combined among a number of parties over the borders. We will discuss three big issues on the information sharing process. Each issue is described below.

2.1   Context-Dependent Values of the Information

A wide variety of data are exchanged and combined on the information sharing platforms. The iKaaS project aims to produce a service by creating new knowledge based on a combination of data among different industries, the combinations of which have not been imagined so far. Attempts to combine these various data open new possibilities of data utilization. However, a new combination of various data may reveal

---

[2] See. Investigative report which was written by a third-party committee (Only in Japanese), http://www.jreast.co.jp/information/aas/20151126_torimatome.pdf. This is the report about the disclosure of the data of Suica outside JR East. The third-party committee didn't mention illegality of the disclosure. JR East planned to disclose boarding history data on Suica, where only names of the card holder were removed. This procedure was criticized because a person who holds the Suica can be estimated by the boarding history data.

unexpected values. For example, some combination of data proved to cause privacy infringements which the platformer had not expected. A simple sensing data or statistical data that have not been treated as a privacy or personal information may trigger privacy invasion. The JR Suica case showed a card holder may be identified based on the combined boarding histories. The JR EAST had explained SuicaIDs (identifier of Suica service) had become irreversible by the number conversion. However, even in such a case, some researchers has pointed out it is possible to re-identify the holder. Also, individual living area of the holder can be almost uniquely estimated from the recorded histories of departure stations and arrival stations. Pseudonymised (including linkable anonymous data) or anonymized method for the data is not effective for preventing such re-identification trials. When we consider more complex context, we have to take into consideration more increased risks of privacy infringements.

When we review international situation on privacy protection, we clearly recognize discussions on privacy matters go deep in the future. Here we show two examples of ongoing discussions. One is the draft of General Data Protection Regulation[3], where "Personal data" is defined as "'personal data' means any information relating to a data subject". The other example is the draft: Consumer Privacy Bill of Rights Act of 2015[4], where "personal data" is defined as "In General— 'Personal data' means any data that are under the control of a covered entity, not otherwise generally available to the public through lawful means, and are linked, or as a practical matter linkable by the covered entity, to a specific individual, or linked to a device that is associated with or routinely used by an individual, including but not limited to—..". In both case, the definitions of personal data has wide meanings.

2.2 The Information Sharing Parties

If the data is processed only within individual party, it is not difficult to define the domain of data utilization. On the other hand, when we consider a situation where the information is shared among several parties, we point out two issues. The first issue presents difficulty of defining information sharing parties. It is unclear whether we are able to itemise all the parties which shares information at present or in the future. Failure of showing all the relevant parties violates against the following law requirements: requirements: in Act on the Protection of Personal Information[5] in Japan, article 17[6]

---

[3] See. Proposal for a REGULATION OF THE EUROPEAN PARLIAMENT AND OF THE COUNCIL on the protection of individuals with regard to the processing of personal data and on the free movement of such data (General Data Protection Regulation)/* COM/2012/011 final - 2012/0011 (COD)*/ http://eur-lex.europa.eu/legal-content/en/TXT/?uri=CELEX:52012PC0011.

[4] See. Administration Discussion Draft: Consumer Privacy Bill of Rights Act of 2015 https://www.whitehouse.gov/sites/default/files/omb/legislative/letters/cpbr-act-of-2015-discussion-draft.pdf.

[5] See. Act on the Protection of Personal Information (translated in English) http://www.japaneselawtranslation.go.jp/law/detail_main?id=130&.

[6] (Proper Acquisition) Article 17 A business operator handling personal information shall not acquire personal information by a deception or other wrongful means deception or other wrongful means.

ordains "Proper Acquisition", and in EU Data Protection Directive[7], article 7[8] ordains "CRITERIA FOR MAKING DATA PROCESSING LEGITIMATE". The second issue is difficulty in defining the purpose of data processing. This difficulty opposes law requirements which demands other purpose than the four conventional purposes (collection, storage, usage, and disclosure) should be explicit and legitimate. However, through trials of combinations of data processing whose purpose is unpredictable, our project is expected to deliver a novel knowledge and service. In order for our project to be legally conformant, explicit informed consent is the only reasonable solution.

2.3   Cross Border Transfer

In EU Data Protection Direction, article 25[9] ordains cross border transfer of personal data. If a third country is to be assessed as an adequate level of protection, it must satisfy article 29. In this project, we plan to transfer data from EU to Japan, but Japan has not the adequacy. If the third country does not have the adequacy, it needs other options (including "SCC" (Standard Contractual Clauses), "BCR" (Binding Corporate Rules) or other international agreement like Safe Harbour agreement between EU and US). At present, Japan does not have international agreement with EU. In addition, both SCC and BCR are too difficult to be certificated for academic research projects. By the way, In EU Data Protection Direction, article 26[10] ordains "Derogations". When the data subject has given his consent to the proposed transfer without clear refusal, Japanese parties can transfer data from EU.

3   Proposal

To solve these problems, we would like to introduce the definition of stakeholders and the internal audit organisation "DPEC".

3.1   Definition of Stakeholders on the Processes

Conventionally, the scheme of the personal data transfer and utilization has been classified as four stages: data collection, storage, usage and disclosure (provision to a

---

[7] See. Directive 95/46/EC of the European Parliament and of the Council of 24 October 1995 on the protection of individuals with regard to the processing of personal data and on the free movement of such data http://eur-lex.europa.eu/legal-content/en/TXT/?uri=CELEX:31995L0046.

[8] Article 7 clarifies the conditions for consent to be valid as a legal ground for lawful processing.

[9] Article 25 1. The Member States shall provide that the transfer to a third country of personal data which are undergoing processing or are intended for processing after transfer may take place only if, without prejudice to compliance with the national provisions adopted pursuant to the other provisions of this Directive, the third country in question ensures an adequate level of protection.

[10] Article 26 Derogations 1. By way of derogation from Article 25 and save where otherwise provided by domestic law governing particular cases, Member States shall provide that a transfer or a set of transfers of personal data to a third country which does not ensure an adequate level of protection within the meaning of Article 25 (2) may take place on condition that: (a) the data subject has given his consent unambiguously to the proposed transfer;.

third party). Many conventional services already obtain the user consent including the first three (from collection to usage) or all the four (from collection to disclosure) of the scheme. However, in our project, the conventional scheme fails to work, as in our project different parties are responsible for each data processing. We had to redefine each process and stake holder to acquire precise user consent through showing exact architecture of the service we are going to provide. Redefined stake holders are shown as follows.

Lead operator: The responsible operator for the iKaaS project in Japan.

System management operator: The responsible operator for the iKaaS platform (design, development, maintenance, operation and security issues etc.).

Data management operator: This operator will collect the information from the participants. It shall be as a responsible operator for collecting and preserving the information.

Data utilization operator: This operator will use the information preserved in the iKaaS platform. It shall be as a responsible operator for using the data.

We have also defined the process of obtaining user consents as follows.

1. Identify individual data to be collected (particle size of type and the data of the data).
2. When collecting the individual data, obtain the explicit consent from the data subject.
3. Define the way to combine what data for what purpose.
4. For the purposes shown above, obtain explicit consent from the data subject. In such consent acquisition process, obtain the consent of the clear opt-in type.

We would like to introduce this "Double informed consent" in order to strengthen user consents.

3.2   DPEC

The iKaaS project implements three use cases. One of the use cases in Japan will include field tests with citizens and procedures under ethical considerations. In the EU, the ethical issues are considered based on the EU data protection legal framework by the Project partners. Since there is no independent data protection authority in Japan at present 5 by contrast to the EU legal framework which has independent privacy commissioners, a self-regulated "Data Projection and Ethical Committee" (DPEC) has been set in the iKaaS Project. DPEC shall clarify legal protection and ethical treatment of personal information gathered and shared among iKaaS Consortium Partners for research and development through iKaaS Platforms, especially concerning the use case which needs ethical considerations, and also the cross-border applications.

DPEC shall draft a privacy policy and a written consent forms and other appropriate guidelines (called "privacy protection documents") in accordance with existing Japanese governmental guidelines, laws and regulations protecting personal information in

Japan. DPEC shall timely review the privacy protection documents depending on the legal amendments by government authorities. DPEC shall monitor the implementation by iKaaS Project Partners of privacy protection documents for adequate treatment of personal information gathered through iKaaS platforms. In the event of infringement of personal information, DPEC shall promptly advise corrective measures to iKaaS Consortium Partners. DPEC shall consult as appropriate legal counsels for getting independent advices as to the privacy protection documents and these implementations.

In the actual evaluation cycle, DPEC shall review the applications from each project partner. The application process shall start in advance of collection, storage, usage and disclosure of the data (including personal data) in the project. The applications shall be reviewed by the factors[11].

4 Conclusion

In this paper, we have introduced the definition of stakeholders on the information sharing platform and internal audit organisation "DPEC". The range of each law was confirmed through comparative law study. Furthermore, our self-regulation provides higher quality of privacy protection beyond the required level by the law. Our self-regulation scheme has proved to be friendly to the consumer rights to privacy and personal data.

In the next step, we plan to demonstrate practical experiments with the actual data collecting from the data subjects. We carefully observe any issue which may arise in performing the actual operation of the platform.

---

[11] We have defined 14 factors.

A Transparent Home Sensors/Actuators Layer for Health and Well-Being Services

Philippe Tanguy$^{(\boxtimes)}$, Christophe Lohr, and Jérôme Kerdreux

Telecom Bretagne, Technopôle Brest-Iroise, CS 83818, 29238 Brest Cedex 3, France
{philippe.tanguy,christophe.lohr,jerome.kerdreux}@telecom-bretagne.eu

Abstract. Risks factor leading to type 2 diabetes and cardiovascular diseases can be reduced by a preventive care infrastructure able to modify the habits toward healthier lifestyles, including more exercise, a better diet and a reduced stress. Accessing the home space is important not only to monitor indoor environment quality (IEQ) but also to provide relevant user's feedback and engage users towards a healthy life style. This paper present a new preventive care infrastructure composed of a distributed infrastructure for heterogeneous devices in the home local area network (named xAAL) in conjunction with a machine to machine protocol (MQTT) to external health & well-being services.

Keywords: Indoor environment quality · Ambient assisted living · User feedback

1 Introduction

Noncommunicable diseases (NCD), for instance diabetes, cardiovascular or respiratory are the leading cause of mortality in the world, representing 60% of all deaths according to the program chronic diseases and health promotion of the World Health Organization [13]. Modifying the habits toward healthier lifestyles, including more exercise, a better diet and reduced stress is associated with the reduced risk of diseases such as type 2 diabetes and cardiovascular diseases. In this context, the PREventive Care Infrastructure based On Ubiquitous Sensing (PRECIOUS [4]) project targets to develop a preventive care system to promote healthy lifestyles with specific focus on the following risk factors: environmental, socio-psychological and physiological. The PRECIOUS[1] system proposes services to end users: monitoring of the home environment factors (e.g., air quality), gathering data from "health & well-being" devices (e.g., body weight scale) and sending feedbacks through multimodal interfaces. In this paper, we focus on the user context related to environmental factors and how we can gather long-term data in the home user space. Particularly, we discuss an infrastructure and a new

---

[1] This project has received funding from the European Union's Seventh Framework Programme for research, technological development and demonstration under grant agreement no 611366.

© ICST Institute for Computer Sciences, Social Informatics and Telecommunications Engineering 2017
K. Giokas et al. (Eds.): eHealth 2016, LNICST 181, pp. 29–35, 2017.
DOI: 10.1007/978-3-319-49655-9_5

protocol to seamlessly integrate home automation devices and data in a health & well-being care system. Moreover, we also address user feedbacks in the home environment to support health & well-being recommendation on different user interfaces.

2   Related Works

The indoor environment quality (IEQ) is most of the time studied from an occupant comfort perspective and/or to reduce energy consumption of buildings [11,14]. Nevertheless, Kim *et al.* in [9] proposed a system to measure, visualize and learn about indoor air quality. The study showed that the inAir system motivates user to improve their indoor air quality. This means that visualization of data related to home comfort needs to be considered in order to engage user change habits. Then, Kim *et al.* in [8,10], presented a sensor network infrastructure for real time monitoring of several gases. The contribution is focused on data acquisition and sensor network infrastructure. The authors show that real-time monitoring is necessary as well as the use of pre-processing algorithm on data to reduce temporary errors. Interoperability issues related to different protocols using by sensors is not addressed. Furthermore, the integration in a smart home and health infrastructure is not considered.

Different vertical domains are present in the home environment: personal health devices, home automation devices, entertainment devices, etc. Recent works about IoT domain architecture proposed horizontal interoperability between vertical silos: eHealth, home automation, agriculture, etc. One can cite the HYDRA [1], IOT-A [2] or BUTLER [6] European projects. There is also a recent effort to standardize machine to machine (M2M) communication with the OneM2M initiative. Gateways between constrained network, e.g. BAN/PAN, HAN and WAN are still needed. Even if protocols like CoAP or MQTT are dedicated to small devices, there is still a gap because of device: power consumption, memory foot print, etc.

3   System Description

The user context awareness (UCA) at home should be a key objective of a system trying to assist user in its daily life. We defined the following environmental variables: thermal comfort (temperature and humidity), noise quality, light quality. To achieve the UCA, a transparent sensors/actuators layer using xAAL [12] has been proposed to fight interoperability issues in the home automation domain. xAAL allows to seamlessly integrate TAN/BAN/PAN/LAN devices from different protocols. The xAAL infrastructure offers access with WAN interfaces (WAN-IF) to use MQTT M2M communication as shown Fig. 1. MQTT is lightweight enough to be used on different communication links such as 3G/4G (cellular), Fiber, ADSL. Then, thanks to the selected M2M protocol, sensors data are exported and stored in a database to be used by health & well-being service. Data are processed and, according to a rules engine, user feedbacks will be sent

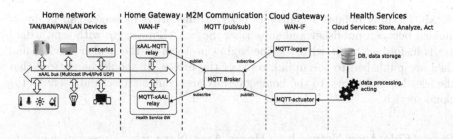

Fig. 1. System overview.

to home. Basically, those feedbacks can take the form of messages, notifications, or devices actions at home (according to user's preferences).

3.1 Home Area Network and External Services

Context Acquisition. xAAL [5, 12] is an open-source distributed infrastructure for heterogeneous ambient devices. The communication between devices is realized by a lightweight event-based messaging protocol working on the so-called xAAL bus. Devices are described by a schema, which provides a first level of semantic. IEQ variables are then related to the following schemas: "thermometer.basic", "hygrometer.basic", "luxmeter.basic", "loudness.basic".

xAAL allows us to reuse traditional home automation devices (e.g., thermometer, luxmeter, soundmeter, Tv, etc.) to set up a pervasive health system. Data are automatically associated by the xAAL system to the location of sensors in various rooms (e.g. bedroom, living room).

From Home Area Network to Wide Area Network. xAAL and external health services are inter-connected with the MQTT protocol. It is a lightweight protocol dedicated to M2M communications and is now an open standard [3]. It is based on a publish/subscribe model and TCP/IP. The home gateway publishes relevant home data to the external health services. It allows to move the management of data storage & analytics over long term and unstructured data in the cloud. According to the MQTT architecture, a broker is needed between publisher & subscriber. This allows multiple publishers to communicate to multiple subscribers in so-called topics. However, this is an additional component to administrate. But, robust open-source implementations exist today.

The infrastructure Fig. 1 is composed by the following components:

- xAAL-MQTT relay: a component of the home gateway which publishes sensor data to the cloud;
- MQTT Broker: dispatches published data to the corresponding subscribers;
- MQTT-logger: a component of the external home service that subscribes to data sent by the smart home and stores them to the health service database.

MQTT only defines a transport layer. Transported messages can be freely defined between publisher and subscriber. So, xAAL messages with sensor data are transformed to fit with the messaging protocol of the health service, and then are published to the uplink topic of the broker. It should be noticed that the user has full access to the home gateway and control/select data sent to the cloud service.

From Wide Area Network to Home Area Network. A preventive health-care system should consider the user feedback. This offers a way to engage and motivate users toward a healthy life style. The home gateway subscribes to the downlink topic of the broker. Figure 1 is composed by the following components:

- MQTT-actuator: a component of the external home service which publishes feedback to home;
- MQTT Broker: the same broker is used to dispatches published messages to subscribers;
- MQTT-xAAL relay: a component of the home gateway that subscribes to feedback and sends xAAL commands.

From the Home Area Network to the Attention of the User. Feedbacks are sent to home over MQTT in the form of JSON messages. Then, they are dispatched to the right actuators according to user preferences and home capabilities. The xAAL infrastructure provides multimodal interaction between home, health systems, and the user. The scenarios addressed in our study consider different kind of users from young to elderly people, from individual to family units, with different needs/wishes/habits regarding uses of devices. The following notifications media are currently available: "Lamp blinking", "Lamp color", "Haptic/Motor vibration", "Message on smartphone" (textual & voice message), "Text message on desktop computer", "Text message on Tv". The definition of each notification depends of the home capabilities. Thanks to xAAL and its discovery mechanism, the health service gateway (at home) is aware of home capabilities. Finally, users can define the appropriate notification type according to their preferences and current home actuators.

3.2 Security & Privacy

xAAL. Firstly, xAAL is working on the local area network (LAN) and is protected by the mechanism that still exists to protect user LAN network. Secondly, with the version 0.5 a security layer has been added to the xAAL protocol [5]. Basically, it is based on a pre-shared private key, Poly1305/Chacha20 algorithm, a timestamp to avoid replay attack. The protocol version, the targets addresses and the timestamp are public. Only the payload is ciphered by the Poly1305/Chacha20 algorithm with "targets" for additional data and a "timestamp" playing the role of nonce.

MQTT. Section 5 of the OASIS MQTT v3.1.1 standard is dedicated to security (for guidance only, non-normative). Four security levels (or profiles) are described: Level 4: Unsecured; Level 3: Base Secured; Level 2: Industry Secured (Base + Industry customizations), Level 1: Cyber Critical Secured. According to guides of the OASIS MQTT security subcommittee, we will match the level 2 security profile. Indeed, TLS provides authentication, integrity and privacy. Moreover, the TLS client authentication will be used in addition to the MQTT client authentication (username/password).

4 Implementation and Discussion

This paper describes an infrastructure aiming to ensure engagement and mid-long term adherence to health & well-being service. The idea is to collect environment parameters at home, to send them to a decision engine, and then to provide feedback and recommendations to users, in a smart and confident way.

xAAL has been deployed and tested [5] in the Experiment'HAAL living lab. Now xAAL includes support for the following home automation technologies: KNX, Zwave, Oregon Scientific, Delta Dore. A dedicated xAAL device have been developed which embed multiple sensors: a Raspberry Pi model B with a grovepi shield, a digital light sensor, a loudness sensor and a vibration motor for notifications. For the temperature and humidity sensor, we reused a "classical" sensor dedicated to a weather station (Oregon Scientific THGR810). This use case particularly shows all the opportunity offered by xAAL to integrate and re-use "classical" home automation sensors/actuators for health application.

xAAL is enough flexible to allow several kind of users feedback in order to target their needs, their preferences, a handicap, the specificity of their ages and their wishes. The following xAAL notifications have been implemented: blink a lamp and/or color lamp, Tv (HTTP protocol according to HbbTV standards), laptop (Use Mac Osx or Gnome notification center), Android smartphone (text & voice), noise with a vibration motor. This offers many alternatives compared to smartphone-centric solutions.

The home gateway offers to users the possibility control on data they accept to share: temperature, humidity, body weight, notifications, etc. The gateway is the place for processing a first level of data fusion, adding a context (e.g., localisation) before to send them to the cloud service. The location information is symbolic and defined by a tag, e.g. *bedroom*. On the other side, the home gateway dispatches feedbacks to rendering devices (smartphone, Tv, lamp, etc.) according to user preferences: the time of the day, the type of device, etc. Feedbacks are predefined messages, with internationalisation (I18n) to fit user language for use cases involving text and voice messages.

In terms of ethics, security & privacy, the external services in the cloud cannot access directly the home devices. What enter at home are just informative notifications whose rendering is controlled by the user, not direct commands for home devices.

From a technical point of view, xAAL allows us to add new low level protocols and devices, such as promising EnOcean or Zwave, thanks to independent software components translating messages to xAAL. Indeed, the integration of low level protocol is done by the xAAL bus itself. Moreover, with the schema modelling, a lamp is a lamp whatever the underlaying protocol. This new lamp is transparent for the health service, developers and users.

Finally, xAAL is an event bus and the association with a pub/sub pattern remains a good combination. The fact that messages between the house and cloud services are not standardized could be a drawback. But new health & well-being services providers are free to design their own gateway to be installed at the patient's home. They can define their own topics and message format.

5   Conclusions and Future Work

This paper proposed an infrastructure using xAAL and MQTT in order to offer the possibility to use home automation sensors/actuators in future health and well-being services. It offers access to home environment data in order to have a better understanding of the user context, i.e. environmental factors such as thermal comfort, noise and luminosity levels. But, it also gives capabilities to developer of health applications to integrate feedbacks in order to engage users and help them to change their behaviour [7]. Healthcare systems need to use existing standards and MQTT combined with xAAL appears to be a well adapted candidate for M2M communication between home automation networks and external health & well-being services.

As future work, end-user tests will be conducted in the Experiment'HAAL living lab according to the Wizard-of-Oz principles. The objective is to collect user recommendations regarding acceptance on the overall functionalities, interfaces, data visualization & consultation, ethics & privacy.

References

1. Hydra project. http://www.hydramiddleware.eu/news.php
2. IOT-A project (2009). http://www.iot-a.eu/public
3. Mqtt (2014). https://www.oasis-open.org
4. The PRECIOUS project (2016). http://www.thepreciousproject.eu/
5. Bretagne, T.: xAAL project (2016). http://recherche.telecom-bretagne.eu/xaal/
6. BUTLER project (2011). http://www.iot-butler.eu/
7. Helf, C., Hlavacs, H.: Apps for life change: critical review and solution directions. Entertainment Comput. 14, 17–22 (2015)
8. Kim, J.-Y., Chu, C.-H., Shin, S.-M.: ISSAQ: an integrated sensing systems for real-time indoor air quality monitoring. IEEE Sens. J. 14(12), 4230–4244 (2014)
9. Kim, S., Paulos, E.: inAir: measuring and visualizing indoor air quality. In: Proceedings of the 11th International Conference on Ubiquitous Computing, pp. 81–84. ACM (2009)
10. Kim, S., Paulos, E.: inAir: sharing indoor air quality measurements and visualizations. In: Proceedings of the SIGCHI Conference on Human Factors in Computing Systems, pp. 1861–1870. ACM (2010)

11. Lai, A., Mui, K., Wong, L., Law, L.: An evaluation model for indoor environmental quality (IEQ) acceptance in residential buildings. Energy Build. **41**(9), 930–936 (2009)
12. Lohr, C., Tanguy, P., Kerdreux, J.: xAAL: a distributed infrastructure for heterogeneous ambient devices. JISYS **24**(3), 321–331 (2015)
13. World Health Organization: Global status report on noncommunicable diseases 2014: attaining the nine global noncommunicable diseases targets; a shared responsibility. World Health Organization (2014)
14. Pitt, L., Green, P.R., Lennox, B.: A sensor network for predicting and maintaining occupant comfort. In: 2013 IEEE Workshop on Environmental Energy and Structural Monitoring Systems (EESMS), pp. 1–6. IEEE (2013)

Augmenting Object with IoT to Enhance Elders' Social Life

Tiago Franklin R. Lucena$^{(\boxtimes)}$, Vinicius Oberleitner, Marcos Demétrius Barbosa, and Hygor Vinícius P. Martins

Unicesumar, Health Promotion Graduate Program,
1610, Guedner Avenue, Building 7, room 12, Maringa, Parana, Brazil
tiagofranklin@gmail.com, viniober@gmail.com,
marcosdemetrius@gmail.com, hvpmar@gmail.com

Abstract. We describe an IoT system composed by a thermos flask with embedded sensors, microprocessor and network interface. The system connects to the internet after recognizing activity and sends a message over online social network-OSN (e.g. Twitter/Facebook) when hot coffee is brewed. The idea is to create a device that engage people to interact face-to-face, bringing old habits of drinking coffee as an excuse to socialize. Drinking coffee with friends is a world habit; in the south of Brazil the tradition to cultivate and drink coffee is very strong (especially in elderly people's life). The device is set to an ideal scenario and we can collect data from user's brewing coffee and therefore his daily consuming habits. The prototype is being improved before testing it with a large number of users and has providing new perspectives about the concept of "OSN based on IoT" and IoT to promote social interaction.

Keywords: Internet of Things · Online social network · Thermos flask · Social interaction

1 Introduction

The pervasive and ubiquitous technology present worldwide has been benefited by reducing small components that can be embedded in objects [1]. Many factors contribute to this increasing number of connected objects including size, price, communication protocols and computational power of electronic components, as a phenomenon observed since Moore [2]. Nowadays, this integration of electronic and smart sensors in objects has received the name of Internet of Things or IoT [3]. Applications of IoT vary from entertainment, economy, communication, security and surveillance. IoT is also applied in health fields, such as monitoring, accessibility, orientation, promotion and prevention. The idea behind IoT is not to build a single object with large computational power but to distribute this power into small and connected objects. This tendency confirms the legacy of Mark Weiser on calm technologies [4].

In relation to health, we can see an increasing number of elderly people [5]. Besides the impact of the growing number of elderly people on economy and public and private sector, the loss of cognitive functions and other chronic and age-related diseases have been pushing forward researches that pay attention to this part of population, to the

© ICST Institute for Computer Sciences, Social Informatics and Telecommunications Engineering 2017
K. Giokas et al. (Eds.): eHealth 2016, LNICST 181, pp. 36–41, 2017.
DOI: 10.1007/978-3-319-49655-9_6

wellbeing and quality of life [6, 7]. The terms of assistive technology, smart houses, or domotics for health are linked to *IoT for health* [8] or their variations: *IoTcare* or u-health.

We will describe an IoT system that takes advantage of the unobtrusive presence of an object in the kitchen of most families in Brazil, especially in elders' houses. The object is a thermos flask with embedded sensor, microprocessor and network interface. The system can connect to the internet after sensing hot coffee is in the thermos flask and the device sends a message over online social network – OSN (e.g. Twitter/Facebook) inviting friends to drink it at their house.

From many other possibilities, we are committed to discuss about how IoT brings people together. We know that IoT can help people in everyday activities [9], including people with disabilities [10], however less attention has been given to IoT regarding social interaction. Our basic questions are: How can we stimulate social interaction among old people who live alone? How can we augment an ordinary object transforming it into a communication tool in order to enhance social life [11]? These questions have pushed us in direction of a "Social Internet of Thing" [12], and other researchers have been challenged to create a smart architecture to integrate all sorts of objects, including those that mediate a context for social interaction [13, 14].

2   IoT and Healthcare: Wellbeing

The expectation of life has been growing over the past years worldwide. Technology, better healthy habits, sanitary condition and prevention programs contribute to a greater number of old people. In Europe and Japan, this large number of old people is addressing political investments which contributes to higher rates in life expectancy [15].

Many researchers pointed out the necessity to lead old people into a social integration and this is an important element to promote health and wellbeing [16]. Old people who live by themselves may lose the sense of community, autonomy and social participation. On the other hand, young people are the majority of OSN users and this mediated communication help them maintain connection with other friends, even if they are physically distant. Based on this, we aim to integrate a common act executed by an elder at home (making coffee) with a device that invites closer users to have coffee at their home.

An example of IoT technology in the health field is an IoT system described by Carmen Domingo related to people with disabilities [10]. The system uses sensors, actuators and monitoring stations (such as cell phones, smartphone, tablet PC, etc.), nano-nodes, RFID tags and readers/writers in order to help and guide users with visual, hearing and physical impairing.

We daily interact with many objects in different places and context. For instance, kitchens have several manually operated devices. In this way, designers and technologists are bringing affordable objects to make life easier. The integration of technology in the kitchen is a natural movement, especially in the field of domotics [17, 18] and experimental works as mentioned by Spence [19].

Some examples confirm the idea of "smart" objects in the kitchen as a way to facilitate life. There are coffee machines, refrigerators, microwave ovens connected and activated from a distance. These "magical" things remind us the objects talking and acting with us, usually seen in the imaginary and creative world of cartoons. Somehow, IoT makes inanimate objects alive. In the real kitchen environment today, we can see ideas like "*HAPIfork*", a fork that counts the time you spend during meals, how many times you take the fork into your mouth and the gap between chews [20]. Another idea is "*Liftware*", a fork designed for people with Parkinson that tries to stabilize the hands tremors [21]. "*Pred Pad*" is a weight scale that measures the food weight and shows, in real time, some nutritional data with an app [22]. Some other ideas create smart objects with online social networks, not addressing directly to health topic, but it can be useful to understand the variety of approaches. For example, "*Whirlpool Co*" is a cooker with an interactive touchscreen cooktop that displays recipes, Facebook/Twitter updates, News and weather forecast. Finally, "*Smart Fridge*" can "see" the products inside the fridge, helping the user identify when the food is expiring [23].

Based on this background and observing elderly people from a city in the south of Brazil, we prototyped a system that helps us identify when an old user brewed coffee. By taking this into consideration, it is possible to know the frequency coffee is made and infer about time spent at home and social life.

3   Description of the System

The thermos flask we are designing is going in a different direction from researches on automatic or "smart" coffee machines – which are more common in developed countries. Many of these promising "smart" coffee machines are addressing to brewing control and yet need improvements [24]. Our focus is on storing coffee rather than making coffee, once it is made the interaction may occur through internet.

Cultural aspects of consuming and sharing coffee with friends and family using a thermos flask to maintain the hot temperature of the beverage for long periods is commonly observed in Brazil. While in other countries the machine keeps the temperature, in Brazil the choice of the majority is usually a thermos flask.

We took an ordinary thermos flask and embedded it with temperature sensor, microcontroller, processor and communication module that logs in an OSN account inviting closer friends to drink coffee and make company to the old users. The system has an LM35 (small temperature sensor) that is placed on the top of a commercial device (Fig. 1) and it is connected to an Arduino Uno R3 microcontroller.

A communication module "Ethernet Shield" is responsible for connecting the system to the internet, and to request permission to post a message on the users' Twitter account. The sensor is responsible for checking when the temperature is equal ($=$) or higher ($>$) than 80°C inside the flask so then the system sends a single tweet. Thus, it is noticeable that coffee was brewed with boiled water. As a first version, a LED was installed to give a feedback when communication is made. After that, the tweet is sent, e.g.: "*Come over and have some coffee with me!*". After the message was posted, Twitter blocked further

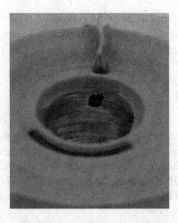

Fig. 1. LM35 sensor embedded inside the container of the flask. It was prototyped with Arduino UNO R3 and Ethernet Shield module and it was attached using a nylon body band. Photo: Authors.

tries to post again for over 12h, that happened because we were using a single message, and due to it being equal to the other previously posted and also due the short time between them, Twitter considered it as a spam.

In order to get past this problem, a "database". The system, after sending a message, skips to another one and this way Twitter won't consider it as a spam, which will allow us to tweet at any time. Generating different contents permits us to give the system a sense that the messages were posted by humans. Every random number is linked with a different message.

4 Conclusion and Further Developments

It is important to highlight that in most part of the world, when age comes, people start losing their autonomy. It becomes bad for the elderly, once that most part of them tend to live by themselves, showing difficulty in accomplishing basic daily activities. Having said that, it is possible to introduce the concept of IoTCare for supporting communication and interaction, especially for those who live alone. It consists of improving the quality of life by promoting social interaction between users who are losing social communication opportunities.

Considering it, the idea of the thermos flask came as a life changing landscape. Analyzing some life styles of elderly people it is possible to say that most of them feel alone and most part of the time, they have no one to share their experiences with. With an embedded technology, the thermos flask helps them connect with people around; making not only some shorts connections with people, but inviting them to personally come to their place. It is important to remember that interaction is not the only role of the object (which is making coffee), but tracking some routines as well. This tracking can be useful to the family, for example, where they can see if their beloved relatives are keeping with their daily activities.

Further test in a bigger group of users will point to other directions; improvements in the system are needed in order to resist impact or water. It is also on the list the necessity to test and validate the architecture of the system with many thermos flasks working simultaneously.

References

1. Weiser, M.: The computer for the 21st century. Sci. Am. **265**, 94–104 (1991)
2. Moore, G.E.: Cramming more components onto integrated circuits. Proc. IEEE **86**, 82–85 (1998). (Reprinted from Electronics, pp. 114–117, 19 April 1965)
3. McEwen, A., Cassimally, H.: Designing the Internet of Things. Wiley, Chichester (2014)
4. Weiser, M., Brown, J.S.: The coming age of calm technology. In: Beyond Calculation, pp. 75–85. Springer, New York (1997)
5. WHO: Active Ageing: A Police Framework, Geneva (2002)
6. Baldoni, A.O., Pereira, L.R.L.: O impacto do envelhecimento populacional Brasileiro para o sistema de saúde sob a óptica da farmacoepidemiologia: Uma revisão narrativa. Rev. Ciencias Farm. Basica e Apl. **32**, 313–321 (2011)
7. Barbosa, B.R., de Almeida, J.M., Barbosa, M.R., Rossi-Barbosa, L.A.R.: Avaliação da capacidade funcional dos idosos e fatores associados à incapacidade. Cien. Saude Colet. **19**, 3317–3325 (2014)
8. Oswald, F., Wahl, H.-W.: Housing and health in later life. Rev. Environ. Heal. **19**, 223–252 (2004)
9. Philipose, M., Fishkin, K.P., Perkowitz, M., Patterson, D.J., Fox, D., Kautz, H., Hähnel, D.: Inferring activities from interactions with objects. IEEE Pervasive Comput. **3**, 50–57 (2004)
10. Domingo, M.C.: An overview of the Internet of Things for people with disabilities. J. Netw. Comput. Appl. **35**, 584–596 (2012)
11. Gourley, M.M.: Activities of daily living evaluation. Encycl. Nurs. Allied Heal. **24**, 1–3 (2010)
12. Atzori, L., Iera, A., Morabito, G., Nitti, M.: The Social Internet of Things (SIoT) – When social networks meet the Internet of Things: concept, architecture and network characterization. Comput. Netw. **56**, 3594–3608 (2012)
13. Nitti, M., Atzori, L., Cvijikj, I.P.: Network navigability in the social Internet of Things. In: 2014 IEEE World Forum, pp. 405–410. Internet Things (WF-IoT) (2014)
14. Kranz, M., Roalter, L., Michahelles, F.: Things that Twitter: social networks and the Internet of Things. What can Internet Things do Citiz. Work. In: Eighth International Conference on Pervasive Computing, (Pervasive 2010), pp. 1–10 (2010)
15. Cain, G.: Why the Japanese live so long? http://www.salon.com/2014/06/17/why_the_japanese_live_so_long_partner/
16. WHO: WHO | The Ottawa Charter for Health Promotion. In: First International Conference on Health Promotion Ottawa, 21 November 1986, pp. 3–5 (2013)
17. Meulendijk, M., Van De Wijngaert, L., Brinkkemper, S., Leenstra, H.: Am I in good care? developing design principles for ambient intelligent domotics for elderly. Inform. Heal. Soc. Care. **36**, 75–88 (2011)
18. Grönvall, E., Kyng, M.: On participatory design of home-based healthcare. Cogn. Technol. Work **15**, 389–401 (2013)
19. Spence, C., Piqueras-Fiszman, B.: Technology at the dining table. Flavour **2**, 16 (2013)
20. Hapifork. https://www.hapi.com/product/hapifork
21. Liftware. http://www.liftware.com/

22. Pred   Pad.   https://www.kickstarter.com/projects/chefsleeve/smart-food-scale-less-about-weight-more-about-you/description
23. Itzkovitch, A.: The Internet of Things and the Mythical Smart Fridge. https://uxmag.com/articles/the-internet-of-things-and-the-mythical-smart-fridge
24. Bennet, B.: Why smart coffee makers are dumb but beautiful dream. http://www.cnet.com/news/why-smart-coffee-makers-are-a-dumb-but-beautiful-dream/

ICT Use in Family Caregiving of Elderly and Disabled Subjects

Mia Hautala[1,2(✉)], Niina S. Keränen[1,2], Eeva Leinonen[3],
Maarit Kangas[1,2], and Timo Jämsä[1,2,4]

[1] Research Unit of Medical Imaging, Physics and Technology (MIPT),
University of Oulu, Oulu, Finland
{mia.hautala,niina.s.keranen,maarit.kangas,
timo.jamsa}@oulu.fi
[2] Medical Research Center (MRC), Oulu University Hospital
and University of Oulu, Oulu, Finland
[3] Faculty of Information Technology and Electrical Engineering,
University of Oulu, Oulu, Finland
eeva.leinonen@oulu.fi
[4] Department of Diagnostic Radiology, Oulu University Hospital, Oulu, Finland

Abstract. This study examined the use of ICT in caregiving as assessed by family caregivers of disabled or elderly subjects (N = 53). The results showed limited current use of ICT-based technologies either for on-site or remote assistance. However, perceived usefulness was evaluated as high when these technologies were used. The factors for the use of ICT were different for on-site assistance or remote assistance. The data obtained can be used in the development of future ICT and IoT –based assistive technologies.

Keywords: Caregiver · Assistive technology · Remote care · eHealth · ICT · IoT

1 Introduction

Persons with disabilities use assistive technology to increase, maintain, or improve their functionality and performance in daily tasks and activities. Assistive technology can be a service, device, application or tool that helps the elderly, disabled person or their caregiver to maintain functional ability of the care recipient [1–3]. Assistive technology can consist e.g. of mechanical and electrical devices, sensors, IoT applications, and cloud services. Assistive technologies have been found to have ability to improve user's activity and participation, and also to reduce the functional decline of the user [2, 4, 5].

Assistive technologies can also be seen as a solution to reduce caregiver's burden. ICT devices and applications can decrease the demands related to care and supervision of the care recipient. In addition, those can be used to monitor any unexpected needs of assistance, i.e. accidents and injuries [2, 6]. Caregivers, either family members or others who provide care for those who need supervision or assistance in illness or disability [7], are seen as a valuable resource for elderly care in their unpaid contribution for the ageing society [8].

© ICST Institute for Computer Sciences, Social Informatics and Telecommunications Engineering 2017
K. Giokas et al. (Eds.): eHealth 2016, LNICST 181, pp. 42–48, 2017.
DOI: 10.1007/978-3-319-49655-9_7

ICT and IoT solutions might be increasingly valuable in assisting elderly and disabled persons in future. The aim of this study was to examine to what extent the family caregivers utilize ICT-based assistive technologies in their caregiving work, and what are the needs for and perceived usefulness of assistive technologies.

2 Materials and Methods

An online survey was implemented through the Finnish Society for Caregivers (Omaishoitajat ry) webpage. The survey was open for responses from September 30th to October 25th 2015 and at the same time it was advertised through social media as well. A pilot survey was carried out with two caregivers and one researcher before the implementation. The caregiver answered both to the questions for him/herself and to the questions related to the care recipient.

The survey consisted of five main categories: Background, Assistive technologies and tools, Time utilization, Burden, and Coping. The response to the questions related to Assistive technologies and tools are presented in this paper (Table 1).

Table 1. Questions related to background information and assistive technology and tools.

Content
Caregiver and care recipient characteristics
Demographics of the caregiver
Relationship between the caregiver and the care recipient
Demographics of the care recipient
Need of assistance
Caregiver's contribution on care
Assistive technologies and tools
Use of ICT equipment to help the care recipient from distance
Use of ICT equipment while assisting
Other assistive technologies and tools used as help when assisting
Most common assistive tools and ICT equipment used by the caregiver or by the care recipient
Experience with telemonitoring (i.e. door alarm, GPS tracking device, fall detector)
Willingness to use telemonitoring application
Need of assistive tools or devices
Pre-agreed terms for caregiving
Availability (times of day) when the caregiver could give remote help if technology existed

The survey contained both qualitative and quantitative questions. Qualitative methods were used for questions about assistive tools and ICT equipment to collect information about the needs and expectations assigned for the technology.

Five-point Likert scale was used to score the perceived usefulness of assistive tools and ICT equipment as a Perceived Usefulness Score (PUS), 1 referring to Never, 2 to Rarely, 3 to Sometimes, 4 to Quite Frequently and 5 to Nearly always. The respondent was allowed to list and score a maximum of 5 tools or equipment for evaluation.

Results are expressed as mean ± standard deviation (SD). Statistical analysis were performed in IBM SPSS 22.

3   Results

In total there were 53 caregiver respondents, mostly female (n = 46), with average age of 54.3 years. Characteristics of the caregivers and care recipients are presented in Table 2. There were 31 male and 22 female care recipients with an average age of 48.7 years. Most of the care recipients lived with the caregiver and only three of them lived alone. Forty-seven of the caregivers had made informal care agreement. Seventy percent of the care recipients needed assistance around the clock and 26% daily. Assistance was also needed when moving outdoors or indoors. Caregiver's contribution on care were typically between 81 and 100% of the total care need.

The care recipients had also need for help in bathing (53 respondents; 100%), using the toilet (48; 91%), getting dressed (53; 100%), cooking (53; 100%), and keeping

Table 2. Characteristics of the caregiver and care recipient (N = 53). N (%) if not otherwise stated.

Characteristics	
Demographics of the caregivers	
Age ± SD (range) (years)	54.3 ± 13.5 (27–82)
Female	46 (87%)
Caregiver agreement	47 (89%)
Relationship to care recipient	
Spouse	25 (47%)
Parent	20 (38%)
(Grand-) Children	7 (13%)
Demographics of the care recipients	
Age ± SD (range) (years)	48.7 ± 29.9 (3–92)
Female	22 (42%)
Living alone	3 (6%)
Living with caregiver	49 (92%)
Need of assistance	
Around the clock	37 (70%)
Daily	14 (26%)
When moving outdoors	48 (91%)
When moving indoors	39 (74%)
Caregiver's contribution on care	
81–100% of total care need	35 (66%)
61–80% of total care need	10 (19%)
41–60% of total care need	6 (11%)
20–40% of total care need	2 (4%)

SD standard deviation

contacts (e.g. using telephone or computer) (49; 92%). Caregivers mentioned that care recipients may also need help with medication (48; 91%), daily chores (24; 45%), eating (43; 81%), hobbies or school (38; 72%), communicating, or in social situations (32; 60%).

Fifteen (28%) of the respondents used ICT equipment to help care recipient from distance (teleassistance), whereas 12 (23%) had used ICT equipment when assisting on-site. Tablets and other devices with internet access had been used to search information, to study (e.g. Papunet, papunet.net), to stay in touch with friends and relatives, and to support and learn communication skills (e.g. DialoQ, www.dialoq.com).

Caregivers had also used other assistive technologies and tools when assisting. Wheelchair was mentioned as the most used when asked for listing five most common technologies (Table 3). Perceived usefulness as scored by the caregivers ranged from 5.0 to 3.6 (scale 1–5) for different assistive tools and equipment.

Table 3. Most common assistive tools and ICT equipment listed by the caregivers and the Perceived Usefulness Scores (PUS). (Open question, N = 53)

Tools	N	PUS
Wheelchair/Stroller	16	4.9
Lifting device/subsidies	12	4.5
Computer/Tablet	11	4.2
Hospital bed	10	4.9
Mobile phone/Security phone	10	4.2
Washing/Shower chair	9	4.7
Rollator	6	3.6
Toilet rack	5	5.0
Electric/Bedsore mattress	4	4.9

Eight caregivers (15%) had some experience with telemonitoring their care recipient (i.e. door alarm, GPS tracking device, fall detector). Additional 14 (26%) would be willing to use telemonitoring applications. Personal emergency response systems, fall detectors, security phones, baby monitors, motion sensors and radar light had been used so far. GPS tracking devices, door alarms and security or web cameras seemed to be most requested in future.

Table 4. Times of day for the availability of the caregiver for teleassistance (i.e. by computer or phone) if the technology existed (N = 23).

Hours	6–9	9–12	12–15	15–18	18–21	21–24	24–3	3–6
Available	78%	78%	78%	87%	100%	87%	74%	74%
Limited availability	17%	4%	4%	4%	0%	9%	4%	4%
Not available		4%	13%	13%	9%	0%	0%	17%	17%

Thirty-four (64%) of the caregivers were unwilling to use telemonitoring applications because they felt there was no need, such applications would not help them, they were not familiar with the applications, or the care recipient needed caregiver's physical presence.

From the respondents seven (13%) had a pre-agreed terms about caregiving, for example about allowing care recipient to do as much as possible on his/her own and

Table 5. Factors related to ICT use in on-site and remote caregiving.

Factors	N	Have used ICT while assisting on-site	Have used ICT for teleassistance
Caregiver's age (years)			
30–39	7	17%	7%
40–49	13	8%	33%
50–59	11	33%	33%
60–69	15	25%	27%
70–79	5	17%	0%
80–	1	0%	0%
Care recipient's age			
1–9	7	33%	33%
10–29	11	33%	17%
30–49	7	0%	43%
50–69	12	25%	33%
70–89	12	25%	0%
90–100	4	0%	0%
Primary disability			
Memory disorder	12	23%	23%
Mental retardation	9	40%	10%
Old age	1	0%	0%
Physical disability	6	0%	57%
Parkinson's disease	3	17%	0%
Brain injury	5	33%	17%
Need of assistance			
Several days (4–6) in a week	2	0%	50%
Daily	14	7%	50%
Around the clock	37	30%	19%
Caregiver's contribution on the care			
20–40%	2	0%	50%
41–60%	6	33%	33%
61–80%	10	0%	60%
81–100%	35	29%	17%
Another work of the caregiver			
Has other work	19	21%	42%
Has no other work	34	24%	21%

assisting only when needed. Also there were terms about the responsibilities, such as who will take care of finances, groceries and medication. Occasionally terms and assistance were dependent on the schedules. Table 4 presents the times of day when the caregivers could help their care recipient from distance, assuming that suitable technology existed.

Table 5 presents factors related to ICT use in on-site and remote caregiving. The factors partly differed between on-site assistance and remote assistance. E.g. physical disability and mid-age of the care recipient were related with increased use of teleassistance.

4   Discussion

This survey presented limited current use of ICT of assistive technologies by family caregivers of disabled or elderly subjects. However, perceived usefulness was evaluated as high when these technologies were used. Additionally, there was some willingness to use assistive technologies if those existed or were available. The factors for the use of ICT were partly different for on-site assistance or remote assistance, e.g. physical disability and mid-age of the care recipient being related with increased use of teleassistance. The data obtained can be used in the development of future ICT and IoT –based assistive technologies.

Acknowledgments. The authors acknowledge the persons participating in the survey, and the Finnish Society for Caregivers (Omaishoitajat ry) for their help. Dr. Jorma Riihijärvi is acknowledged for statistical analyses. The study was supported by the ASTS (Assistive Technologies for Seniors, Teleassistance for seniors with Dementia – A Novel Concept for Safety) joint project by Academy of Finland (grant nr 270816) and Japan Science and Technology Agency; the iKaaS joint project by the European Union (grant nr 643262) and the Ministry of Internal Affairs and Communication, Japan; Infotech Oulu; and the Finnish Cultural Foundation.

References

1. McKeon, H.P.: Assistive Technology Act of 2004 (2004)
2. Mortenson, W.B., Demers, L., Fuhrer, M.J., Jutai, J.W., Lenker, J., DeRuyter, F.: Development and preliminary evaluation of the caregiver assistive technology outcome measure. J. Rehabil. Med. **47**, 412–418 (2015)
3. Administration on Aging. Assistive Technology. Fact Sheet. U.S. Department of Health and Human Services (2003)
4. Wilson, D.J., Mitchell, J.M., Kemp, B.J., Adkins, R.H., Mann, W.: Effects of assistive technology on functional decline in people aging with a disability. Assist. Technol. **21**, 208–217 (2009)
5. Salminen, A.L., Brandt, Å., Samuelsson, K., Töytäri, O., Malmivaara, A.: Mobility devices to promote activity and participation: a systematic review. J. Rehabil. Med. **41**, 697–706 (2009)
6. Aloulou, H., Mokhtari, M., Tiberghien, T., Biswas, J., Phua, C., Lin, J., Yap, P.: Deployment of assistive living technology in a nursing home environment: methods and lessons learned. BMC Med. Inform. Decis. Mak. **13**, 42 (2013)

7. National Center for Biotechnology Information. MESH-term: Caregiver. http://www.ncbi.nlm.nih.gov/mesh/68017028
8. Feinberg, L., Reinhard, S.C., Houser, A., Choula, R.: Valuing the Invaluable: The Growing Contributions and Costs of Family Caregiving (2011 update). American Association of Retired Persons, Washington (2011)

Self-aware Early Warning Score System for IoT-Based Personalized Healthcare

Iman Azimi[1]([✉]), Arman Anzanpour[1], Amir M. Rahmani[1,2], Pasi Liljeberg[1], and Hannu Tenhunen[1,2]

[1] Department of Information Technology, University of Turku, Turku, Finland
{imaazi,armanz,amirah,pakrli}@utu.fi, hannu@kth.se
[2] Department of Industrial and Medical Electronics,
KTH Royal Institute of Technology, Stockholm, Sweden

Abstract. Early Warning Score (EWS) system is specified to detect and predict patient deterioration in hospitals. This is achievable via monitoring patient's vital signs continuously and is often manually done with paper and pen. However, because of the constraints in healthcare resources and the high hospital costs, the patient might not be hospitalized for the whole period of the treatments, which has lead to a demand for in-home or portable EWS systems. Such a personalized EWS system needs to monitor the patient at anytime and anywhere even when the patient is carrying out daily activities. In this paper, we propose a self-aware EWS system which is the reinforced version of the existing EWS systems by using the Internet of Things technologies and the self-awareness concept. Our self-aware approach provides (i) system adaptivity with respect to various situations and (ii) system personalization by paying attention to critical parameters. We evaluate the proposed EWS system using a full system demonstration.

Keywords: Early warning score · Internet-of-Things · Self-awareness system · Personalized monitoring

1 Introduction

Patients suffering from life-threatening diseases have a high risk for a sudden clinical deterioration. Research on cardiac arrests shows that indications of deterioration are visible in patients vital signs several hours (often up to 24 h) prior to occurrence [1]. Therefore, prediction of imminent clinical deterioration is possible by paying enough attention to patient status [2,3]. Continuous patient monitoring in such a situation bring forth early detection and rapid response in a form of early treatment and prevention of fatal cases. It can also decrease the stress on hospital resources, reduce the associated costs and, most importantly, decrease mortality. Several scoring methods have been proposed based on vital signs to classify the risk level of patient status and to find the severity of the medical condition. Such methods are mostly scoring methods developed by emergency

© ICST Institute for Computer Sciences, Social Informatics and Telecommunications Engineering 2017
K. Giokas et al. (Eds.): eHealth 2016, LNICST 181, pp. 49–55, 2017.
DOI: 10.1007/978-3-319-49655-9_8

Table 1. A modified early warning score model [4]

Physiological parameters	3	2	1	0	1	2	3
Respiration rate (breaths/minute)		0-8		9-14	15-20	21-29	30+
Oxygen saturation (%)	0%-84%	85%-89%	90%-94%	95%-100%			
Temperature (oC)		0-35		35.1-38.0		38.1-39.5	39.6+
Systolic BP (mmHg)	0-69	70-80	81-100	101-149	150-169	170-179	180+
Heart rate (beats/minute)	0-39	40-50	51-59	60-100	101-110	111-129	130+
Level of consciousness				A	V	P	U

* A=Alert, V=response to voice, P=response to pain, U=unresponsive

departments or intensive care units in hospitals in which fast and dependable values are required.

Early warning score is the most prevalent method in medicine which has been in use for several years as a tool for predict the risk level of patients. This model was proposed for the first time by Morgan et al. in 1997 [5] as a paper-based method needing periodical checkups to assign a score based on patients vital signs (i.e., heart rate, respiration rate, body temperature, blood pressure, blood oxygen saturation). The score of each medical sign depends on the deviation from predefined normal limits, and the summation of all scores reflects the patients risk level [4]. Table 1 shows a Modified Early Warning Score guide. Manual data collection is a major drawback of this approach considering the unreliable results due to errors in recording and late response to deterioration due to the manual intervention. This has recently give pressure for hospitals to move towards electronic, computerized, and more intelligent solutions. Another drawback of current EWS systems is the dependency of the medical parameters to environmental conditions making the system limited to hospital strictly controlled environment.

Internet of things [6], as a network of connected physical and virtual things, is propagating in every corner of the world and leading us to smart solutions by constructing a new insightful medium. It enables the things with unique identities to satisfy common goals more efficient by interacting with each other. Considering a wireless body area sensor network (WBAN) for reading patients vital signs and an intelligent cloud service for processing the patients medical information, utilizing the Internet of Things is applicable for continuous patient monitoring to solve the drawbacks of current manual Early Warning Score systems both for eliminating the errors in recording and extending the solution to out of hospital.

We recently presented an IoT-based early warning system and demonstrated the feasibility of remote EWS monitoring using a full system implementation. More details are available in [7,8]. In this paper, we introduce a self-aware EWS system to personalize the system for remote monitoring scenarios and to provide intelligence in decision making process for patients at different situations. In addition, we utilize the *Attention* property of self-aware systems [9] to improve the energy efficiency, sensitivity and specificity of the system via adjusting the priorities of the heterogeneous sensory data w.r.t. changes in the environment or patients state.

2   Self-aware Early Warning Score System

Individuals suffering from acute diseases, such as cardiovascular diseases, might have several physical activities (e.g. sleeping, running and eating) and encounter diverse environments during a day. Unlike the EWS system in stationary hospital situation, the EWS results outside hospital environment might not be that accurate in many situations due to the susceptibility of vital signs to variations. A consistent heart rate more than 100 times per second in hospital might indicate a serious medical state whereas a healthy adult heart may beat 120 times per second during outdoor exercises. Hence, an adaptive and personalized system is required to consider the variants in the analysis and adapt the EWS score for the situation at hand.

Self-awareness can be utilized to reinforce the EWS system to tackle the daily monitoring obstacles. Self-awareness is defined as the ability of a system to be aware its state and surrounding environment and to adapt to new situations [10]. This knowledge enables a system to implement reasoning and intelligent decision making [11]. Similar to the available self-aware computing systems [9,12], the EWS system can be boosted to behave intelligently with respect to diverse situations. This can be realized by enhancing the score calculation process to consider patient state parameters. Moreover, as introduced in [9], Attention is an advantageous property in self-awareness which can provide efficient data acquisition and processing w.r.t. the instantaneous requirements of the system, and subsequently improve data analysis to obtain better results in terms of ambiguity, sensitivity and specificity of the results and energy efficiency of the system. In the following, we introduce our proposed IoT based self-aware EWS system (Fig. 1) constituting situation awareness and attention.

2.1   Situation Awareness

Situation awareness is utilized in our self-aware EWS system to provide adequate information about the patient. It enables the system to detect and predict patient deterioration regardless of the patient condition during daily activities. It can be achieved by considering the dependency of medical parameters to the variations, and intelligently respond to the changes. In this regard, patient state is defined to indicate the situation of the monitored person. It includes constant and variable parameters.

Constant parameters are defined as patient specification. Age, body mass index (BMI), and gender are main examples of such parameters influencing the average vital signs in different group of people [13] and their estimated scores in the EWS system. Physical condition and activity type of the patient are examples of variable parameters. We collect parameters such as position, altitude and pace in order to let the system determine the patient's current state. Machine learning algorithms can be utilized to recognize activity types such as sitting, running and sleeping and, subsequently, the related score ranges are adjusted.

2.2   Attention

Constant system functionality (e.g., data collection and data analysis rate) during the monitoring not only can lead to energy inefficiency and increased decision making latency, but also make the system susceptible in case of emergency because of not paying enough attention to critical parameters. Providing feedback from heterogeneous data coming from the sensory level, our self-aware EWS system is able to implement Attention property. To this end, the system determine priorities for different parameters in order to set a balance for data acquisition, analysis, and decision making.

The priorities make the system personalized with respect to the patient requirements at a time. For example, in case of a patient with a cardiovascular disease, the system should assign higher data collection rate and processing power to heart-related computations while reducing attention to non-related parameters. Moreover, patient state need to be considered in the priority calculation. Monitoring during an exercise makes the system more sensitive and subsequently increases the priorities. Other variables such as a high warning score for a long time and feedback from medical experts can also affect the priorities during the monitoring.

In addition, the attention unit adjusts the data collection for situation awareness enhancement. It eliminates the ambiguity of the results by adding more parameters to the calculation to improve situation awareness and consequently the sensitivity and specificity of the system. On the other hand, it removes the unnecessary data collection having insufficient correlation with the obtained results to enhance energy efficiency and latency of the system.

3   Demonstration and Evaluation

Our implemented IoT-based self-aware EWS system comprises three main components entitled as EWS, Situation Awareness and Attention (Fig. 1). The first part is the IoT-based EWS system including sensor network layer, a gateway and the cloud server. The sensor network layer acquires vital signs via wearable devices (i.e., BioHarness 3 chest strap, iHealth PO3 finger grip and iHealth BP5 device). In the gateway layer, we utilized a smartphone to receive data from sensors via Bluetooth. The score calculation and related emergency notifications are implemented in the server.

The second and third components are specified to implement the two self-awareness properties for the reinforcement of the basic IoT-based EWS system. The situation awareness includes data collection from activity-related sensors and analysis in the cloud. In the analysis, the situation is detected and consequently the related adjustments are applied to the score ranges. In addition, the third component (i.e., attention) considers the system feedback. Attention contributes to removing ambiguity in situation detection by adjusting data collection and updating the importance of each vital sign and encountered situations during the monitoring.

As a case study, the system continuously monitored a 35 years old healthy male subject (BMI = 28.3) for 8 h which in practice should get score 0. As shown in Fig. 2, incorrect (i.e., falsely calculated as high) scores in EWS while subject

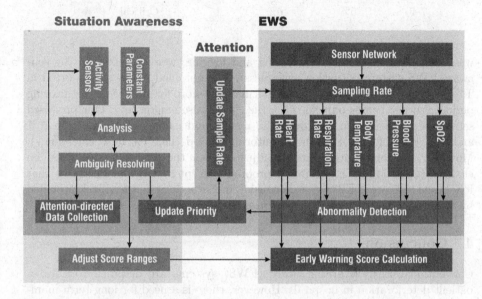

Fig. 1. Diagram of the proposed self-aware EWS system.

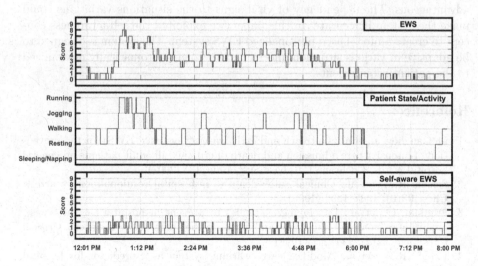

Fig. 2. Self-aware EWS adjustment according to the patient state (activity)

Table 2. A comparison on calculated scores between traditional EWS and self-aware EWS systems

Final score	EWS results	Self-aware EWS results	Emergency level
0	15%	46%	No action
1–3	50%	53%	Low
4–6	30%	1%	Equivocal
7–9	5%	0%	Critical

was having activities such as running and jogging, were corrected in the self-aware EWS system (situation awareness). The obtained scores are reported in Table 2. Conventional EWS system calculated 0 score for 15% of the monitoring period and 0–3 scores only for 65% (i.e., 35% false emergency). Our proposed self-aware EWS system improved the results and calculated 0 score for 46% and 0–3 scores for 99% of the monitoring period (i.e., 1% false emergency). Moreover, the computation rate are adjusted when the vital signs shows sudden changes (attention). The proposed proof-of-concept system demonstrates that IoT-based self-aware EWS system considering situations and feedback provided by attention can offer promising features and enhancements.

4 Conclusions

Conventional Early Warning Score (EWS) systems are designed to address patient deterioration in hospitals. However, there is a need for long-term monitoring of patients with serious diseases outside the hospital environment. Hence, automated EWS systems that can be continuously used in daily life would be advantageous. The dependency of vital signs to the situations variations could make the system inaccurate. In this paper, we exploited the self-awareness concept to create an IoT-based personalized EWS system. The system is designed to be adaptive in various situation and to be able to get automatically customized to the patient requirements.

References

1. McGaughey, J., et al.: Outreach and early warning systems (EWS) for the prevention of intensive care admission and death of critically ill adult patients on general hospital wards. Cochrane Database Syst. Rev., (3) (2007)
2. Schein, R.M., et al.: Clinical antecedents to in-hospital cardiopulmonary arrest. Chest **98**(6), 1388–1392 (1990)
3. Franklin, C., et al.: Developing strategies to prevent in hospital cardiac arrest: analyzing responses of physicians and nurses in the hours before the event. Critical Care Med. **22**(2), 244–247 (1994)
4. Urban, R.W., et al.: Modified early warning system as a predictor for hospital admissions and previous visits in emergency departments. Adv. Emerg. Nurs. J. **37**(4), 281–289 (2015)

5. Morgan, R.J.M., et al.: An early warning scoring system for detecting developing critical illness. Clin. Intensive Care **8**(2), 100 (1997)
6. Atzori, L., et al.: The internet of things: a survey. Comput. Netw. **54**(15), 2787–2805 (2010)
7. Anzanpour, A., et al.: Internet of things enabled in-home health monitoring system using early warning score. In: MobiHealth 2015 (2015)
8. Anzanpour, A., et al.: Context-aware early warning system for in-home healthcare using Internet-of-Things. In: HealthyIoT 2015 (2015)
9. Preden, J.S., et al.: The benefits of self-awareness and attention in fog and mist computing. Computer **48**(7), 37–45 (2015)
10. Lewis, P.R., et al.: A survey of self-awareness and its application in computing systems. In: SASOW, pp. 102–107 (2011)
11. Jantsch, A., Tammemae, K.: A framework of awareness for artificial subjects. In: CODES+ISSS, pp. 1–3 (2014)
12. Agarwal, A., et al.: Self-aware computing. Technical report, MIT (2009)
13. Ostchega, Y., et al.: Resting pulse rate reference data for children, adolescents, adults. United States, 1999–2008. National Health Stat Report (41) (2011)

Towards Longitudinal Data Analytics in Parkinson's Disease

Nikos F. Fragopanagos[1], Stefan Kueppers[2,3]([⊠]), Panagiotis Kassavetis[4],
Marco U. Luchini[3], and George Roussos[2]

[1] Retechnica Ltd., London, UK
[2] Birkbeck College, University of London, London, UK
stefan@dcs.bbk.ac.uk
[3] Benchmark Performance Ltd., London, UK
[4] Boston University, Boston, USA

Abstract. The CloudUPDRS app has been developed as a Class I medical device to assess the severity of motor symptoms for Parkinson's Disease using a fully automated data capture and signal analysis process based on the standard Unified Parkinson's Disease Rating Scale. In this paper we report on the design and development of the signal processing and longitudinal data analytics microservices, developed to carry out these assessments and to forecast the long-term development of the disease. We also report on early findings from the application of these techniques in the wild with a cohort of early adopters.

1 Introduction

The CloudUPDRS app and its associated information management and analytics platform, have been designed and developed to meet the standards set for medical devices. CloudUPDRS achieves the accurate, precise, and repeatable assessment of motor symptoms for people with Parkinson's (PwP), which clinicians can use with confidence. The app itself is employed as a data capture device relaying captured information to a service back-end developed following the microservices pattern [4] incorporating a so-called signal processing service that converts raw observations to motor performance metrics and a data analytics service that carries out longitudinal analyses revealing the pattern of development of the disease over time.

CloudUPDRS capitalises on the observation that it is possible to employ certain aspects of movement that are disrupted in Parkinson's as surrogate biomarkers of dopamine levels, a fact that forms the basis for Part III of the MDS-UPDRS. Previously, we investigated the possibility to precisely quantify and implement the MDS-UPDRS methodology as a smartphone app to enable the assessment of motor performance through tremor, gait and bradykinesia measurements obtained from standard sensors embedded in smartphones within a clinical setting [2]. Extending this approach, we currently focus on capturing in-depth medical intelligence supporting the discovery of longitudinal trends,

© ICST Institute for Computer Sciences, Social Informatics and Telecommunications Engineering 2017
K. Giokas et al. (Eds.): eHealth 2016, LNICST 181, pp. 56–61, 2017.
DOI: 10.1007/978-3-319-49655-9_9

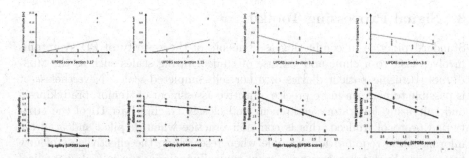

Fig. 1. Correlation between CloudUPDRS metrics and the corresponding sections of MDS-UPDRS.

promoting deeper understanding of the patterns of normal daily symptom variations, and predicting the onset of dyskinesias thus facilitating high-precision personalised targeting of treatment. A key ingredient of this work is that we have successfully transferred the process that until recently was available only in the clinical setting so that PwP and their carers can administer the tests unsupervised at home. We anticipate a significant reduction of the number of emergency hospital visits while considerably increasing data availability through high-frequency assessment of a large population of PwP (Fig. 1).

2 The CloudUPDRS App and Service Platfrom

Overall, the CloudUPDRS system consists of the following elements:

1. PD patient smartphone apps for Android and iOS that carry out motor performance measurements and wellness self-assessment; conduct session management; securely transfer captured data to the CloudUPDRS service; and, present an interface providing guidance and feedback.
2. Cloud-based scalable data collection engine that safely and securely collects data from patients' smartphones; ensures secure data management; and applies the MDS-UPDRS signal processing pipeline.
3. A data analytics toolkit for medical intelligence incorporating quantitative and semi-structured data, and longitudinal analyses, clustering and classification; and a clinical user interface incorporating visualisation.

The CloudUPDRS service platform enables the secure capture, management and analysis of data collected by the app and provides effective communication of insights generated to clinicians enabling them to explore alternative treatment scenarios. To cater for the diverse needs of the PwP population in the UK, the platform has been engineered to facilitate scalable performance by adopting the microservices architecture [6]. The microservices architectural style is set in contrast to traditional monolithic web applications and aims to maximise opportunities for vertical decomposition and scaling-out, which are critical for high performance and service resilience in data intensive situations.

3   Signal Processing Toolkit

Standard practice in conducting assessments of the severity of PD symptoms involves visit to a clinic and the use of clinical rating scales such as the MDS-UPDRS [1], using patient diaries or other self-completed scales. Nevertheless, it is possible to perform more precise objective assessment of tremor, bradykinesia and gait using laboratory equipment and closely tracing Part III of the MDS-UPDRS protocol. Indeed, this is common practice when detailed and accurate information is required for example when researching the effectiveness of new treatments. Such laboratory equipment typically includes specialised biomedical data acquisition systems incorporating transducers such as high-frequency/high-accuracy accelerometers and gyroscopes, signal amplifiers and filters and high-performance analog-to-digital converters as well as advanced single processing software. These systems are obtained by specialist commercial providers such as Cambridge Electronic Design Ltd. in the UK, currently the market leader, with the total cost of a complete system rising to tens of thousands.

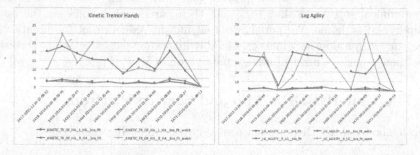

Fig. 2. Individual patient longitudinal analysis of kinetic tremor of the left hand and left leg agility showing significant daily variations.

3.1   Tremor

Tremor measurements are recorded for both hands at rest, at posture and in action. For rest tremor measurements, users are asked to relax their hands on their lap in a supine position while the phone is lying in their palm. For the postural tremor measurements patients are guided to keep their arm outstretched directly at their front while holding the smartphone. Finally, for action tremor measurements they are required to hold the phone and move it between the chest and the fully outstretched position at their front. In all cases, acceleration is recorded along three axes in m/s^2 at the maximum supported sampling rate and timestamped at maximum resolution (typically microseconds).

Tremor is calculated as the cumulative magnitude of the scalar sum acceleration across three axes for all frequencies between 2 Hz to 10 Hz. To obtain this power spectrum the signal is first filtered with a Butterworth high-pass second order filter at 2 Hz and the Fast Fourier Transform (FFT) subsequently applied to the filtered waveform data.

3.2 Bradykinesia

MDS-UPDRS assess bradykinesia, or else the slowness of movement, through three different factors: (i) pronation-supination movements, (ii) leg agility, and (iii) finger tapping. In the first test patients are asked to hold the phone and perform alternating pronation-supination movements, that is rotating the palm of the hand toward the inside so that it is facing downward and then toward the outside so that the palm is facing upward, as fast and as fully as possible. Leg agility measurements require the phone to be placed on the thigh of the patient while seated, holding the phone lightly with the ipsilateral hand, while raising and stomping the foot on the ground as high and as fast as possible. During both tests the phone is recording acceleration data in a manner similar to the tremor tests.

The assessment of the pronation-supination movements and leg agility tests requires the estimation of the frequency and power of movement. To obtain these, the toolkit first removes DC and applies a Butterworth low-pass second order filter at 4 Hz in order to exclude most of the tremor. Subsequently, the power of the movement is calculated as the total amplitude between 0 Hz and 4 Hz and the frequency derived from the power spectrum.

Finger tapping performance is assessed in two tests using single and dual targets presented on the screen of the phone at set locations with patients attempting to tap them as fast and as accurately as possible (alternating between targets in the dual-target case). When tapping accidentally occurs outside the screen area the test is repeated. The touch-sensitive screen of the smartphone is used to collect the information used for performance calculations, specifically the timing of each touch event, its duration, the direction of movement (upwards or downwards), the coordinates on the phone screen, and the amount of pressure applied are recorded. For the two-target variant it is necessary that the distance between targets be at a specific distance irrespective of the size of the screen or of the device.

To estimate finger tapping performance the analytical functions first identify all touch events and employ the associated timestamps to estimate tap frequency (expressed as number of taps per second), the mean hand movement time between taps (in milliseconds), and the actual movement distance between alternative tappings in the dual-target case (in centimetres). The calculation of distance requires scaling of measurements expressed in screen pixels to account for the pixel density characteristics of to particular smartphone model. Similar to tremor, bradykinesia functionalities in the CloudUPDRS analytics toolkit are implemented in python incorporating features from NumPy and SciPy.

3.3 Gait

MDS-UPDRS assesses gait by considering multiple behaviours including stride amplitude and speed, height of foot lift and heel strike, and turning and arm swing. The CloudUPDRS variant of this test requires the patient to walk along

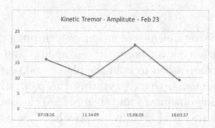
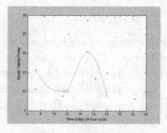

Fig. 3. Patterns of daily variation during a typical day of bradykinesia symptoms. The graph on the right displays a smoothed curve representing fine grain progression and offers a measure of variation between days.

a straight line for five meters, turn around and return to the point of departure, while the smartphone is positioned either in their belt or trousers pocket. Since it is only possible to measure acceleration data from a single point at the waistline it is realistic to attempt the estimation of only stride frequency and length, velocity and turning time. The estimation of these measurements in CloudUPDRS follows the techniques suggested [3] using PyWavelets for their implementation in python.

4   Testing

The performance of the CloudUPDRS signal processing toolkit was validated on a bespoke data set comprised of 20 complete sets of measurements. Results obtained from its application were compared against the same calculations implemented using Spike2 and matlab and compared against the UPDRS score provided for each test and patient by an experienced clinician after carrying out their standard assessment during a hospital consultation. This study [2] confirmed the consistent performance of CloudUPDRS against the golden standard i.e. clinical result and indeed indicated consistent accuracy exceeding 10^{-3} relative error suffices for MDS-UPDRS assessment.

5   Longitudinal Data Analytics

Having established the capability to conduct motor performance assessments at home and in the community using the CloudUPDRS app we have now developed a community of early adopters to develop and test a data analytics framework to study the longer-term development of the disease. Of particular interest is the investigation of ways to cluster patients in smaller groups that have similar progression patterns and are responsive to similar treatment. Indeed, symptoms vary greatly independent of treatment and PD progresses at different rates in different individuals, it requires regular clinical monitoring and medication adjustment. Our specific aim to develop novel opportunities to precisely quantify PD progression and the effectiveness of patient stratification [5]: the wider availability of data concerning individual variability and actual symptom trends provided by CloudUPDRS is expected to identify opportunities to adapt care to the needs of a particular individual at a specific time.

The first stage of this work is the identification of daily, weekly and longer patterns of variation in symptoms which would provide the baseline for adaptation. Figure 2 shows how upper and lower body performance varies during a period of weeks – clearly the day-to-day variation is significant and more importantly this variation is not typically captured by UPDRS scores that smooth out differences. Further, Fig. 3 shows an aggregate pattern of performance variation for bradykinesia thus providing an early result towards the development of characteristic patterns of disease variation for the individual.

6 Work in Progress

The longitudinal analysis presented in the previous Section has been based on data collected during a period of four months and while further improvements were implemented in both analytics and app. In particular, we are now able to identify a subset of tests that are specifically selected for each patient matching their particular symptoms. This allows a considerable reduction in the time required to carry out the test thus allowing even more frequent assessments. We anticipate that in the coming six month period we will have collected adequate information to be able to create progression profiles and in particular conduct reliable trend analysis on individual performance. This will further enable experimentation with clustering and classification techniques towards our objective of patient stratification.

Acknowledgments. Project CloudUPDRS: Big Data Analytics for Parkinson's Disease patient stratification is supported by Innovate UK (Project Number 102160).

References

1. Goetz, C.G., et al.: Movement disorder society-sponsored revision of the unified Parkinson's disease rating scale (MDS-UPDRS): scale presentation and clinimetric testing results. Mov. Disord. **23**(15), 2129–2170 (2008)
2. Kassavetis, P., Saifee, T.A., Roussos, G., Drougkas, L., Kojovic, M., Rothwell, J.C., Edwards, M.J., Bhatia, K.P.: Developing a tool for remote digital assessment of Parkinson's disease. Movement, Disorders Journal (2015)
3. Martin, E., et al.: Determination of a patient's speed and stride length minimizing hardware requirements. In: Proceedings of Body Sensor Networks, pp. 144–149 (2011)
4. Marz, N., Warren, J., Data, B.: Principles and Best Practices of Scalable Realtime Data Systems. Manning Publications, Shelter Island (2013)
5. Matthews, P.M., Edison, P., Geraghty, O.C., Johnson, M.R.: The emerging agenda of stratified medicine in neurology. Nat. Rev. **10**, 15–27 (2014)
6. Newman, S.: Building Microservices. O'Reilly Media, San Francisco (2015)

GOWELL 2016

Cultures of Participation in the Healthcare Field: Could a VideoGame-Based Perspective Be Useful?

Ines Di Loreto[(✉)]

TechCICO, ICD-Université de Technologie de Troyes, Troyes, France
ines.di_loreto@utt.fr

Abstract. The games for health field links many actors with many complementary roles. In an ideal world, all the stakeholders participate to each Participatory Design loop and all continue to participate meaningfully as the design is specified, implemented, delivered, installed, and used. In this paper we argue that before a successful Participatory Design session can take place all the stakeholders need to construct a common Culture of Participation. In order to construct this shared Culture of Participation we propose to use games (in place of Participatory Design sessions) to reach a sufficient level of shared understanding that will allow to improve rehabilitation methods and treatments.

Keywords: Participatory design · Games for health · Serious games · Culture of participation

1 Introduction

In a 2007 paper, Carroll and Rosson [1] observed that Participatory Design integrated two radical propositions about design at its origins. The first is the moral proposition that the people who will be affected most directly by a design outcome should have a say in what that outcome is. This leads to the assumption that users *have a right* to be directly included in the design process. The second is the pragmatic proposition that the people who will need to adopt, and perhaps to adapt to an artefact, should be included in the design process, so that they can offer expert perspectives and preferences regarding the activity that the design will support, and most likely transform. The pragmatic proposition leads to the assumption that the direct inclusion of the users' input will *increase the chances of a successful design outcome.*

In an ideal world, all the relevant stakeholders participate to each design loop and all continue to participate meaningfully as the design is specified, implemented, delivered, installed, and used. The Participatory Design (PD) process becomes a social negotiation among partners, and the designer's responsibility in this process is to faithfully translate, collaborate, and respond to the concerns of the other stakeholders [1].

We would like to argue that, for this social negotiation to be fruitful, all the stakeholders need to construct a common Culture of Participation [2], which will create the shared background on the top of which Participatory Design can take place. A Culture of Participation (CP) describes how participants will act and react to

© ICST Institute for Computer Sciences, Social Informatics and Telecommunications Engineering 2017
K. Giokas et al. (Eds.): eHealth 2016, LNICST 181, pp. 65–74, 2017.
DOI: 10.1007/978-3-319-49655-9_10

Participatory Design. It reflects the values that underpin participatory practice and the reasons for involving and being involved, when and how participation is used, and the extent to which the different actors are listened to and appropriate action is taken [3]. Cultures of participation require contributors with diverse background knowledge who require different support and value different ways of participating. The difficulty to make all these different contributors work together is particularly evident in the games for health field.

The health field (excluding for the moment the gaming part) links many actors with many complementary roles. At the centre is the patient, the person whose health will be considered. Around her, people whose numbers and richness of roles vary gravitate. Doctors, specialists, auxiliary nurses and other therapists, spouse and family are all people who interact with the patient, and can influence in one way or another (i.e., more or less directly) her health. The scenario becomes increasingly complex when we add to the scene also the professionals who will develop the games for health. While this inclusion allows for taking into account not only the health aspects but also the playful mechanisms linked with video games, doctors and game developers rarely share a common Culture of Participation. If we consider Participatory Design in terms of who should sit around the table during the design phase, we are tempted to look only at the primary circle represented in Fig. 1: the patient, the healthcare staff, and the game designers. However what happens is more similar to the secondary circle. Sitting around the table are not only the primary stakeholders, but also the beliefs they have, their cultural background, their habits in participation, and we could go on adding the

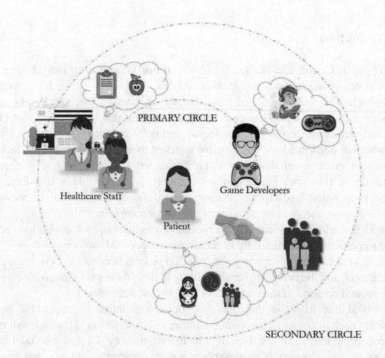

Fig. 1. The Game for health ecosystem

sociopolitical and technical structure (such as the hospital, the game studio where the game will be developed and so on) surrounding each of these actors.

In addition, health professional are adopting new collaborative practices to handle cost-containment policies and the need to take care of increasing numbers of patients and elderly people staying at home; collaborative practices that are more similar to Engestrom knotworking [32] – where people are loosely connected - than classical structured healthcare collaborative practices [33].

To better understand if and how the actors and elements in the secondary circle can participate in creating a common Culture of Participation for the games for health domain, we will first look at the cultures of participations for each different stake-holders and then try to understand where these cultures could meet. At the end of the paper, we will give a suggestion for a possible reversal of perspective. It is worth to note that this work does not pretend to be exhaustive. It will not take into account for example the socio-technical and political implication of a shared Culture of Partici-pation, elements that will need to be taken into account for a real application of the proposed approach.

2 Culture of Participation in the Healthcare Field: The Health Personnel and the Patient

When we talk about Culture of Participation (CP) in the healthcare domain, we first think about humanitarian assistance, particularly during a crisis. During a period of humanitarian crisis, hundreds or thousands of people around the world organize themselves to provide logistical, food or medical support for local people in need. Many organizations like the *Red Cross* or *Médecins Sans Frontières* are able to quickly provide emergency medical assistance across the world. However, humanitarian aid is increasingly structured and professionalized, with humanitarian organizations now looking for professionals and specialists from diverse professions. Laypeople across the world support these humanitarian organizations mostly thorough financial participa-tion. On a local level, medical institutions and services – through their health personnel – constitute complex systems. They include highly specialized knowledge and skills aimed to treat the higher number of people possible. They form what can be called an expert group, using their special skills on a second group, the laypeople (patients and relative), which is inherently in a subordinate position: this second group is requesting care and is usually devoid of health competencies. The relationship between the health personnel and patients and families is thus an asymmetrical one. On the opposite side there is peer communication between colleagues, where health professionals (we are using here health professional as a generic term, even if the relationship between e.g., doctors and nurses should be further expanded) turn to each other for information and decision support. It is through the multitude of conversations scattered during the clinical day, for example, that clinicians examine, present, and interpret clinical data and ultimately decide on clinical actions [4]. Social interaction between peers is composed of sharing and interpreting information as an interactive process that emerges out of communication. Discussing a medical problem with a clinical colleague or with a patient results thus in very different conversations. Unsurprisingly, human agents communicate more easily with others of similar occupation and educational background, since they have similar experiences, beliefs, and knowledge [5]. Still, these kind of conversation are local and time limited, constructed around a particular patient or case, and thus very dependent on the context and on the people participating in the conversation.

Not only do patients and health personnel not share a common knowledge, but neither do they share a common Culture of Participation. For example, cultural issues play a major role in patient compliance, and in her willingness to participate to the Participatory Design culture [6]. Patients and their families bring culture specific ideas and values related to concepts of health and illness, reporting of symptoms, expectations for how health care will be delivered, and beliefs concerning medication and treatments. In addition, culture specific values influence patient roles and expectations, how much information about illness and treatment is desired, how death and dying will be managed, bereavement patterns, gender and family roles, and processes for decision making. Unfortunately, in the asymmetric relationship described above, the expectation of many health care professionals (that patients will conform to their health values) have frequently created barriers to care that have been compounded by differences in language and education between patients and providers from different backgrounds. In this scenario, the *faith* the patient has in her doctor, could influence the acceptance of the therapy. During a project on the usage of mixed reality and games for post stroke rehabilitation, the author of this paper heard more than once (from patients not used to playing video games) statements such as: "if my doctor says it is useful, then I will do it" [7]. The acceptance/resistance to the usage of the proposed tools was thus subordinated to the confidence relationship between the patient and the doctor. In this setup is kind of improbable that the designer, the patient, and the doctor, will be on the same level while doing PD sessions.

The scenario becomes more and more complicated if we analyze the implementation of a shared Culture of Participation between health institutions. While from an insider perspective the above mentioned culture of information sharing and discussion is the norm, between hospitals it involves mostly information sharing (when it is not clearly hampered by the *publish or perish* factor[1]). Finally, the healthcare sector is known to be relatively change resistant (e.g. [8]), and with a reason. Introducing new technologies and treatments usually involves going through long and complicated approval processes as the risks associated with healthcare are extremely high. A wrongfully applied treatment or a poorly designed technology might at best not help a patient's recovery, but potentially leads to worsening of a patient's condition, or even death.

Still, healthcare is one of the most promising domains for the application of end-user development [9] and cultures of participation [10]. In many cases, patients have such specific conditions that they are in a 'universe of one' [11]: a unique case. Therefore, standardized technologies and treatments might not deliver an optimal solution and it seems only logical to allow doctors, therapists, caregivers and even patients to adjust these technologies to better fit the needs of the individual patient [12].

---

[1] Publish or perish" is a phrase coined to describe the pressure in academia to rapidly and continually publish academic work to sustain or further one's career.

Different attempts to create formal practices for Participatory Design in the health domain have been proposed. Arstein [13] described the different possible interactions between the power holders and the powerless, and proposes a 8 levels ladder of participation from "citizen control" to "manipulation". Each rung corresponds to the extent of citizens' power in determining the end product. Tritter et al. [14] judge Arstein's ladder not adapted for health and too power oriented which limits effective responses and undermines the potential of the user involvement in the process. For this reason they propose a new model and argue that user involvement in improving health services must acknowledge the value of the process, and the different knowledge and experience of both, health professionals and laypeople.

In recent decades, a number of user-centered approaches have been introduced for the development of health information systems, like usability engineering [15] or contextual design [16]. In particular, PD methods have widely been applied in the field of health informatics [17–19]. Indeed, Clemensen [18] adapted PD adding a clinical trial phase to take the experiment into a real life situation, testing the idea with health care workers and patients who have not participated in the project. They conclude that PD provides an effective means for researchers from the seemingly disparate worlds of health science and computer science to work together.

Still, we should keep in mind that whatever designed artefact (and thus also computer based systems as games) conveys a cultural message and that technology and its adoption are not neutral phenomena that give equal chance to concordance and dissent: through the design of an artefact, the invisible work of 'others', alternative cultures and sciences (and thus alternative solutions) are receding [20].

3   Culture of Participation in Game and Serious Game Design

By observing the practices of the gaming industry we realize very quickly that every game studio (and we could say each team–artists, game designers, developers-in a studio) sets up its own strategy for game design and game development. As in the game market originality is the factor that can give a competitive advantage, information sharing between studios is not the norm (with a dynamic that is not different from the scientific publish or perish one). Inside each studio, information and conversation sharing vary depending on the size of the studio, the type of product, and the inter-action that developers have with their gaming community (that, in the case of Serious Games for health, could be brought back to patients and family).

Still, sectors of the game development market share a common culture, a game culture based on the games they played as children plus the game culture of the studio they are currently working in. In game developers conferences- GDC[2] for example –it wasn't unusual some years ago to hear discussions on if or not casual gaming should be considered a real form of gaming. The logical structure of those discussions wasn't far from the one used in the artistic domain when evaluating if a particular form of art – graffiti for example- should be considered art; and concerned categories such as the

---

[2] http://www.gdceurope.com/.

artistic value of the final game, the time spent developing it, and so on. While at first glance it could seem that the Game Development field does not involve a Culture of Participation, things change when we look at the relationship developers/players. Opposite to what happens in the healthcare field, where the patient is not consulted about the diagnosis or the creation of a new therapy, in the last ten years the game development field has seen many initiatives promoting broad participation and reconciliation between game designers and players. Not only we assist to the practice of beta testing, in which early version of the games are released to get costumer advices on future developments, but also crowd-funding has been a key driver for video game creation (for more information see e.g., [21]). Many projects were possible only thanks to this participatory funding system. In this way consumactors (a term defining users that are consumers and actors at the same time) could define the major trends to be followed by the industry[3].

In the same way, game jams (i.e., gathering of game developers for the purpose of planning, designing, and creating one or more games within a short span of time) take now place on a planetary scale and help further democratize video games creation.

Hence, the video game industry has taken advantage of its Culture of Participation to bring closer game creators and players, increasing its own potential and diffusion.

In what concerns the Serious Game for health field, the Culture of Participation of this domain is more similar to the scientific one, in particular through the usage of Participatory Design. Different specific approaches have been created to integrate the serious and playful dimensions, in particular, giving the final user (in most cases doctors) power on the content of the Serious Game. In his analysis work, Djaouti [22] reviews a dozen of different design tools and methods for conceiving educational serious games, such as the one focused on the usage of technical tools [23], the content centered model [24], design patterns for serious games [25] or the DODDEL model [26]. All these methods aim to enable people new to game creation, but with competences on the serious domain, to make pedagogical games aimed to transmit knowledge or skills. This kind of approach allow the designer to understand the needs of patients and therapist without becoming an expert of the domain.

4 Discussion: Is It Possible to Create a Shared Culture of Participation in the Games for Health Domain?

The actors we described until now have thus very different Cultures of Participation that are not always compatible. In addition, even if we did not address the PD expert's Culture of Participation, it is worth to note that saying that it is the designer's responsibility in the PD process to faithfully translate, collaborate, and respond to the concerns of the other stakeholders is not neutral on consequences. In some way we are saying that the designer is an expert of expert, someone with a meta-knowledge who will know what is better to take and what to leave from the PD session with the concerned actors. This assumption - not necessarily false and surely useful to have a

---

[3] The pertinence and openness of this approach has still to be proved.

final artefact by the end of the process - could lead to adoption problems if the artefact wasn't created in a shared CP [34]. In our specific context, the risk is amplified by the kind of tools we are designing: serious games in the health field. These tools require a high level of acceptance by two stakeholders, the healthcare professionals and the patients, of a tool that is not devoid of stigmatization [27]. Still, considering the point of views of a maximum of different types of actors during design phases could potentially lead to better solutions and offer patients the best possible treatment for their situation.

Even if from our discussion, it seems difficult to reconcile the video games and the healthcare worlds, there is a notable example proving that it is not only possible but also profitable to make the video games and the medical worlds to cooperate through technology: *Foldit*. *Foldit*[4] is a puzzle video game invented to imagine protein folding possibilities in order to improve the knowledge about proteins and their modeling. Thanks to this experience that brought together more than 200 000 *non-expert* users, players and researchers have been able to find the 3D structure of a retroviral HIV protease, a necessary step in the development of a treatment drug.

Games for health are still recent and, as seen above, very few methods or tools exist in order to improve communication and collaboration between all the different concerned actors. Donnellon et al., [28, p.44] explain that when groups of participants do not have «shared meanings» or shared interpretations, they may engage in coordinated action by engaging in a set of communication practices that enable them to create "equifinal meanings." Equifinal meanings, they explain, are "interpretations that are dissimilar but that have similar behavioral implications." Achieving equifinal meanings does not require that participants achieve equal or overlapping understandings but rather that they develop a set of complementary understandings that lead to coordinated actions. If we look attentively, this is exactly what happened in the *Foldit* example, where people worked together in a loosely way, without necessarily sharing a common objective. The collective work in the *Foldit* project however, could potentially lead to a community who shares a common Culture of Participation that could be re-instantiated in other occasions. We believe that not starting from Participatory Design sessions but from videogames play is exactly the means we should exploit to create a common CP between health professionals, patients, and game designers. The act of playing together could thus be used as a pretext to create a shared language and a common understanding.

A first attempt by the authors to devise a coherent approach with various stake-holders through game play could be read in [29]. The game described in the paper had as aim to help with the rehabilitation of equilibrium disorders. It was however designed with the goal of adoption not only by patients and therapists, but also by the general public (for example, to be able to involve the family in the therapy). In order to achieve this goal, an incremental approach was put into practice, with game sessions (not necessarily involving the designed game) with all the different stakeholders. We tried thus to introduce the different actors to the game culture, and not only asked game designers to appropriate the healthcare one. This approach forced us to rethink Participatory Design sessions and the shift of perspective showed interesting results in a first experiment for the video game event MIG -Montpellier in Games.

---

[4] http://fold.it/portal/.

5   Conclusions

Participatory design is both a moral proposition where users *have a right* to be directly included in the process of design, and a pragmatic proposition *to create better arte-facts*. Still, there is a lack of a common Culture of Participation that could prevent implementing both propositions when doing Participatory Design. We nevertheless believe that an increased Culture of Participation in this area would strengthen the creation, use, and potential of games for health [30]. Therefore, a fundamental challenge for supporting cultures of participation should be to conceptualize and create socio-technical environments able to take into account the different cultures of participation. We proposed to use games (in place of Participatory Design) to reach a sufficient level of shared understanding that will allow to create a shared Culture of Participation, thus allowing to improve rehabilitation methods and treatments.

References

1. Carroll, J., Rosson, M.B.: Participatory design in community informatics. Des. Stud. **28**, 243–261 (2007)
2. Fischer, G.: End user development and meta-design: foundations for cultures of participation. J. Organ. End User Comput. **22**(1), 52–82 (2010)
3. Kirby, P., Lanyon, C., Cronin, K., Sinclair, R.: Building a Culture of Participation. Involving children and young people in policy, service planning, delivery and evaluation (2003). Retrieved May 2016. http://resourcecentre.savethechildren.se/sites/default/files/documents/1259.pdf
4. Coiera, E.: When conversation is better than computation. J. Am. Med. Inform. Assoc. JAMIA **7**(3), 277–286 (2000)
5. Lazarsfeld, P.F., Merton, R.K.: Friendship as social process: a substantive and methodological analysis. In: Berger, M., et al. (eds.) Freedom and Control in Modern Society, p. 1964. Octagon, New York (1964)
6. EuroMed Info: How culture influences health beliefs (2014). Retrieved May 2016. http://www.euromedinfo.eu/how-culture-influences-health-beliefs.html/
7. Di Loreto, I., Dokkum, L., Gouaich, A., Laffont, I.: Mixed reality as a means to strengthen post-stroke rehabilitation. In: Shumaker, R. (ed.) VMR 2011. LNCS, vol. 6774, pp. 11–19. Springer, Heidelberg (2011). doi:10.1007/978-3-642-22024-1_2
8. Boonstra, A., Broekhuis, M.: Barriers to the acceptance of electronic medical records by physicians from systematic review to taxonomy and interventions. BMC Health Serv. Res. **10**(1), 1–17 (2010)
9. Costabile, M.F., Lanzilotti, R., Piccinno, A.: Analysis of EUD survey questionnaire (2003). http://giove.isti.cnr.it/projects/EUD-NET/d4.2.htm
10. Fischer, G.: Understanding, fostering, and supporting cultures of participation. ACM Interact. **18**(3), 42–53 (2011)
11. Carmien, S.P. Fischer, G.: Design, adoption, and assessment of a socio-technical environment supporting independence for persons with cognitive disabilities. In: Proceedings of CHI 2008, pp. 597–606. ACM (2008)

12. Tetteroo, D., Markopoulos, P.: Cultures of participation in healthcare: a healthy idea? Cultures of participation in the digital age. In: International Workshop at Advanced Visual Interfaces, AVI 2014 (2014)
13. Arnstein, S.R.: A ladder of citizen participation. J. Am. Inst. Planners **35**(4), 216–224 (1969)
14. Tritter, J.Q., McCallum, A.: The snakes and ladders of user involvement: moving beyond Arnstein. Health Policy **76**(2), 156–168 (2006)
15. Malhotra, A., Laxmisan, A., Keselman, J., Zhang, V.L.: Patel designing the design phase of critical care devices: a cognitive approach. J. Biomed. Inform. **38**(1), 34–50 (2005)
16. Martin, J.L., Murphy, E., Crowe, J.A., Norris, B.J.: Capturing user requirements in medical device development: the role of ergonomics. Physiol. Meas. **27**(8), R49–R62 (2006)
17. Sjöberg, C., Timpka, T.: Participatory design of information systems in health care. J. Am. Med. Inform. Assoc. **5**(2), 177–183 (1998)
18. Clemensen, J., Larsen, S.B., Kyng, M., Kirkevold, M.: Participatory design in health sciences: using cooperative experimental methods in developing health services and computer technology. Qual. Health Res. **17**(1), 122–130 (2007)
19. Pilemalm, S., Timpka, T.: Third generation participatory design in health informatics— making user participation applicable to large-scale information system projects. J. Biomed. Inform. **41**(2), 327–339 (2008)
20. Locoro, A., Cabitza, F.: Should the culture of participation inform a new Ethics of Design? Cultures of participation in the digital age. In: International workshop at Advanced Visual Interfaces, AVI 2014 (2014)
21. Melia, G., Di Loreto, I.: Participatory design in the games for health domain: why and for whom? Cultures of participation in the digital age. In: International workshop at Advanced Visual Interfaces, AVI 2014 (2014)
22. Djaouti, D., Alvarez, J., Jessel, J.P., Rampnoux, O.: Origins of serious games (2010). Retrieved May 2016. http://bit.ly/11Kxa5x
23. Robertson, J., Howells, C.: Computer game design: opportunities for successful learning. Comput. Educ. **50**(2), 559–578 (2008)
24. Moreno-Ger, P., et al.: A content-centric development process model. Computer **41**(3), 24–30 (2008)
25. Marne, B., Huynh-Kim-Bang, B., Labat, J-M.: Articuler motivation et apprentissage grâce aux facettes du jeu sérieux. In: Actes de la conférence EIAH 2011 (2011)
26. McMahon, M.: Using the DODDEL model to teach serious game design to novice designers. In: ASCILITE (2009)
27. Newman, J.: Playing with Videogames. Routledge, London (2008). Everybody hates videogames, Chap. 1, pp. 1–20
28. Donnellon, A., Gray, B., Bougon, M.G.: Communication, meaning, and organized action. Adm. Sci. Q. **31**(1), 43–55 (1986)
29. Di Loreto, I., Lange, B., Seilles, A., Andary, S., Dyce, W.: Game design for all: the example of hammer and planks. In: Ma, M., Oliveira, M.F., Petersen, S., Hauge, J.B. (eds.) SGDA 2013. LNCS, vol. 8101, pp. 70–75. Springer, Heidelberg (2013). doi:10.1007/978-3-642-40790-1_7
30. Barricelli, B.R., Fischer, G., Mørch, A., Piccinno, A., Valtolina, S.: Cultures of participation in the digital age: coping with information, participation, and collaboration overload. In: Díaz, P., Pipek, V., A, C., Jensen, C., Aedo, I., Boden, A. (eds.) IS-EUD 2015. LNCS, vol. 9083, pp. 271–275. Springer, Heidelberg (2015). doi:10.1007/978-3-319-18425-8_28
31. Herold, D.K., Sawhney, H., Fortunati, L.: Introduction to Understanding Creative Users of ICTs: Users as Social Actors. Routledge, London (2012)

32. Engeström, Y., Engeström, R., Vähäaho, T.: When the center does not hold: the importance of knotworking. In: Activity Theory and Social Practice: Cultural-Historical Approaches, pp. 345–374 (1999)
33. Abou Amsha, K., Lewkowicz, M.: Shifting patterns in home care work: supporting collaboration among self-employed care actors. In: De Angeli, A., Bannon, L., Marti, P., Bordin, S. (eds.) COOP 2016: Proceedings of the 12th International Conference on the Design of Cooperative Systems, 23–27 May 2016, Trento, Italy, pp. 139–154. Springer, Switzerland (2016)
34. Schaper, L.K., Pervan, G.P.: ICT and OTs: a model of information and communication technology acceptance and utilisation by occupational therapists. Int. J. Med. Inform. **76**, S212–S221 (2007)

Exploiting Users Natural Competitiveness to Promote Physical Activity

Matteo Ciman and Ombretta Gaggi[✉]

Department of Mathematics, University of Padua, Padua, Italy
`Matteo.Ciman@unige.ch`, `gaggi@math.unipd.it`

Abstract. *ClimbTheWorld* is a *serious game* to promote physical activity, by asking users to climb stairs, simulating the climbing of a real building. In this paper, we describe the complete redesign of the game to improve its persuasion capability, by adding collaboration and competition between users, and micro-goals to encourage the user to do not give up. Our experiments show that the game is really effective in incentivizing people in taking stairs, in particular singleplayer modes increased the average amount of stairsteps made of about 61%, while multiplayer modes of about 64%.

Keywords: Persuasive technology · Serious games · Mobile computing

1 Introduction

The reduced or insufficient amount of physical activity is a well-known problem of modern society, which spreads across different ages, since in the recent years also children suffer from some of its consequences, e.g., obesity [2,3]. Many figures, e.g., doctors, teachers and personal trainers, constantly warn population against risks connected to physical inactivity, but they are often unsuccessful.

In the recent years, researchers have explored the possibility to use smartphones as a sort of *digital personal trainer*, since they are equipped with a set of sensors which allows to analyze and recognize users' activity. Moreover, they are already present in most users' pockets, therefore there is no need for the user to buy other expensive devices.

Many applications have been developed with the aim of persuading people to increase their physical activity. Some examples of *digital personal trainer* are "Runtastic" [11], "FitBit" [4] and "Nike + Running" [9], which propose a set of exercises, record the user performances and, sometimes, share them with users friends. Their biggest problem is that they have a very specific target users, that are people already healthy and that want to keep themselves active.

A different approach is the usage of the *serious game paradigm* to persuade users to perform physical activity while having fun. A *seriuos game* [15] is a game whose principal intent is not fun, but to hide under fun an activity which is useful for the user. In this case, the application transforms physical exercises in games. As an example, "Zombies, Run!" [12] asks to the user to run away from

K. Giokas et al. (Eds.): eHealth 2016, LNICST 181, pp. 75–83, 2017.
DOI: 10.1007/978-3-319-49655-9_11

a group of zombies following him/her; the "Piano stairs" Project [14] transforms stairs climbing into music playing since each stairstep is a key of a piano.

Another example is *BeatClearWalker* [6], a smartphone Android application that asks people to do 8000 steps/day, walking in a moderate intensity. This *serious game* helps users to walk at the right cadence by reducing the audio quality of the music when the target walking cadence is not respected. *Fish'n'Steps* [8] is a *serious game* that links the walking activity with the growth and moving activity of a fish in a fish tank. Moreover, a kind of social function of the game has been introduced, since it is possible to create a sort of environment with other participants both for competition and collaboration. After the first two weeks of experiment, players' enthusiasm for the game decreased. Nevertheless, this was a really good result since the participants changed their habits and lifestyle in the meanwhile and they did not need any more the *serious game*.

In this paper we present the redesign of our application *ClimbTheWorld*, a *serious game* to promote physical activity. It is an Android application which is able to recognize and count stairsteps. Each stairstep in a *real* building corresponds to a *virtual* stairstep. In this way the user simulates the climbing of a building each time he/she, chooses the stairs instead of elevators or escalators. Figure 1a shows the user interface of the game. When the user reaches the top of a building, he/she gains the access to a gallery of pictures about the building and the view from the top of it, as shown in Fig. 1b.

A first version of this game was presented in [1]. We aimed at understanding if it was possible to recognize stairsteps using only smartphone sensors and its limited computation capability. In this paper, we focus on improving its persuasive capability. In particular, we have added collaboration and competition between users, implementing challenges between single users or group of users. Players can also collaborate to reach the top of a very high building. We analyzed the game using the Fogg Behaviour Model (FBM) [5], and we implemented a system to provide *Trigger* at the right moment. Then, we added micro-goals to encourage the user to do not give up.

2   Modelling Persuasiveness

The Fogg Behavior Model (FBM) [5] is a model to design tools with a good chance of persuading users to do something. Three elements must converge at the same moment for a behavior to occur: *Motivation*, *Ability* and *Triggers*. *Ability* is not a problem for our target audience, since the game is not intended for impaired users, so our target user is considered able to climb the stairs. Clearly, climbing stairs can become tiring or even frustrating. For this reason, we added *sub-goals* so that the goal is not too far away. In Fig. 1a, the stars on the bar on the left side of the interface denote the sub-goals. They are used to encourage users to never give up.

Each stairstep in real life corresponds to one (or more) stairstep in the game, according to the difficulty level. Different difficulty levels also bring different quality and number of provided photos, thus user's satisfaction (see Fig. 1b).

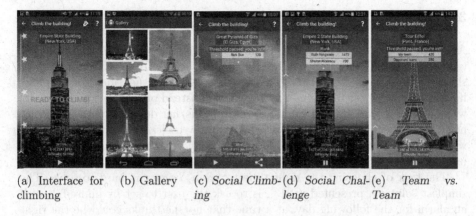

(a) Interface for climbing (b) Gallery (c) *Social Climbing* (d) *Social Challenge* (e) *Team vs. Team*

Fig. 1. *ClimbTheWorld* application.

To improve both *Motivation* and *Ability*, we designed four different game modes: we call "social" the game modes which involve user's friends[1].

The "Solo Climb" game mode requires the user to climb a building alone (Fig. 1a). Figure 1c shows a screenshot of the "Social Climb" game mode, where the user has invited one of his/her Facebook friends to help him/her to reach the top of the Pyramid of Giza. This game mode improves *Ability*, since it lowers the required number of stairsteps. *Motivation* is strongly affected by two other game modes, "Social Challenge" and "Team vs. Team", by exploiting the natural competitiveness of the users. The first one implements a challenge between two (or more) players. Differently from "Social Climb", the players do not collaborate but compete. The winner is the first user that reaches the top of the building. Figure 1d shows a screenshot during a challenge between two players. Similarly, the "Team vs. Team" game mode (Fig. 1e) implements a challenge between teams of an equal number of players.

The game also considers the problem of the management of *freeloaders*, i.e., players who join a team or a "social" climb but do not contribute to the climb with stairsteps. To avoid this kind of players, *ClimbTheWorld* imposes a threshold (see Fig. 1c and e): players who do not contribute with a minimal set of stairsteps are not rewarded even in case of victory.

Triggers are implemented by a push notification that remembers the player to play the game and take stairs. According to the FBM, this type of *Triggers* are called *signals* and are discussed in details in Sect. 3.

To increase the engagement of the user, the game provides some bonuses, to constantly encourage and help the user. Each bonus depends on user's performance: if the user improves his/her performance with respect to the day before, he/she gets a 30% increase on the total number of stairsteps made.

---

[1] These modes require the user to connect to Facebook and to give the application the right to explorer his/her network of friends.

3 Design of the Trigger

According to FBM, one of the key elements that influences the possibility or not to change people' behavior are the so called *Triggers*. To be efficient, *Triggers* should happen at the right time. This is a very difficult issue, since, for example, if we want to suggest to the user to take stairs instead of elevators or escalators while he/she is working and cannot move from his/her desk, or simply there are no stairs in the area, these *Triggers* are absolutely useless, if not disturbing, and will not help in behavior change. Moreover, *Triggers* can also be used to keep users involved in the game.

The task of choosing the right time to fire a *Trigger* is hard to solve. The simplest solution, presented in [13], is to ask the user to set by himself/herself an alarm for the following day, at a time that he/she thinks could be the right moment to perform the target activity or, in general, some physical activity. This solution has some drawbacks: it is not ubiquitous, and it is boring for the user since it requires the person to set every day the alarm for the day after. We propose a solution which is able to automatically adapt itself to user habits, showing *Triggers* only when it is supposed to be the best moment of the day. This solution is to silently sense user's activity, in order to learn user's habits. It is not intrusive, since it requires only an initial setup, and afterwards is able to understand user habits and the best moments to show *Triggers*.

We were inspired by genetic algorithms [10]: we consider a population in which each individual corresponds to an interval of time of one our. At the first run, the user has to indicate in which time slots performs/probably performs/do not perform physical activity. Figure 2 shows the user interface to give this initial knowledge: time slots in which the user declares to perform physical activity are marked as green, the slots in which he/she declares a probability to perform some physical activity are marked as yellow, and the slots in which the user does not perform physical activity are marked as red and are not considered by the algorithm. The stairstep classifier, which is more expensive in terms of energy consumption, is used to sense the user activity during the green intervals of time,

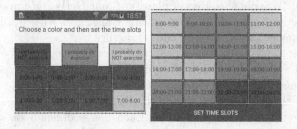

Fig. 2. Initial setup of time slots to provide initial information to the algorithm (Color figure online)

while the Google Activity Recognition service[2] is used to understand if, and in which measure, some physical activity is performed during the yellow intervals.

The algorithm senses the user activity for a week and then decides when to listen user's activity in the next weeks and when to fire the *Triggers*. How the population (intervals) evolves is easy: (1) if during a yellow time slot the Google Service returns an evaluation $v(x)$ so that $0 \leq v(x) < 0.5$, i.e., the user performed no or very few physical activity, the time slot is marked as red, (2) if the evaluation $v(x)$ is $0.5 \leq v(x) < 1$, i.e., some physical activity was performed, the time slot becomes green and (3) a green slot remains green if more than one stairstep is performed by the user, otherwise it is marked as yellow.

The use of a genetic algorithm is important since the user can change his/her behavior during time, or the initial description about his/her habits can be inaccurate. To allow an automatic adaptation to changes in user's behavior, a random exploration of the time slots marked as red is needed. According to genetic algorithms, a random probability of mutation is introduced: a red interval can be mutated into a yellow one. In this way, Google Service is used to analyze physical activity, and the same interval can be better analyzed the following week if the user performs a sufficient amount of physical activity.

Triggers notifications are implemented considering intervals marked as green. First of all, to avoid to disturb too much the user, we decided to notify at most two *Triggers* during the day, separated by, at least, 6 h. Moreover, we do not notify the user if he/she is already playing with *Climb The World* in the same temporal interval. If these conditions are satisfied, the *Trigger* is notified if the number of stairsteps made so far that day does not overtake the number of stairsteps done the day before plus 10. In this way, we aim at keeping constantly active the user and try to increase his/her performance among the days.

4   Users Tests

Climb The World was tested with a users study to evaluate its persuasive power with real users. We selected 13 participants, 8 females and 5 males, and we asked them to use the game and to answer to a small questionnaire. Players involved aged between 24 and 30.

The experiment lasted 9 days, and each participant used his/her own smartphone. We did not ask participants to change their daily routine, we asked them to freely use the application whenever they could or wanted.

Players were randomly divided into two different groups of 7 and 6 users. We used these two groups to randomize our test, changing the order in which each group used the singleplayer or the multiplayer modes (see Table 1). The first two days we asked all the participants to use the "Step counter" mode to record a baseline about the number of stairsteps made without a *serious game*.

---

[2] https://developers.google.com/android/reference/com/google/android/gms/location/ActivityRecognitionApi.

Table 1. Game mode order for each of the two groups. (MP) denotes the multiplayer mode.

Day	Group A	Group B
1	Stairstep counter	Stairstep counter
2	Stairstep counter	Stairstep counter
3	Singleplayer	*Social Climb* (MP)
4	Singleplayer	*Social Challenge* (MP)
5	*Social Climb* (MP)	*Team vs Team* (MP)
6	*Social Challenge* (MP)	Singleplayer
7	*Team vs Team* (MP)	Singleplayer
8	Stairstep counter	Stairstep counter
9	Stairstep counter	Stairstep counter

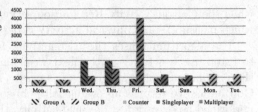

Fig. 3. Number of stairsteps made by both groups each day of the test.

At the end of the experiment, each participant completed a 5-point Likert questionnaire, based on the *IBM Computer Usability Satisfaction Questionnaires* [7], with possible answers ranging from "Strongly disagree" to "Strongly agree". Our questionnaire was divided into two different main sections: the first one to describe the participants that took part to the experiment, e.g., what they think about physical activity and being physically active, and the second one contained questions about *ClimbTheWorld*, the different game modes and their experience during the days. Thanks to a background logger, during the experiment we collected objective data about the number of stairsteps made by participants.

Data about users showed that our participants were a difficult test case, since they already preferred to take stairs and have an active life, meaning that, actually, they do not need a *serious game* to increase their physical activity. In fact, even if 77% of participants have positive feelings about being physically active, 54% of them think they do not need any form of external stimulus to be active, and about 61% does not frequently use elevators or escalators, but prefers to take stairs in order to be more active. Moreover, 53% of participants does not play any sport and the other 47% performs an individual sport. They were mainly "casual players" (69%), that play almost alone (61.5%) or with another player in the same room (46.2%). Finally, only 23% of participants frequently plays with mobile games. These data are confirmed also from the second part of the questionnaire: about 70% of participants preferred to play in single mode, while only 38.5% preferred to play with his/her friends. Moreover, 92.2% of participants liked the "Solo Climb" mode.

The multiplayer mode obtained less appreciation. In particular, the most preferred multiplayer mode was the "Social Climb" mode, since all the participants used it at least one time and 92.3% of them ranked it positively. The second preference was "Social Challenge", played by 77% of participants and 80% of them liked it. Finally, "Team vs. Team" mode was played by 61.5% of participants and 63.6% would play again with it. This rank can be explained by the fact that this mode, that should be the most challenging and engaging one, has the drawback that it is difficult to set up: it is necessary to find at least 4 users, active in the same interval of time, to be able to start the game (and this could take time that not all users are happy to wait for).

The last part of the questionnaire asked an evaluation of *Triggers* notification and battery life. The majority of the users declared that *Triggers* did not disturb them (70% of the users) and were able to motivate them to take the stairs (only 38.5% of the users declare to not be motivated). Moreover, only 30.8% of the users reported a drop in the battery lifetime. Therefore, we can argue that the *Triggers* implementation was well tolerated by the users and also the system to save energy power worked well.

Analyzing data acquired with the data logger, we evaluated the number of stairsteps participants made, and the game mode used during all the days. We compared answers provided with the questionnaire with objective data, and performance of participants depending on the game mode used. Figure 3 shows the number of stairsteps made by all the participants during the experiment. Together with Table 1, the figure also shows the number of stairsteps made by participants depending on the game mode used: the number of stairsteps made using the *serious game* (both in singleplayer or multiplayer) is higher with respect to the number when using simply the counter. In particular, singleplayer modes increased the average amount of about 61%, while multiplayer of about 64%. This means that the game is effective in incentivizing people in taking stairs, and this is even more important since our test groups were made by people that think that they do not need to be incentivized to be physically active.

A very important result is about efficacy of the "Team vs. Team" game mode that, when used, allows to reach the highest number of stairsteps made. This probably comes from the fact that this game mode combines both collaboration and competition among users, a combination that is able to engage participants and create high motivation. On the other side, the big difference between the two groups even shows the limitation of this game mode, since the setup phase is longer than the other ones and could reduce users' interest.

There is another important difference in the behavior of the two groups. In fact, the second group, the one that used the "Team vs. Team" game mode, approximately doubled the number of stairsteps made with the simple counter in the last two days, while the first group lowered the number of stairsteps made without the game in the last two days with respect to the first two days of the experiment. This means that the "Team vs. Team" game mode is not always accepted by the users due to the initial setup phase, but, if used, is able to obtain good results in persuading people to change their behavior, and this result remains also in absence of the game. On the other side, singleplayer games were able to engage both groups, showing how an easy entry setup of the game makes it more engaging.

As we can see from these results, it is clear that *ClimbTheWorld* is really effective in incentivizing people in taking stairs, and both singleplayer and multiplayer modes are engaging and appreciated by users.

5   Conclusions

In this paper we presented the redesign of our smartphone application, *ClimbTheWorld*, to improve its persuasiveness. To incentivize people in taking stairs instead of elevators or escalators, we used the Fogg Behavior Model and we exploited natural competitiveness between people creating competition and collaboration, to increase users' engagement and so the power of the game to correct a bad behavior. Moreover, we introduced an algorithm that is able to understand user's habits and automatically determines when it is the best moment during the day to fire a *Trigger* to remember the user to perform some activity (in particular, to take stairs).

Our tests showed that the game was effective in incentivizing people in taking stairs (about 61% of increase with singleplayer modes and 64% with multiplayer modes). Even notifications provided were considered not intrusive and helpful.

In the future, we plan to increase persuasiveness of our system adding more game modes to *ClimbTheWorld*, and more challenges between users. Moreover, we plan to increase the precision of the algorithm that defines *Triggers* timing, in order to make them even more useful and less intrusive. We will study other approaches, like the use of artificial neural networks [10].

References

1. Aiolli, F., Ciman, M., Donini, M., Gaggi, O.: ClimbTheWorld: real-time stairstep counting to increase physical activity. In: Proceedings of the 11th Conference on Mobile and Ubiquitous Systems: Computing, Networking and Services (2014)
2. Centers for disease control, prevention. Childhood obesity facts (2015). http://www.cdc.gov/healthyyouth/obesity/facts.htm
3. de Onis, M., Blössner, M., Borghi, E.: Global prevalence and trends of overweight and obesity among preschool children. Am. J. Clin. Nutr. **92**, 1257–1264 (2010)
4. Fitbit Inc. Fitbit (2015). http://www.fitbit.com/
5. Fogg, B.J.: A behavior model for persuasive design. In: Proceedings of Persuasive 2009, New York, NY, USA, pp. 1–7. ACM (2009)
6. Komninos, A., Dunlop, M.D., Rowe, D., Hewitt, A., Coull, S.: Using degraded music quality to encourage a health improving walking pace: BeatClearWalker. In: Proceedings of PervasiveHealth (2015)
7. Lewis, J.R.: IBM computer usability satisfaction questionnaires: psychometric evaluation and instructions for use. Int. J. Hum. Comput. Interact. **7**(1), 57–78 (1995)
8. Lin, J.J., Mamykina, L., Lindtner, S., Delajoux, G., Strub, H.B.: Fish'n'Steps: encouraging physical activity with an interactive computer game. In: Dourish, P., Friday, A. (eds.) UbiComp 2006. LNCS, vol. 4206, pp. 261–278. Springer, Heidelberg (2006). doi:10.1007/11853565_16
9. Nike, Inc. Nike + runing (2015). https://itunes.apple.com/us/app/nike-gps/id387771637?mt=8
10. Rajashekaran, S., Vijayalksmi, G.A.: Neural Networks, Fuzzy Logic and Genetic Algorithms: Synthesis and Applications. Prentice-Hall of India Private Limited, New Delhi (2004)
11. Runtastic GmbH. Runtastic (2015). https://www.runtastic.com/

12. Six to Start. Zombie, Run! (2015). https://zombiesrungame.com/
13. van Eijk, R.M.: Requirements for relaxation coaching - a formalization of the Fogg behavior model. In: Proceedings of ICT for Ageing Well and e-Health, Lisboa, Portugal, pp. 31–36 (2015)
14. Volkswagen. The Piano stairs. http://www.youtube.com/watch?v=2lXh2n0aPyw
15. Zyda, M.: From visual simulation to virtual reality to games. IEEE Comput. 38(9), 25–32 (2005)

A Location-Based Game for Two Generations: Teaching Mobile Technology to the Elderly with the Support of Young Volunteers

Wiesław Kopeć[1]([✉]), Katarzyna Abramczuk[2], Bartłomiej Balcerzak[1],
Marta Juźwin[1], Katarzyna Gniadzik[1], Grzegorz Kowalik[1],
and Radosław Nielek[1]

[1] Polish-Japanese Academy of Information Technology,
Koszykowa 86, 02-008 Warsaw, Poland
{wieslaw.kopec,bartlomiej.balcerzak,
marta.juzwin,katarzyna.gniadzik,
grzegorz.kowalik,nielek}@pja.edu.pl
[2] Institute of Sociology, University of Warsaw,
Karowa 18, 00-927 Warsaw, Poland
k.abramczuk@uw.edu.pl

Abstract. This paper presents a cooperative location-based game for the elderly with the use of tablets equipped with mobile application. The game was designed to tackle at once several crucial topics related to the issue of aging, namely the social inclusion, education in the field of modern technology, motivation for learning as well as physical activity. Mixed-aged teams consisting of two players: a junior and a senior took part in the game. The preliminary results suggest that the game can successfully address a number of issues including improving the elderly technical skills, increasing the elderly physical activity as well as positive intergenerational interaction. The paper describes the game setup in details and presents some initial data gathered during the gameplay.

Keywords: Location-based games · Elderly · Intergenerational cooperation · Mobile games and applications

1 Introduction

The process of aging accelerates in European societies and becomes one of the greatest social and economic challenges. Specialists in the field of demographics predict that by 2050 over a quarter of the EU population will be composed of people that will be 65+. Therefore, it is of the highest importance for us to learn how to include this demographic in various activities, facilitate their participation in modern technology-based world, and ultimately apply their strength for the benefit of the society at large. This objective cannot be achieved without solid knowledge about the psychological and sociological processes associated with aging. Modern ways of dealing with the problem are inevitably related to the Information and Communication Technologies (ICT).

© ICST Institute for Computer Sciences, Social Informatics and Telecommunications Engineering 2017
K. Giokas et al. (Eds.): eHealth 2016, LNICST 181, pp. 84–91, 2017.
DOI: 10.1007/978-3-319-49655-9_12

The location-based-game research case described in this paper is a part of the project called Living Laboratory (LivingLab) initialized, developed and implemented at Polish-Japanese Academy of Information Technology (PJAIT) located in Warsaw, Poland. It is run in cooperation with the Municipality of Warsaw. Its goals are related to the vital problems of social informatics and are connected with a broad range of GOWELL topics including research and development of solutions for active aging and healthy living, game application for better lifestyle and well-being, positive gaming, stress management and technologies enhancing social well-being. Currently it is in testing stage, with over 200 hundred elderly participants, most of whom are seniors who completed the basic computer course provided by the City of Warsaw.

In this paper we describe one of the LivingLab PJAIT attempts to tackle at once several crucial topics related to the aging issue, namely improve social inclusion of the elderly, their technological skills in the field of mobile technologies, motivation for learning as well as physical well-being, due also to a positive intergenerational inter-action. The tool that allowed us to combine all those issues was a location-based game "Stroll Around Yesterday" which joined historical knowledge with the use of tablets and interaction in mixed-age teams of two players (a senior and a PJAIT student of the computer science track). We also chose this form of activity to help a IT student to understand the requirements that should be taken into account in the process of creating software applications for senior citizens.

2 Related Work

The multidisciplinary research approach mentioned above implies the necessity of considering various perspectives related to a broad range of topics including social inclusion of elders, intergenerational interaction and stereotypes, ICT skills and barriers as well as well-being of the elderly. The problem analysis leads us from the motivation and social activities of older adults to the use of location-based games and modern ICT technology.

A general model for changes in social activities at different stages of life was proposed by Carstensen [1], who suggested that limited activity among older adults may be an adaptive mechanism for coping with changing environment. Previously, models of motivation of the elderly were also studied by Vallerand [2], where moti-vation was divided into measurable mechanisms. Similar measures for apathy among older adults were proposed by Resnick [3]. Motivation has ramification in many fields of social activity. Hence, researchers conducted studies about the interaction between the elderly motivation and their purchase decisions [4], physical and sport activity [5, 6], psychological adjustment in nursing homes [7], family interactions [8] and work-place performance [9, 10], volunteering for social activities and leisure participation [11, 12], and, what is particularly important for the scope of our paper, use of internet-based communication and use of computing technologies [13–18]. A separate aspect of this research is also connected to investigation into the use of ICT resources in medical treatment of older adults [19].

During all of these studies the observation was made that older adults suffer from a decrease of motivation, and the results suggested the active role of the elderly in restoring the lost motivation and activity. This makes reaching out and providing support for the elderly crucial.

Many methods for achieving this objective have been suggested and tested. Casati et al. [20, 21] have built an on-line platform which encompasses various application designed to motivate older adults to participate in various physical activities. They emphasize the importance of social cues, such as communication with other users, and a coherent narrative for improving the overall performance of the older adults.

Combining location-based games and mobile technologies has also been studied. Avouris [22] reviewed 15 location-based games where mobile technologies were applied and described the impact of the technology on the general performance. Kiefer [23] proposed a classification of different designs of location-based games. Intergenerational aspects of location-based games were considered for example by Charness [9], who studied how participation in such activities differs among younger and older adults. The findings suggested that older adults, while more cooperative, were equally motivated as their younger counterparts.

Another important field of scientific research is related to the intergroup relations and intergenerational interactions. In connection with outdoor activities and location-based games they are sometimes referred to as hybrid reality games [24]. There are some studies on the impact of negative stereotypes on the attitude and performance of the elders. They reveal an interference with intergenerational communication [25], show that stereotypes can both impair and enhance older adults' memory [26], and indicate that the direct, personal contact with members of a different age group can be more effective in improving the intergroup relations than indirect contact [27, 28].

3 Gameplay

The game setup was inspired by the study of related work and literature supported by a set of best practices conveyed by external consultants experienced in location-based game design and elderly outdoor activities (e.g. city tour guides). The game "Stroll Around Yesterday" joins historical knowledge with the use of tablets and interaction in mixed-age teams of two players: a senior and a junior. The study concept was to stimulate interaction and cooperation between the team partners: on the one hand, the elderly participants were using the device and mobile apps with an indirect assistance of the younger tech-savvy team member, on the other hand the elderly should be more familiar with the historical and cultural context of the game (location descriptions and hints based on the literature and photos from the past).

Since every successful location-based game needs a good storyline with an alluring plot, we developed a story about a mad scientist, dr von Gestern, who had built a machine disturbing the space-time continuum and bringing back buildings from the past, namely from the communist era. The task for each team was to find all locations, close the wormholes and restore the contemporary buildings. The corresponding promotional materials were created (movie trailer, website, press release, Facebook profile etc.) in order to support the recruitment process of game participants. The preliminary expert consultation along with field tests provided valuable insight and led us to refine the scenario before conducting the first research gameplay. The route was simplified and tailored to the capabilities of the elderly. Finally, the game consisted of four stages, with total route of about 2 km length and duration of about 1,5 h including mid-time coffee break.

The initial gameplay "Stroll Around Yesterday" was held in Warsaw in the area of the Constitution Square (Southern part of the city center) on October 4th 2015. It was during Warsaw Senior Week, as a part the of the local International Day of Older Persons celebration (UN established, observed on October 1st).

The teams consisted of two people: a senior (the user of the LivingLab PJAIT platform) and a junior (PJAIT student of the computer science track). They were all equipped with space-time fixing modules i.e. tablets provided by the LivingLab team with preloaded software including the special game application.

The tablets could only be operated by the older team member. Directions to the next location were provided by our mobile application. The application was displaying current GPS position on the map alongside with the additional destination hints: textual (based on literature and cultural context) and visual (old B&W depiction gradually transforming into contemporary colorful location photograph). Having reached the location players were obliged to close a wormhole by completing certain task, which always included using the tablet. The tasks were connected to the storyline and related to various activities usually performed on mobile devices. On the first location the task was to connect to the Wi-Fi hotspot and scan the QR code. On the second station the task was to take a panoramic picture. On the third location players were to search the information on the Internet. The game ended at the starting point with playing a puzzle game on the tablet. The gameplay was accompanied by the pre- and post-game evaluation as well as in-game observation.

The follow-up game (shortened demonstration version) was held on October 9th as a subject of a field visit of the "AFE-INNOVNET: Towards an Age-Friendly Europe" international workshop.

4 Results

The game was played by 30 participants organized in 15 two-person teams. The general impression was very positive. All participants enjoyed the event and we received many requests for continuation. The older people were satisfied with their performance and pleased with cooperation with the junior counterparts. Both groups claimed that during the game there was a true cooperation were both sides had an opportunity for an initiative and contributed nearly equally to the success of the team (all the teams completed the game).

Below we present some preliminary statistics obtained in surveys that were deployed before and after the gameplay. Due to limited space we only present the most basic results. First, we describe shortly the elderly participants' profile. Then we move on to the performance evaluation. Finally we are signaling some findings concerning intergroup relations.

An average senior player was almost seventy-year-old retired woman from a large city (73% female participants, average age 69, youngest 60, oldest 86), rather well

educated (60% of higher education) with basic computer skills and motivation to learn
how to use tablets. She uses smartphones rather regularly (60%) and considers mobile
devices very useful (75% before the game, 87% after the game), but has a limited
knowledge about using it (40% of younger participants evaluated their older counterpart as having little knowledge about how to use tablet; some participants claimed
that it was the first time they used the tablet, nevertheless they managed to complete the
game). From additional surveys performed on the LivingLab platform we also know
that our senior is rather independent: 50% live on their own, without family members,
75% have a PC, and 63% use it without any assistance. They have a broad variety of
interests from cooking and crosswords to chemometrics and fitness.

To evaluate the performance, we asked both groups (seniors and juniors) to choose
the most accurate description of what had happened in each game task on a 5-point
scale from "junior completed the task" to "senior completed the task without any
assistance". The reports were rather consistent within most pairs. In very few cases the
evaluations by two parties differed by more than one category, which demonstrates
their reliability. According to the participants' evaluations in most cases the senior
completed the tasks instructed by her/his partner. The most problematic task was
establishing Wi-Fi connection where oftentimes-direct junior assistance was needed.

We asked both parties to indicate which game task in their view could be performed
again by senior without any assistance. The results are presented in Fig. 1. An interesting conclusion is that seniors generally underestimate their performance in comparison with the external estimate of their capabilities. This refers particularly to those
tasks that are relatively unfamiliar to their experience such as taking a panoramic photo,
scanning a QR code or playing a mobile game. On the other hand, seniors overestimate
their competence in more common tasks such as establishing a Wi-Fi connection or
searching the Web.

According to the contact theory [29, 30], if certain conditions are met, contact
between different groups can improve their attitudes towards each other. As our game
fulfilled most of the criteria for a successful contact, we decided to explore whether we

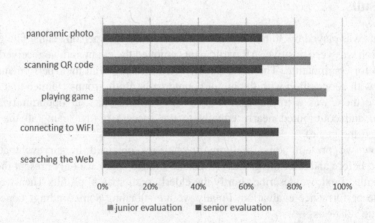

Fig. 1. The game tasks evaluation by both groups of participants indicating which tasks could
be performed again by senior without any assistance.

Table 1. List of 12 dimensions for intergroup evaluation.

Positive	Negative
productive	unproductive
active	passive
aggressive	defensive
independent	dependent
organized	disorganized
decisive	indecisive
cooperative	uncooperative
flexible	inflexible
hopeful	dejected
trustful	suspicious
pleasant	unpleasant
exciting	dull

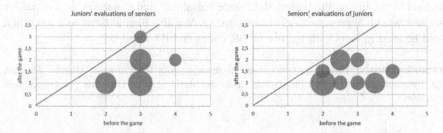

Fig. 2. Median evaluations of general other before and after the game.

can observe some shift in attitudes. We asked both seniors and juniors to evaluate members of the other age group with the use of a set of 12 antonyms selected from Aging Semantic Differential by Rozencranz and McNevin [31]. The list of the antonyms can be found in Table 1.

Before and after the game the participants were asked to evaluate a general other (some unspecified member of the other age group) using the antonym pairs. The chart below shows the median evaluations of the general other from the other age group for junior and senior evaluators.

The larger values indicate less favorable opinions. The size of the circles matches the number of antonyms with the corresponding coordinates. For example, the outermost left circle on the left hand side graph corresponds to 3 antonyms for which the median evaluations of the general older other was 2 before the game and 1 after the game. The straight lines indicate equal medians. This is where all the circles would lie, was there no shift in attitudes. As virtually all of the circles in Fig. 2 are below that line, we can hypothesize that for almost all the dimensions the perception of the outgroup improved for both juniors and seniors. A more detailed statistical analysis is needed to validate this claim.

Summing up, we have reasons to believe that this kind of activity is a very promising tool for improving intergroup relations, and diminishing age-based stereotypes. We plan to conduct additional gameplays to verify this result.

5 Summary and Future Work

The game described in this paper proved to be promising in several ways. It can increase the technical skills of the elderly, improve their physical activity and enhance positive intergenerational interaction.

Apart from the scientific results, the outcome from the initial gameplay was lots of hands-on experience. Unfortunately the initial game setup was very demanding and turned out to be resource intensive and time consuming. On the whole, there were dozens of people engaged from actors and movie crew to software developers, testers and gameplay staff.

In the nearest future we plan to retake the original game to verify the outcome, as well as to continue the struggle in order to prepare more concise and robust setup of the game which could be replayed automatically by a larger group of participants without the need of relying on the human staff, since reusability and scalability are crucial for various research approaches, i.e. crowdsourcing. We also plan to develop a setup that could be used indoors with the use of QR codes and BT beacons.

Acknowledgments. This project has received funding from the European Union's Horizon 2020 Research and Innovation Programme under the Marie Skłodowska-Curie grant agreement No 690962.

References

1. Carstensen, L.L.: Motivation for social contact across the life span: a theory of socioemotional selectivity. Nebr. Symp. Motiv. **40**, 209–254 (1993)
2. Vallerand, R.J., O'Connor, B.P.: Motivation in the elderly: a theoretical framework and some promising findings. Can. Psychol./Psychol. Can. **30**(3), 538 (1989)
3. Resnick, B., et al.: Use of the apathy evaluation scale as a measure of motivation in elderly people. Rehabil. Nurs. **23**(3), 141–147 (1998)
4. Kim, Y., Jikyeong, K., Minsung, K.: The relationships among family and social interaction, loneliness, mall shopping motivation, and mall spending of older consumers. Psychol. Mark. **22**(12), 995–1015 (2005)
5. Mullen, S.P., et al.: Measuring enjoyment of physical activity in older adults: invariance of the physical activity enjoyment scale (paces) across groups and time. Int. J. Behav. Nutr. Phys. Act. **8**(1), 1–9 (2011)
6. Dacey, M., Baltzell, A., Zaichkowsky, L.: Older adults' intrinsic and extrinsic motivation toward physical activity. Am. J. Health Behav. **32**(6), 570–582 (2008)
7. O'Connor, B.P., Vallerand, R.J.: Motivation, self-determination, and person-environment fit as predictors of psychological adjustment among nursing home residents. Psychol. Aging **9**(2), 189 (1994)
8. O'Connor, B.P.: Family and friend relationships among older and younger adults: Interaction motivation, mood, and quality. Int. J. Aging Human Dev. **40**(1), 9–29 (1995)

9. Charness, G., Villeval, M.C.: Cooperation and competition in intergenerational ex-periments in the field and in the laboratory. Am. Econ. Rev. **99**, 956–978 (2009)
10. de Lange, A.H., et al.: Dominant achievement goals of older workers and their relationship with motivation-related outcomes. J. Vocat. Behav. **77**(1), 118–125 (2010)
11. Okun, M.A., Barr, A., Herzog, A.: Motivation to volunteer by older adults: a test of competing measurement models. Psychol. Aging **13**(4), 608 (1998)
12. Losier, G.F., Bourque, P.E., Vallerand, R.J.: A motivational model of leisure participation in the elderly. J. Psychol. **127**(2), 153–170 (1993)
13. Ng, Ch.: Motivation among older adults in learning computing technologies: a grounded model. Educ. Gerontol. **34**(1), 1–14 (2007)
14. Wagner, N., Khaled, H., Head, M.: Computer use by older adults: a multi-disciplinary review. Comput. Human Behav. **26**(5), 870–882 (2010)
15. González, A., Ramírez, M., Viadel, V.: Attitudes of the elderly toward information and communications technologies. Educ. Gerontol. **38**(9), 585–594 (2012)
16. Selwyn, N., et al.: Older adults' use of information and communications technology in everyday life. Ageing Soc. **23**(05), 561–582 (2003)
17. Neves, B.B., Amaro, F.: Too old for technology? How the elderly of Lisbon use and perceive ICT. J. Community Inform. **8**(1) (2012)
18. Naumanen, M., Tukiainen, M.: Guided participation in ICT-education for seniors: motivation and social support. In: 39th IEEE Frontiers in Education Conference, FIE 2009, (2009)
19. Heart, T., Kalderon, E.: Older adults: are they ready to adopt health-related ICT? Int. J. Med. Inform. **82**(11), e209–e231 (2013)
20. Far, I.K., Silveira, P., Casati, F., Baez, M.: Unifying platform for the physical, mental and social well-being of the elderly. In: (Jong Hyuk) Park, J.J., Jeong, Y.-S., Oh Park, S., Chen, H.-C. (eds.) EMC Technology and Service. LNEE, vol. 181, pp. 385–392. Springer, Netherlands (2012). doi:10.1007/978-94-007-5076-0_46
21. Silveira, P., et al.: Motivating and assisting physical exercise in independently living older adults: a pilot study. Int. J. Med. Inform. **82**(5), 325–334 (2013)
22. Avouris, N.M., Yiannoutsou, N.: A review of mobile location-based games for learning across physical and virtual spaces. J. UCS **18**(15), 2120–2142 (2012)
23. Kiefer, P., Matyas, S., Schliede, C.: Systematically exploring the design space of location-based games. In: 4th International Conference on Pervasive Computing, 2006, pp. 183–190 (2006)
24. de Souza e Silva, A., Delacruz, G.C.: Hybrid reality games reframed: potential uses in educational contexts. Games Cult. **1**, 231 (2006)
25. Pinquart, M., Wenzel, S., Sorensen, S.: Changes in attitudes among children and elderly adults in intergenerational group. Educ. Gerontol. **26**, 523–540 (2000)
26. Barber, S.J., Mather, M.: Stereotype threat can both enhance and impair older adults' memory. Psychol. Sci. **24**(12), 2522–2529 (2013)
27. Couper, D.P., Sheehan, N.W., Thomas, E.L.: Attitude toward old people: the impact of an intergenerational program. Educ. Gerontol. **17**(1), 41–53 (1991)
28. Dovidio, J.F., Eller, A., Hewstone, M.: Improving intergroup relations through direct, extended and other forms of indirect contact. Group Processes Intergroup Relat. **14**(2), 147–160 (2011)
29. Allport, G.W.: The Nature of Prejudice. Addison-Wesley, Cambridge/Reading (1954)
30. Pettigrew, T.F.: Intergroup contact theory. Annu. Rev. Psychol. **49**, 65–85 (1998)
31. Rozencranz, H.A., McNevin, T.E.: A factor analysis of attitudes toward the aged. Gerontologist **9**(1), 55–59 (1969)

Ring a Bell? Adaptive Auditory Game Feedback to Sustain Performance in Stroke Rehabilitation

Kasper Hald[✉] and Hendrik Knoche

Department of Architecture, Design and Media Technology,
Aalborg University, Aalborg, Denmark
{kh,hk}@create.aau.dk

Abstract. This paper investigates the effect of adaptive auditory feedback on continued player performance for stroke patients in a reaction time tablet game. The feedback sound pitch followed a saw-tooth shape that cumulatively increased for fast reaction times and flying back to the base pitch after a single slow reaction time. The analysis was based on data obtained in a field trial with lesion patients during their regular rehabilitation. The auditory feedback events were categorized by feedback type (positive/negative) and the associated pitch change of either high or low magnitude. Both feedback type and magnitude significantly affected on players performance. Negative feedback improved patients reaction times in subsequent hits by $0.42\,s$ and positive feedback impaired their performance by $0.15\,s$.

Keywords: Stroke patients · Rehabilitation · Attention · Hemi-spatial neglect · Serious games · Adaptive difficulty · Non-speech audio · Adaptive audio feedback · Sonification

1 Introduction

Self-rehabilitation initiatives place emphasis on the growing responsibility that patients have for improving their own well-being and progress. Stroke rehabilitation is a lengthy and expensive process. However, it leaves time for pátients to improve their situation on their own time, even while in rehabilitation centers. Games are now being sought as a means to tap into the intrinsic motivation they promote and research has started investigating to what degree, for example, causal games train cognitive abilities [1]. We believe that purpose-built games that provide more feedback and are simple for patients to understand are better suited for rehabilitation. But the literature is scant on how to challenge players adequately and give in-game feedback on performance for individual interactions and how negative or positive feedback influences patient performance. We focus on brain lesion patients who suffer from hemi-spatial neglect or other types of attention deficiency disorders.

Inspired by the Whack-a-Mole arcade game, we designed a tablet game that adapted target positions to the player's performance to sustain engagement [11]

© ICST Institute for Computer Sciences, Social Informatics and Telecommunications Engineering 2017
K. Giokas et al. (Eds.): eHealth 2016, LNICST 181, pp. 92–99, 2017.
DOI: 10.1007/978-3-319-49655-9_13

and emphasized how they excelled [16] through incremental auditory feedback. The auditory feedback adapted by increasing pitch by 10% on each consecutive quick hit while resetting the pitch on slower hits. We evaluated the game in a field study with patients at a neuro-rehabilitation center whom we encouraged to play the games three time a day while undergoing regular therapy. The results showed that negative feedback yield faster subsequent hits while hit time increases after positive feedback.

2 Background and Related Work

Patients suffering from hemi-spatial neglect, as a result of a stroke or lesion, fail to respond to stimuli on the contra-lateral side of their lesion, despite having the motor and sensory capacity to do so. Most common, persistent, and severe after right hemisphere lesions, neglect affects visual sensory input, resulting in left-side visual neglect affecting daily living [3]. Patients may for example only groom or dress the right side of their body, or only eat from the right half of a plate. In addition to ignoring sensory input, patients can be expected to have a lowered capacity for sustained attention according to feedback from rehabilitation center staff.

Cognitive training has been proven to be effective, but research has yet to determine, which regimen and conditions result in the best transfer effect [7]. Video games for rehabilitation and cognitive training based on standardized tests have been implemented [6,9] and positively received by users [5,12]. The methods used to engage and intrinsicly motivate players may address the problem of the intensive and repetitive rehabilitation activities [2].

Malone distinguished between two types of user interfaces: toys and tool. People use toys or games for their own sake whereas they use tools as a means to pursue external goals [13]. Good toy should be easy to learn and hard to master while a tool should be easy to both use and master. However, in cases where the external goal is not motivating enough on its own, tools can benefit from having toy-like features. In our case, the game constitutes the tool with the toy-like qualities to help the patient overcome the repetitive nature of rehabilitation.

However, despite the novelty of the game format patients need different challenge levels to remain engaged [11], which research in dynamic difficulty adjustment (DDA), both within and outside the subject and rehabilitation, has started addressing [10]. Mainetti et al. designed a home-based motion-controlled game for rehabilitation of hemi-spatial neglect with increasing difficulty levels by removing visual and auditory cues and hints [12] and found continued engagement and positive responses from one patient using the game in half hour sessions on weekdays for a month.

Non-speech auditory feedback have previously been used in the context of rehabilitation systems. Masiero et al. [14] utilized auditory feedback in a robotic-assisted motor rehabilitation system, which kept patients' attention throughout a training session. In stroke rehabilitation, Wallis et al. [18] used musical sonification of movement as well as discrete sounds for positive feedback and sustained audio indicating poor performance. Similarly, Newbold et al. [15] investigated musically-informed movement sonification and found that harmonic stability useful in a physical rehabilitation context, as stable and unstable cadences encouraged either ending or continuing stretching movements. Cockburn and Brewster [4] researched feedback modalities in the context of acquisition of small targets and discovered that auditory feedback reduces targeting time significantly.

Rabbitt conducted a study on how positive or negative feedback impact performance focusing on error correction in a continuous-performance choice-response task involving signal lamps as feedback. On correct responses the lit lamp would turn off and another lit up delivering positive feedback. Errors yielded negative feedback through the lack of changes. Response times before negative feedback were not different from the mean response times of all correct responses. However, errors as well as subsequent responses to correct errors after negative feedback were significantly faster ($\sim$500 ms) than equivalent correct responses either before or after the error and correction ($\sim$600 ms) [17].

3   Game Design

Drawing on the eponymous arcade game, our Whack-a-Mole (WAM) game focused on hemi-spatial neglect patients. Following clinical staff recommendations, a game lasted for 8 min to maintain on-task attention. In WAM, the player presses a large center sphere, upon which one or several six millimeter targets (with 12 mm touch collision area) appear around it (see Fig. 1). The player has to hit targets before they disappear again. After such timeouts or successful hits another center sphere hit makes new targets appear. The distance at which new targets appear depends on player performance. Expired targets reduce while hit targets increase the distance. We used the delay between tapping the center and hitting the targets as a reaction time performance measure to evaluate the effect of feedback.

A chime sound plays upon pressing the center sphere and coincides with target appearance. Target hits provide audio-visual feedback in the form of a bell sound paired with an animation. Hits targets fly with a visual trail in a direct line into the center, which responds with a bouncing animation, a small particle explosion, and turning green again. All cues aim at grabbing attention and guiding to press the center sphere for new targets. Auditory feedback upon target expiration played at most twice within 20 s to reduce potential frustration in case of poor performance. An initially low pitched bell like sound plays upon successful hits. Hits below one second reaction time increase the current feedback pitch by 10% resulting in no pitch ceiling for consecutive fast hits. The audio feedback on center sphere taps remains unchanged, providing an audible baseline with increasing contrast between center and fast target hits. This adaptive positive feedback aimed at providing motivational feedback for sustained high performance. WAM gave negative feedback for slow target hits by resetting the feedback pitch to the starting pitch. This resulted in high contrasts to what the players hear before, especially in cases of long streaks of fast hits. We categorized

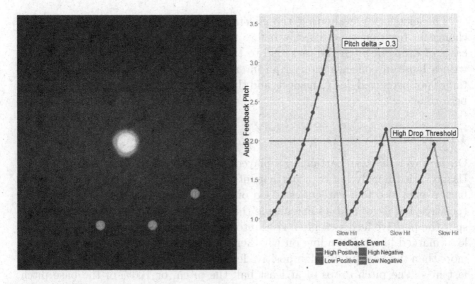

Fig. 1. Left: Cropped 16/10 landscape screenshots of multi-target events requiring hitting all three before tapping the center. Right: Illustration of the accumulating pitch on fast hits and drops in pitch on slow hits. (Color figure online)

audio feedback based on the magnitude of pitch changes (see Fig. 1, right). We categorized increases to pitches higher than 30% from the baseline pitch as high, drops in pitch of at least 100% of the baseline pitch as a high negative feedback event. The asymmetry in the thresholds is due to the nature of the patients participating in the study: because each participant needs to contribute samples to each of the four feedback event, the thresholds are set as to include as many participants as possible.

4   Study

The participants were volunteers from Brønderslev Neurorehabilitation Center recruited by the therapist supervising the experiment. Inclusion criteria for participating were suffering from a form of acquired attention deficit disorder as a results of a brain lesion, being able to use the tablets, and giving informed consent. Forty-two out of fifty-two patients completed the trial. Some patients dropped out early due to moving to a different facility. Regardless, we considered all logged data in the analysis. Thirty-three men and eleven women (63 years on average, SD: 14.5) contributed data. Based on Jehkonen et al's test suite (line bisection, line cancellation and letter cancellation [8]) and their cut-offs from the literature, four participants suffered from neglect. Seven participants had above cut-off scores on both the left and right hand side of the paper tests and the health care professional in charge of conducting all tests classified them as attention deficit cases. During the trial period, participants continued regular rehabilitation in addition to being encouraged to play the game three time a day.

The metric for evaluating the effects of adaptive audio feedback was the change in reaction time directly before and after an audio feedback event. In cases of drops in pitch the task tied to the feedback event would be associated with a lapse in concentration or an interruption in the form of a mistake or a target not perceived due to neglect, and the feedback is there to sustain continued performance.

4.1   Results

On average, the test participants played WAM for 5.6 min per day (SD 1.8). Usage varied hugely between participants. We categorized adaptive audio feedback events into four categories based on two attributes pitch change direction (positive/negative) and its magnitude (high/low). In our analysis we arbitrarily split the positive feedback pitch rises into high (marked green in Fig. 1, right) or low (marked blue) depending on whether the rise yielded an increase of 30% or more than the base pitch. High positive feedback occurred after twelve successive fast hits. The pitch drops of at least half the pitch, or 100% of the base pitch we defined as high (marked red) others as low (orange). High negative feedback drops could occur after at least eight successive fast hits, as illustrated in Fig. 1, right. In order for each participant to contribute their average change in reaction time to each of the four event categories, we excluded thirteen patients, eight men and five women, who did not receive high positive or negative feedback from the analysis. Four suffered from attention deficiency and one suffered from neglect. The subsequent analysis is based on 170 thousand feedback events.

We used a within subjects analysis of variance (ANOVA) to test the effect of *feedbacktype* (positive or negative), *magnitude* (high or low) on the change in reaction time performance surrounding a feedback event. In terms of the reaction time at the feedback events themselves only *feedbacktype* ($F_{1,120} = 929.60$, $p < 0.001$) was a significant factor, meaning that the prior performance and accumulated pitch had no effect on the reaction time at the event. The average reaction time was 1.31 at a negative feedback event and 0.66 s for a positive event. Both *feedbacktype* ($F_{1,120} = 7.95$, $p < 0.01$) and *magnitude* ($F_{1,120} = 6.97$, $p < 0.01$) had a significant albeit small effect on reaction time after a feedback event: The average reaction time after negative feedback was slower (0.89 s) than for positive feedback (0.81 s). Large magnitudes in feedback made people go faster (0.81 s) than low (0.89).

However, if we compare the changes in reaction time between the feedback event hit and the subsequent hit As for the change in reaction time going from the feedback event to the hit directly after, both *feedbacktype* ($F_{1,120} = 762.95$, $p < 0.001$) and *magnitude* ($F_{1,120} = 6.41$, $p < 0.05$) were significant factors, negative feedback improved reaction time on the subsequent hit by 0.42 s and positive feedback impaired performance by 0.15 s.

Another way of looking at performance changes is the comparison between reaction times before and after feedback, similarly to [17]. Both *Feedbacktype* ($F_{1,120} = 88.78$, $p < 0.001$) and *magnitude* ($F_{1,120} = 27.93$, $p < 0.001$) and the interaction between the two ($F_{1,120} = 10.46$, $p < 0.01$) were significant factors in

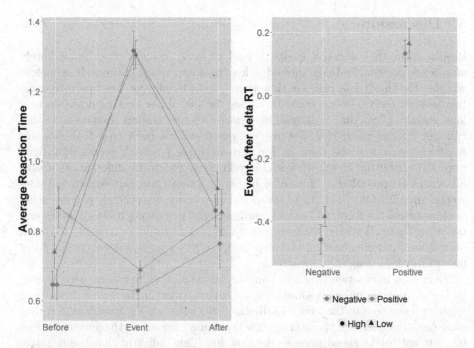

Fig. 2. Left: Average reaction times before, during and after an audio feedback event, including error bars at 95% confidence intervals from per participant averages. Right: The average delta reaction time between an audio feedback event and the next task split between *feedbacktypes* and change *magnitude*, including error bars at 95% confidence intervals from per participant averages.

the delta reaction time between the hits prior to and after the feedback event. However, the reaction time prior to a feedback event was significantly different depending on *magnitude* ($F_{1,120} = 47.83$, $p < 0.001$) in addition to *feedbacktype* and factor interaction, meaning that the base reaction time was not comparable within the *feedbacktypes*. Figure 2 illustrates this in the differences in average reaction times for the low feedback groups (triangles). This difference stems from the order in which feedback could occur in the game: Negative feedback must have been preceded by a quick hit, while a (low) positive feedback event can be preceded by either a quick or a slow hit. In contrast, high magnitude feedback events have to preceded by several positive feedback events, and we can see that the *before* averages of these groups are the same. To remove this difference we averaged the low magnitude feedback groups and reran the analysis on delta reaction time before and after a feedback events. Both *feedbacktype* ($F_{1,120} = 1.040$, $p < 0.01$) and *magnitude* ($F_{1,120} = 11.080$, $p < 0.01$) were significant factors - negative feedback increased reaction time by 0.17 s and positive feedback by 0.085 s compared to average performance before the feedback event.

5   Discussion

Results show that negative feedback lead to faster reaction time immediately after while positive feedback showed to lead to slower reaction times. It is unclear whether the changes in reaction time were caused by players' prior performance: Increases in reaction time could be caused by the player slowing down do to a long streak of hits due to fatigue or lapses in concentration. However, we can rule out fatigue given that the average reaction time prior to a high positive feedback event was the same as for high negative feedback events. If fatigue were a contributing factor we would expect these two to be different, as a slow hit would be preceded by hits of a higher reaction time, but within the one-second margin. Our field study setup did not verify whether all players in all sessions heard the feedback, e.g. by muting sound or putting in headphones and not using them. However, we saw clear differences in response to audio feedback indicative of patients hearing and responding to it, seeing as patients would react faster after high magnitude feedback.

Decreases in reaction time following negative feedback may have been caused by the player continuing at same pace as previous, wanting to recover from their mistake regardless of the audio feedback. Still, what we see from Fig. 2 is that after negative feedback the average reaction time recovers to the speed of a fast hit, but not to the speed prior to the slow hit. This indicates that the negative feedback may contribute to a performance as a reminder in cases of lapses in concentration or other causes for slowing down. The increases in reaction time after both low and high magnitude positive feedback events suggested that continuous positive feedback did not contribute to sustained performance, even though average reaction times remained within the limit of a fast hit. It may, however, serve to motivate to work up the fast pace in the first place.

Whether the recovery time for reaching previous speed after an negative feedback is comparable to [17], where response time after errors were significantly faster than prior or subsequent responses, is inconclusive. This is because reaction time prior to a feedback event varies significantly independently of the subsequent audio feedback. The condition for the reaction time before a feedback event is a mix successful hits, motivated recovery from past mistakes and warming up at the beginning of a session, creating varying baseline performances. Negative feedback does lead to faster reaction time immediately after, but it is not significantly faster than at other events.

6   Conclusion

We created a Whack-a-Mole style game for assessment and rehabilitation of stroke patients suffering from hemi-spatial neglect that patients with attention deficiency disorder found enjoyable, too. Our analysis of the adaptive incremental audio feedback for showed that negative feedback was followed by an improvement in reaction time while positive feedback increased.

References

1. Baniqued, P.L., Kranz, M.B., Voss, M.W., Lee, H., Cosman, J.D., Severson, J., Kramer, A.F.: Cognitive training with casual video games: points to consider. Front. Psychol. **4** (2013)
2. Burke, J.W., McNeill, M.D.J., Charles, D.K., Morrow, P.J., Crosbie, J.H., McDonough, S.M.: Optimising engagement for stroke rehabilitation using serious games. Vis. Comput. **25**, 1085–1099 (2009). Springer
3. Cherney, L.R.: Unilateral neglect: a disorder of attention. Semin. Speech Lang. **23**, 117–128 (2002). Thieme Medical, New York
4. Cockburn, A., Brewster, S.: Multimodal feedback for the acquisition of small targets. Ergonomics **48**, 1129–1150 (2005). Taylor & Francis
5. Connolly, T.M., Boyle, E.A., MacArthur, E., Hainey, T., Boyle, J.M.: A systematic literature review of empirical evidence on computer games and serious games. Comput. Educ. **59**, 661–686 (2012). Elsevier
6. Dalmaijer, E.S., Van der Stigchel, S., Nijboer, T.C.W., Cornelissen, T.H.W., Husain, M.: CancellationTools: all-in-one software for administration and analysis of cancellation tasks. Behav. Res. Meth. **47**, 1065–1075 (2014). Springer
7. Jaeggi, S.M., Buschkuehl, M., Jonides, J., Shah, P.: Short- and long-term benefits of cognitive training. In: PNAS 2011, vol. 108, pp. 10081–10086 (2011)
8. Jehkonen, M., Ahonen, J., Dastidar, P., Koivisto, A., Laippala, P., Vilkki, J.: How to detect visual neglect in acute stroke. Lancet **351**, 727–728 (1998)
9. Knoche, H., Hald, K., Jørgensen, H.R.M., Richter, D.: Playing to (self-)rehabilitate: a month-long randomized control trial with brain lesion patients and a tablet game. In: PervasiveHealth 2016. IEEE (2016)
10. Liu, C., Agraval, P., Sarkar, N., Chen, S.: Dynamic difficulty adjustment in computer games through real-time anxiety-based affective feedback. Int. J. HCI **25**(6), 506–529 (2009). Taylor & Francis
11. Lopez-Samaniego, L., Garcia-Zapirain, B., Ozaita-Araico, A., Mendez-Zorrilla, A.: Cognitive rehabilitation based on working brain reflexes using computer games over iPad. In: Proceedings of CGAMES 2014, pp. 1–4. IEEE (2014)
12. Mainetti, R., Sedda, A., Ronchetti, M., Bottini, G., Borghese, N.A.: Duckneglect: video-games based neglect rehabilitation. Technol. Health Care J. **21**, 97–111 (2013). IOS Press
13. Malone, T.W.: Heuristics for Designing Enjoyable User Interfaces: Lessons from Computer Games. ACM (1981)
14. Masiero, S., Celia, A., Rosati, G., Armani, M.: Robotic-assisted rehabilitation of the upper limb after acute stroke. Arch. Phys. Med. Rehab. **88**(2), 142–149 (2007). Elsevier
15. Newbold, J.W., Bianca-Berthouze, N., Gold, N.E., Tajadura-Jiménez, A., Williams, A.: Musically Informed Sonification for Chronic Pain Rehabilitation: Facilitating Progress & Avoiding Over-doing. In: Proceedings of CHI 2016, pp. 5698–5703. ACM (2016)
16. Przybylski, A.K., Scott, C., Ryan, R.M.: A motivational model of video game engagement. Res. General Psychol. **14**, 154–166 (2010). APA
17. Rabbit, P.M.A.: Errors and error correction in choice-response tasks. J. Exp. Psychol. **71**(2), 264–272 (1966). APA
18. Wallis, I., Ingalls, T., Rikakis, T., Olsen, L., Chen, Y., Xu, W., Sundaran, H.: Real-time sonification of movement for an immersive stroke rehabilitation environment. In: Proceedings of Auditory Display 2007, pp. 26–29 (2007)

Games and Gamification for Healthy Behaviours: The Experience of PEGASO Fit 4 Future

Maria Renata Guarneri[✉] and Paolo Perego

Politecnico di Milano, Milan, Italy
{mariarenata.guarneri,paolo.perego}@polimi.it

Abstract. Challenging teenagers in the context of their own areas of interest, Pegaso Fit 4 Future - aims to promote sustainable behaviours geared towards achieving healthy lifestyles. Behaviour-change techniques are applied as a preventative measure to accomplish positive behaviour change outcomes. Pegaso Fit 4 Future is a EU funded project whose objective is the development of a behaviour change platform targeting teenagers in preventing obesity and related comorbidities. The overall approach is based on three main elements: a Smartphone as central element and agent for behaviour change (through a set of coordinated apps); a sensors system for self-monitoring; games and gamified approach to support user engagement and awareness. The paper describes the project focusing on the gaming aspects. Games have been identified as key element in the PEGASO strategy since its conception. After the initial requirements definition phase, a threefold approach to gaming has been adopted in order to address in an integrated strategy the following dimensions of behaviour change: motivational, social and educational aspects. This paper describes this aspect with three different mini-game developed under the project.

Keywords: Gamification · PEGASO · Health game · Behaviour change · Nutrition

1 Introduction

Funded under the umbrella of the 7th Framework Programme of the European Union, the project PEGASO Fit 4 Future [2,3] has the objective of promoting healthy behaviours and lifestyles in the teenagers population. Objective of the project is the development of a behaviour change system based on a mobile/smartphone platform, integrating a wearable sensing system in a cloud based architecture. In view of such ambitious objectives and the specific target addressed, games - as a way to attract and involve teenagers - have been in the radar of PEGASO since its conception. The specific strategy has evolved with the progress of the project and currently we are working with a multifaceted approach to gaming. This paper provides a recap on the main goals and motivations of the project, a description of the approach to gaming, detailing on some specific aspects and games currently under development. In particular section two

© ICST Institute for Computer Sciences, Social Informatics and Telecommunications Engineering 2017
K. Giokas et al. (Eds.): eHealth 2016, LNICST 181, pp. 100–109, 2017.
DOI: 10.1007/978-3-319-49655-9_14

describes the goals and the rationale behind the project, section three provides an overview of the gaming approach within the behavior change theory adopted and section four provides more detailed information on the educational mini-games, which have been designed and developed by the Politecnico di Milano. Section five provides an overview of the validation and evaluation approach of the overall PEGASO system. Finally section six provides some conclusions and highlights on future work.

2   The PEGASO Goals and Motivations

Challenging teenagers in their own fields and areas of interest, PEGASO Fit 4 Future - aims at promoting a sustainable change towards healthy lifestyles, with an holistic and multidisciplinary approach. Pivotal elements of the PEGASO strategy are:

1. Developing self-awareness
2. Enhancing and sustaining motivation
3. Promoting behavioural change towards a healthy lifestyle

On the technology level, PEGASO is a multi-dimensional and cross-disciplinary ICT-based system that exploiting sophisticated and engaging game mechanics. This will motivate behavioural changes towards healthy lifestyles thus preventing overweight and obesity in the younger population.

Childhood obesity, defined as a body mass index higher than 30 kg/m2 has more than doubled in children and quadrupled in adolescents in the past 30 years [1]. Over 60% of children who are overweight before puberty will be overweight in early adulthood. Childhood obesity is a serious problem because it is not only a predisposition to many other childhood diseases but also to premature death. Moreover, childhood obesity is strongly associated with other conditions like breathing difficulties, hypertension, type 2 diabetes, orthopaedic complications, and mental disorders. However, overweight and obese children not only experience an increased risk of the aforementioned diseases; they are also vulnerable for academic underachievement, social isolation and lowered self-esteem due high body weight and negative self-image. In this situation, a tool for behavioural change for a better healthy lifestyle becomes mandatory. The framework of PEGASO is developed along three main dimensions:

1. **Individual and Environmental Monitoring** - a high level-monitoring platform including wearable sensors, for the acquisition of physical, behavioural and emotional attitude of adolescent.
2. **Feedback System** - providing feedback in terms of "health status" changes, requiring actions to undertake and so on, proposing personalized healthy options for alternative lifestyles.
3. **Social connectivity and engagement** - sharing experiences in a community of peers through different gaming strategies.

PEGASO considers three levels of engagement towards empowerment of teenagers in developing virtuous behaviours: awareness of risks, motivation, affective learning and finally behaviour change.

Develop Awareness: Teenagers need to be aware of what they are doing; what is right and what is wrong for their healthy living. Some of them are unconsciously and automatically acting, and often under estimate or have no clear notion about information they receive. Monitoring lifestyle of teens activity, collecting parameters and integrating their own data will enable self-awareness on their current situation. Through developing self-awareness and self-reflection, teens can frame the problem or the opportunity area to act upon or intervene.

Create Motivation: It is important to motivate teenagers to change their behaviour and sustain motivation in the long-term. This goal is quite challenging, since motivation depends on many factors as well as emotions, psychological environment and personality. The use of games and, even more, the provision of services and opportunities for health with a gamified approach of reality, can support this level of engagement.

Enable Behaviour Change: Once teenagers have awareness and motivation, it is important to support the behaviour change process and reinforce acquired virtuous behaviours. The turn from old unhealthy behaviours into new healthier ones has to be monitored on a longer period.

In order to create prevention, it is important to change or stop old unhealthy habits and develop new healthier ones. In this respect, PEGASO takes a holistic approach involving the teenagers environment and specifically the families, by means of an education process empowered by training that will be provided on location (schools) and on line. The expert team will give feedbacks to the users allowing them to change their behaviour on a long-term basis. The overall system takes advantage of gaming strategies to persuade users to change their behaviour.

3   Gaming Approach in PEGASO

The main element of PEGASO Fit 4 Future interface towards the teenagers is the PEGASO Companion [4]. The Companion is the main interface between the user and the PEGASO system and plays the major role of unifying the user experience within PEGASO. The Companion is the management center of the PEGASO service system and, via the Companion, teenagers seamlessly can access the different apps. The Companion allows PEGASO to appear as a single, modular application. The overall gaming system in PEGASO is managed via the Companion and is based on a three-fold approach, leveraging:

The PEGASO game: A 3D serious game aimed at increasing nutritional awareness and promoting physical activity, providing the motivational component [5,6]. The PEGASO game is developed under the responsibility of the PEGASO partners imaginary srl (Italy) and University of Coventry.

The PEGASO serious game performs a central role as a motivational component of the system. It offers capabilities to entertain and engage the player, whilst the PEGASO sensors system captures information on lifestyle and encourage positive changes. There are two central behavioural mechanisms within the game. The first is an "energy bar", consumed by the player's actions in the game, and replenished by achieving behavioural goals set and monitored according to the behavioural theories of self-determination and nudging [7]. Secondly, the game implements "research" mechanics that require the player to apply and develop their nutritional knowledge of various food sources. Each of the two mechanisms leads to a different scenario for positive lifestyle change involving the game. The first scenario is that the player wishes to replenish them in-game energy to boost her/his abilities and expedite their progress within the game; the second one is that in attempting to complete research tasks successfully and efficiently, the player is required to develop and apply her/his knowledge about nutrition (prior researches show a strong link between lifestyle choices and in-game practices, and in particular there is a correlation between healthier lifestyle and game [8].

The PEGASO gamified approach: Linking **real world** activity with online and gaming applications, providing the social component.

Gamification and serious game are concepts integrated in PEGASO with the aim of enhancing the effect of the behaviour change techniques. Simply stated, these approaches, if correctly designed, can increase the user motivation in doing healthy tasks (or, equivalently, demotivating unhealthy behaviours). Gamification techniques in PEGASO leverage the concept of controlled or extrinsic motivation.

Controlled motivation *reflects engaging in behaviors for externally referenced reasons such as to gain rewards or perceived approval from others or to avoid punishment or feelings of guilt. Individuals engaging in behavior for controlled reasons feel a sense of obligation and pressure when engaging in the behavior and are only likely to persist with the behaviors as long as the external contingency is present. If the reinforcing agent is removed, action is likely to desist. Individuals who are control-motivated are therefore less likely to be self-regulated.* Therefore, controlled motivation, also called *extrinsic motivation* [9], involves doing something for external rewards, like money, services, praise or something else that is tangible. The drawback of this typology of reward is that extrinsically motivated people do not have to like the behaviour that the system is encouraging but the outcome. In the PEGASO context, this means that teenagers may not enjoy eating healthy food or doing sport, they are motivated to continue doing so because of the promise of a reward at the end of the process. And if at a certain point in time the reward is removed, the user will stop the desired behaviour. However, jointly with intrinsic motivation, which may be developed through the development of awareness about the different lifestyles and behaviours, linking individual choices with rewards in the social sphere has the potential of reinforcing motivation. Further through gamification techniques it is possible to develop a positive social ecosystem that will influence the behaviour of the individual and of the group is part of.

The PEGASO partners responsible for the overall approach to gamifications are mainly Neosperience (Italy) and the University of Applied Science of Western Switzerland (HES-SO). Linked to the overall ecosystem sustaining the positive behavioural changes, gamification is also a key element of the definition of the PEGASO value network and the potential business model.

The PEGASO minigames: Addressing specific aspects of healthy behaviour, providing the educational component. The minigames are small games that have very specific goals, that can be completed in a short timespan and that provide information in a playful manner. The main goal is to develop awareness and encourage healthy behavior developing the intrinsic (autonomous) motivation. **Autonomous motivation** *is defined as engaging in a behavior because it is perceived to be consistent with intrinsic goals or outcomes and emanates from the self. In other words, the behavior is self-determined. Individuals engaging in behaviors feel a sense of choice, personal endorsement, interest, and satisfaction and, as a consequence, are likely to persist with the behavior. The behavior is consistent with, and supports, the individuals innate needs for autonomy, the need to feel like a personal agent in ones environment, competence, and the need to experience a sense of control and efficacy in ones actions. Individuals acting for autonomous reasons are more likely to initiate and persist with a behavior without any external reinforcement and contingency. Autonomously motivated individuals are, therefore, more likely to be effective in self-regulation of behavior.* Intrinsic motivation fosters behaviours that result in internal rewards (such as satisfaction, positive feelings and happiness). When people are intrinsically motivated, they have a sincere desire for the activity and behaviour change techniques have mainly to work as facilitators for the target behaviours. The PEGASO minigames are the results of work conducted by Politecnico di Milano (Italy) and are further described in more details.

4   Current Work on Educational Games and Mini-Games

PEGASO system includes mini-games related to different and specific aspects of healthy behavior in order to provide an educational media which involve teenagers in the educational process. We focus onto three aspects of health: Food diversification; Food related to energy intake; Food myths and legends. We developed three mini-games, one for each of these aspects: the Food Quiz, the Calories Quiz and the Food Pyramid.

4.1   The Pegaso Food Quiz

The Pegaso Food Quiz is inspired by very popular games on mobile platform like Trivia Crack or Quizoid. It tries to mix the popularity of these game with food education in order to eliminate false information and myths that our society creates around physical activity and food. As visible in Fig. 1, the game is very

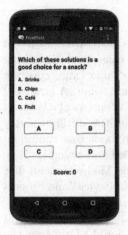 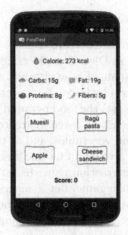 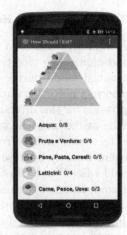

Fig. 1. The three Pegaso mini-games: from left the "Food Quiz" for food diversification, the "Calories Quiz" for food related to energy intake, and How Should I Eat? for Food diversification.

simple; ten multiple choice questions are shown to the player who has to choose the correct answer out of four possibilities. At the end of the ten questions, the game shows the score and the possibility to insert it in a global leader-board. All the questions and leader-board are stored in a cloud-based repository in order to facilitate the insertion of new questions and take a global leader-board. The questions in the game concern many different aspects of health, food and activity. Here are two examples of question with the right answer underlined:

– *All these nutrients are essential for strong bones except ... Calcium - Magnesium - Vitamin D -Sodium.*
– *How many servings of fruits and vegetables should consume per day? zero - four - five - two.*

4.2   The Pegaso Calories Quiz

As the first one, this second mini-game follows the strategy of quiz to teach players the energy content of the different foods. In order to test different user interface, in this second mini-game the graphic is completely different and it is based on Marije Vogelzang food design [11]. The UI (User Interface) is very simple but clear, and the food icon design by Marije Vogelzang help teenagers to easily understand the gameplay. The game shows the amount of calories, fats, carbs, fibers and proteins included in a meal, and the player has to select the correct answer between four different dishes. As for the PEGASO Food Quiz, the score depends on the number of correct answer and it is stored in a global leader-board. The gameplay of this game allows to teach teenagers the food diversification and the content provided by each dish in order to explain the correct association between diet and daily activity. We used different user interfaces in order to test the pleasantness of the two different quiz games.

4.3 How Should I Eat?

The food diversification is one of the main aspects of a correct diet and is the foundation of the Mediterranean Diet. The diversification consists of consuming diversified foods during the span of a week and, at the same time, covering the correct needs for water, carbohydrates, fats, proteins and sugar. A graphical expression for this diversification is the food pyramid [10]. It consists of a triangle having at the basis the foods must be eaten in greater quantities during the day (or the week), such as fruits and vegetables, and at the top foods that should be consumed rarely because they are rich in fat and sugar (fried and sweets). "How should i Eat?" is a physical interaction game based on the Mediterranean diet pyramid. It is not a usual mobile game, but it makes use of devices and objects to involve the player and make the gaming experience more tangible. The game is inspired by Disney Infinity [12] and Tiggly Shapes [13] which use physical object to interact with the mobile phone or tablet. How should i Eat? uses the so called BLE Beacons; they are small devices with Bluetooth® Low Power and iBeacon [14] service which allow measuring approximately the distance between the same and the smartphone/tablet. In this way, the smartphone/tablet is able to trigger action depending on the beacon distance.

We created a table with 35 different dishes and drinks (Fig. 2); each of these is composed by a cardboard disc which includes a beacon specially programmed with the name of the dish/drink. On the mobile device screen a Food Pyramid is shown. The players choose a series of food they usually eat during a day and approach them to the smartphone/tablet. The mobile device automatically recognizes the selected beacons, visualizes the dishes/drinks on the screen (Fig. 2) and insert the relative content in the food pyramid. After the completion of a typical daily food intake, the pyramid can be saved in order to compare it with other pyramids of different players.

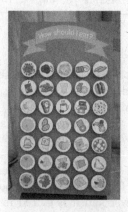 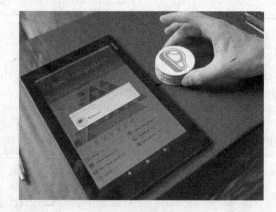

Fig. 2. How should I Eat? Cardboard and an example of use for the iBeacon

5   Evaluation of the PEGASO System

Games and gamification have been identified as key elements of the PEGASO approach since its conception and constitute the main factor for the engagement strategy. The overall system, which includes also a wearable sensors system, for monitoring of current behaviour, and a recommendation system - leveraging the concept of target behaviour and gentle push - will be evaluated by means of three pilot experiments in three countries (Italy, Spain and United Kingdom) enrolling about 400 students in high-schools.

Such evaluation will cover the overall PEGASO platform as a tool aimed to support teen-agers to get aware about their health status. The validation of the PEGASO platform will assess the following factors:

- System and Technology acceptance, usability and long-term use: these will be also a secondary assessment of motivation and engagement;
- Reliability in assessing the teen-agers lifestyles and their changes (with focus on the eating habits and on physical activities) and related efficacy on the sensors network system;
- Efficacy of the system in encouraging lifestyle change;
- Subjective assessment for awareness;
- Systems compliance to Stakeholders needs.

In order to access the efficacy of the system in encouraging lifestyle change, the consortium will use an approach based on pre post assessment of behaviour by means of questionnaires combined with the use of a control group to check efficacy beyond chance. The following existing questionnaires are planned to be used:

- Usability: System Usability Scale (SUS) [15]
- User interaction and experience: Emotional Metric Outcome (EMO) [16]
- Acceptability Technology acceptance model (TAM) [17]
- Desirability: Microsoft Desirability Toolkit [18]

Interventions designed to encourage the adoption of health-promoting behaviours involve a broad spectrum of complexity due to various factors: the number and difficulty of the behaviours required from participants, the coexistence of diverse components that may interact or act independently, the participation of multiple disciplines, and the need for flexibility in adapting to changing contexts. It is essential to gain a deep understanding of the context, which also influences the effectiveness of the intervention. The system PEGASO may be considered as a complex intervention.

The main directives for the design, implementation, and evaluation of this type of interventions were developed by the Medical Research Council (MRC). The MRC Framework [19] promotes research participation by the general public and practicing professionals, which increases the interventions acceptance and feasibility in addition to facilitating participant recruitment and follow-up. This approach also improves the validity and reliability of the assessment tools and ensures the cultural and social relevance of the intervention. These design strengths can also help to increase the sustainability of the intervention, transfer research findings to actual practice, and increase the long-term impact of the health outcomes [20,21].

6   Conclusion

All the games were developed for Android smartphones and tablets. They have been tested on different OS version starting from Android Jelly Bean 4.3. The game are still in the first alpha release, but they have been tested by about 100 teenagers player during two main events ("Wired Next Fest 2015" and "Giovani ambascaitori del cibo @Expo 2015"). After the test all the teenagers were asked to complete a small survey in order to gather opinions regarding the gameplay, the user interface and the user experience. Results of questionnaires show an high acceptability of the games, especially for kids around 10/12 years old. As it might have been expected, the favorite game was "How should I eat?" thanks to both the engaging user interface and the interactivity provided by the ibeacons. For the two quiz games, teenagers underlined the importance to insert more questions and diversifying them inserting grouping (e.g., for Calories Quiz groups foods by Vegetarian, Vegans, Fast-food, Snacks...). Future works aim to insert other features into this game:

- Insert a check on the question already dealt by the player in order to avoid presenting the same questions in a short time;
- Insert the possibility to use a question of the game for unlocking the phone.

As described in the first part of this paper, all these games are part of the Pegaso system of apps. In order to minimize the number of apps to install, quiz games will be merged in the Pegaso Companion main app. In this process they lose their identity of mini-game, but the gamification aspects are maintained.

As indicated earlier, PEGASO is a complex system, of which the game related part constitutes a key component. Other components are the wearable sensors subsystem and the recommendation subsystem. Validation of the system and of the intervention as a whole will be performed by means of pilots involving 400 students in three European countries.

Acknowledgments. This paper is partly based on the work performed within the context of the PEGASO project. The PEGASO project is co-funded by the European Commission under the 7th Framework Programme. PEGASO is part of the cluster of projects in the ICT for health area; it has started in December 2013 and will run for 42 months. The author wishes to thank all the project partners for their contribution to the discussion.

References

1. Childhood obesity. http://www.project-earlynutrition.eu
2. Pegaso fit for future website. http://www.pegasof4f.eu
3. Guarneri, R., Andreoni, G.: Active prevention by motivating and engaging teenagers in adopting healthier lifestyles. In: Duffy, V.G. (ed.) DHM 2014. LNCS, vol. 8529, pp. 351–360. Springer, Heidelberg (2014). doi:10.1007/978-3-319-07725-3_35
4. Carrino, S., Caon, M., Abou Khaled, O., Andreoni, G., Mugellini, E.: PEGASO: towards a life companion. In: Duffy, V.G. (ed.) DHM 2014. LNCS, vol. 8529, pp. 325–331. Springer, Heidelberg (2014). doi:10.1007/978-3-319-07725-3_32
5. Pannese, L., Morosini, D., Lameras, P., Arnab, S., Dunwell, I., Becker, T.: Pegaso: a serious game to prevent obesity. In: Duffy, V.G. (ed.) DHM 2014. LNCS, vol. 8529, pp. 427–435. Springer, Heidelberg (2014). doi:10.1007/978-3-319-07725-3_43
6. Dunwell, I., Dixon, R., Morosini, D.: A mobile serious game for lifestyle change: conveying nutritional knowledge and motivation through play. In: International Conference on Interactive Mobile Communication Technologies and Learning (IMCL) 2015, pp. 259–263. IEEE (2015)
7. Leonard, T.C., Thaler, R.H., Sunstein, C.R.: Nudge: improving decisions about health, wealth, and happiness. Const. Polit. Econ. 19(4), 356–360 (2008)
8. Baranowski, T., et al.: Playing for real: video games and stories for health-related behavior change. Am. J. Prev. Med. 34(1), 74–82 (2008)
9. Ryan, R.M., Deci, E.L.: Self-determination theory and the facilitation of intrinsic motivation, social development, and well-being. Am. Psychol. 55(1), 68 (2000)
10. Willett, W.C., Sacks, F., Trichopoulou, A., Drescher, G., Ferro-Luzzi, A., Helsing, E., Trichopoulos, D.: Mediterranean diet pyramid: a cultural model for healthy eating. Am. J. Clin. Nutr. 61(6), 1402S–1406S (1995)
11. Marije Vogelzang website. http://www.marijevogelzang.nl/
12. Disney Infinity Website. https://infinity.disney.com/it/
13. Tiggly shape website. https://www.tiggly.com/
14. Newman, N.: Apple ibeacon technology briefing. J. Direct Data Digit. Mark. Pract. 15(3), 222–225 (2014)
15. Sauro, J.: A practical guide to the system usability scale: background, benchmarks & best practices. Measuring Usability LLC (2011)
16. Lewis, J.R., Mayes, D.K.: Development and psychometric evaluation of the emotional metric outcomes (EMO) questionnaire. Int. J. Hum. Comput. Interact. 30(9), 685–702 (2014)
17. Davis, F.D.: Perceived usefulness, perceived ease of use, user acceptance of information technology. MIS Q. 13, 319–340 (1989)
18. Benedek, J., Miner, T.: Measuring desirability: new methods for evaluating desirability in a usability lab setting. In: Proceedings of Usability Professionals Association, 8–12 2002 (2003)
19. Medical Research Council (Great Britain). Health Services and Public Health Research Board. A framework for development and evaluation of RCTs for complex interventions to improve health. Medical Research Council (2000)
20. Campbell, N.C.: Designing, evaluating complex interventions to improve health care. BMJ 334(7591), 455–459 (2007)
21. Craig, P., et al.: Developing and evaluating complex interventions. Medical Research Council, UK (2011)

Effect of Different Looting Systems on the Behavior of Players in a MMOG: Simulation with Real Data

Daniele De Felice, Marco Granato, Laura Anna Ripamonti, Marco Trubian, Davide Gadia$^{(\boxtimes)}$, and Dario Maggiorini

Department of Computer Science, University of Milan, 20135 Milan, MI, Italy
{marco.granato,marco.trubian}@unimi.it,
{ripamonti,gadia,dario}@di.unimi.it

Abstract. Massively Multi-player Online Games (MMOGs) are complex and persistent video games developed for a large public of players. The complex relations and dynamics among players represent an interesting research topic not only for developers, but also for experts in social relations and psychologists. Looting Systems (LSs), i.e. the procedure applied to allocate goods or items to a group of players after a successful collaborative activity, can have an important role in the overall satisfaction of a player towards the game and the other players in her group, leading even to the decision to abandon the virtual world. In this work we analyze different types of LSs, and we try to simulate the behavior of different type of players using real data from World of Warcraft, in order to understand which LS can be the more appropriate to maintain a high level of satisfaction and engagement in the players.

Keywords: Videogames · Massively multiplayer online games · Agent base model simulation · Looting system

1 Introduction

Massively Multi-player Online Role-Playing Games (MMORPGs) and Massively Multi-player Online Games (MMOGs) are games where players interact in an online, persistent, and shared virtual world. This game category has gained success and diffusion thanks to Blizzard's World of Warcraft (WoW) [1]: in 2014, WOW could count on 10 million worldwide subscribers [2,3]. The high number of players, and the need of a large scale cooperation, interaction and competition among players have led to a relevant interest not only from the gaming research community, but also from experts in social sciences and psychologists. As a matter of fact, in literature it has been proposed that satisfaction or frustration in video game can modify short-term emotions: "games are generally more or less appealing, and have a greater or lesser influence on player well-being, as a function of the extent to which the in-game experiences they provide fulfill fundamental psychological needs" [18]. In this paper, we aim to investigate

© ICST Institute for Computer Sciences, Social Informatics and Telecommunications Engineering 2017
K. Giokas et al. (Eds.): eHealth 2016, LNICST 181, pp. 110–118, 2017.
DOI: 10.1007/978-3-319-49655-9_15

the role of the Looting System (LS) [5], i.e. the procedure applied to allocate the resources/items won by a group of players after a successful collaborative activity in a MMOG.

Dungeons and *Raids* are two common structures used by almost all MMOs. Usually, *Dungeons* are instanced confined areas designed for a limited number of players at a time. *Raids* are similar to the *Dungeons* but designed for a larger number of players that devote a relevant amount of time in order to accomplish the mission and to obtain, usually, items or objects of higher level than in the Dungeons. In almost all MMOs, there is a *guild* (also named *clan*) system. It unifies different classes of players under the same name and rules, and consequently these players regularly play together creating a bond that allows a better game performance. Once the guild has successfully concluded a Raid, the items obtained during the mission have to be allocated among the players. If this situation is mismanaged, the satisfaction of the players (and their will to continue to participate and play to the game with that guild) can be affected.

Valid LS can contribute to the overall success of a MMOG, by maintaining an appropriate level of satisfaction in the players, by allocating fairly the obtained items, on the basis of well-described and explained rules.

Unfortunately, only a few studies have been conducted on this topic [6,8,11]. In the present work, we try to understand which approach could guarantee an adequate level of satisfaction in the players. To this aim, we show the results of a simulation based on real data from WoW, applied to several LSs described in literature.

2   Types of Looting System

Different approaches to LS are present in literature (for a detailed description and overview see [8–10]).

In this paper, we consider the following methods:

- *Rolling*: this system tries to reproduce the most random action possible. Each player rolls a "dice" for each object (from 1 to 100), and the player with the highest result gets the item.
- *Dragon Kill Points (DKP)*: During various events players can obtain points (called DKP) that are later used as a currency to bid on available items. In the paper, we consider the following variants of the original DKP approach:
  - *DKP fixed*: the item has a fixed price in DKP. Players interested in the loot bid the points. The item is then assigned randomly among them or following a predetermined priority list.
  - *DKP auction*: the item is put up for auction. Different types of auction can be used.
  - *DKP zero-sum*: the points spent on the item are redistributed amongst other participants in the group.
- *Dual Token*: a pair of Tokens is assigned to every player (Need and Greed). Players interested in the item use their Need token: the object is then assigned

randomly among those who used their tokens. In case no Need tokens were used, Greed tokens placement takes place, to assign the item for speculative goals or for a secondary use on the character.

- *Dual Token ordered (hybrid)*: a hybrid looting system proposed in [8]. It combines ideas from both Dual Token and *DKP relational* (where the order in which players are listed is based on the relationship between acquired and spent DKP). The use of tokens is the same as in the Dual Token system, but the priority list on which the item is assigned is based on the relationship between number of missions whose the player has taken part and the value of the items she has already received. In this case, a player with a high number of missions but without many powerful items will have priority on a player with many powerful items already assigned.

3   Looting System Effect Analysis

In the work by *Maggiorini et al.* [8], a preliminary evaluation of different LSs has been presented, and in this paper we expand their approach, basing our analysis on a simulation based on real data regarding WoW players characteristics and classification.

3.1   Players Classification and Data

The analysis is based on a classification of players: the parameters used for the classification are Bartle-Type, Game-Time, and Class.

Bartle classification [4] tries to describe how the players interact with each other. He identifies four main types of players:

- *Killers*: focus on winning, rank up and competition
- *Achievers*: focus on attaining status and achieving pre-set goals quickly
- *Socializers*: focus on socializing and aim at developing a network of friends
- *Explorers*: focus on exploring and aim at discovering the unknown

Another criterion by which players can be classified is how much time they spend playing every week. We can identify three groups: Casual (<20 h), Medium (20–40 h), and Hardcore (>40 h) players.

Finally, we classified players on the basis of their main Class in WoW: tank, healer, melee DPS, and ranged DPS. We limited the classification to 4 classes because the actual class structure in WoW is too complex and redundant to be handled by the simulation.

After a review of the literature [15–17], we determined a set of data related to real players in Wow. The results are summarized, in percentage, in Table 1, and they represents the basis for the overall simulation on LSs effect.

Table 1. Resuming empirical data in percentage [15–17].

Bartle-type	Percentage	Game-time	Percentage	Class	Percentage
Explorer	30%	Casual	50%	Tank	15%
ocializer	25%	Medium	35%	Melee DPS	25%
Achiever	25%	Hardcore	15%	Ranged DPS	40%
Killer	20%			Healer	20%

3.2 Simulation

The simulation model considered is an expansion of the model used by *Maggiorini et al.* [8]. A detailed description of the original model is beyond the scope of this paper. We recall the overall principles of the model, and we describe the extensions and differences introduced to deal with the set of data regarding actual WoW players.

Overall Approach. While the previous method [8] was focused more on the simulation of the possible choice made by a guild to change the adopted LS (the players of a guild use a specific LS, then after each raid vote the effectiveness of the LS and choose if change or keep it), the current approach is focused instead on the possible decision to change the guild, made by a single player, because of dissatisfaction of the current LS. Other differences with the previous model are mainly due to the adoption of real data to set Bartle type and the time spent playing (in the previous model they were calculated in a separate simulation), and in the consideration of a higher number of players (ten times more than in [8]) inserted in a dynamic flow of players composed by newbies and players that abandoned the game.

The presented simulation is based mainly on the mathematical model presented in [8].

In the original model, the players judged the adopted LS, and evaluated if to change or keep it. This decision calculating with the following formula:

$$Change_D = diss(item, player) + change(Ls, tot\_items) \tag{1}$$

Where *diss* is measure of dissatisfaction of the player for the item dropped by the mission, and $change(Ls, tot_i items)$ measures the desire to change the current situation (using LS and the number of objects collected by the player).

In the original model, contribution of each player of a guild to the $Change_D$ parameter is compared with a random number (<100): if the value is bigger, the simulation would force a new LS for the guild, otherwise the current LS is used again for the next mission, and a counter connected to the current LS is increased. The simulation described in [8] would end here, looping for a fixed amount of missions and showing the results, printing the LSs counters and showing which one was kept the longest and voted to be changed the last times.

In the proposed approach, this is not adequate since we are adding guilds and players movements between different guilds instead of a static environment, and as a consequence LS cannot be changed in the same way. Therefore, in our approach a guild never changes its LS: on the contrary, a specific and unchangeable LS is randomly assigned to every guild. In the new model, the evaluation of single $Change_D$ parameter determines whether a player of the guild is more inclined to stay or to change guild. When players are searching for a guild, they will be less interested in guilds with a high number of members because the chance to participate in raids carried out by that guild will be much lower than with a smaller one [12].

Simulation Setup and Parameters. The simulation is initialized with 250 guilds with an average of 16.8 players each [14]. The initial population consists of 5000 players. During the simulation the number of players may fluctuate because there is a process of introduction of newbie players and the elimination of players abandoning the game. The players are simulated through *agents* using [7]: i.e., a software simulation about an entity with its personal goals and behaviors, which adapts and modifies its behaviors according to the environment. Following [13], we set in the simulation a random number between 3 and 6 of players linked to other players, in order to simulate friendship bonds from the real life between players.

During the simulation, the probability that a player attends at one raid is calculated using the amount of time spent playing alone and by his guild, if the guild has enough members. A hardcore player has a higher chance to participate (95%) than medium (70%) and casual (50%). Raids give higher rewards (medium-high power items) and the assigned LS of the guild is used after the mission. Then, a fixed number of dungeons, depending on the total number of players, are simulated: groups of 5 players are randomly created without checking guild membership. However, the simulation tries to have a balanced group with at least one tank, one healer, and one DPS. There is also a 50% probability to choose a hardcore player, 30% a medium, and 20% a casual. Items, of low-medium power, are assigned using a *rolling* LS.

A general loot generated by a dungeon or a raid can fall in 5 groups. The items in the first 4 groups regard only one of the four classes: tank, healer, melee DPS, and ranged DPS (e.g. a special bow usable only by a ranged DPS). In this case the item will interest only players in the same item class. In addition to this, the item can be a no-class item that can be taken by any player (e.g. consumables, recipes, crafting requirements). Every player that plays in the raid group generates a preference value very similar to the model described in [8].

For every simulated day, the simulation checks if a player is unsatisfied with his guild and its LS. The overall behavior of an agent is controlled by 3 parameters: the *guild-satisfaction*, *move-changes*, and *overall-satisfaction*.

Guild-satisfaction defines how much an agent is satisfied by his/her guild and the connected LS. It is formulated using the $Change_D$ value, the threshold of objects satisfaction (*Item won*) described in [8], and data in *Patil et al.* [19].

Table 2. Guild satisfaction changes. For more information on *Item won* see [8]

Event	Guild-satisfaction change
Not raiding	−days since last raid * 0.1%
Guild size > 80	−0.10%
Guild size > 120	Additional −0.10%
Item won	$+item\ satisfaction\ ratio * (\frac{No.\ found\ obj.}{No.\ players\ in\ the\ mission})$
$Change_D$ check passes	−50

The calculation of *guild-satisfaction* is described in Table 2. It generally increases on successful acquisition of items and lowers vice-versa.

When "*guild-satisfaction*" goes under 50, a random check is done to see if the player leaves the guild.

Players that leave a guild, or never had a guild, will try to find a new guild. Every player checks for one guild chosen by one of his friends every day. The simulation calculated an index called "*move-chance*" in order to determine the inclination of the player to join a guild.

It is calculated using different properties:

- if Player game-time == hardcore then *move chance* += 30,
- if Player game-time == medium then *move chance* += 25,
- if Player game-time == casual then *move chance* += 20,
- if Player Bartle == guild Bartle then
  - if Player game-time == hardcore then *move chance* += 50,
  - if Player game-time == medium then *move chance* += 40,
  - if Player game-time == casual then *move chance* += 30,
- if Player game-time == guild game-time then *move chance* += 40,
- if Guild size > 30 then *move chance* += (100 - guild size),
- if Guild size > 70 then *move chance* −= (guild size - 30).

The *move-chance* value is then compared to a random value (<100): if it is bigger, than the player joins the guild adopting its LS.

Finally, "*overall-satisfaction*" checks if a player is playing or being passive. This value is affected by Bartle type and time spent playing. It decreases if the agent does not participate to a raid for several days. In particular, the "*overall satisfaction*" value is changed as:

- if casual: $-0.1\% * day\_since\_last\_raid$,
- if medium: $-0.2\% * days\_since\_last\_raid$,
- if hardcore: $-0.3\% * ticks\_since\_last\_raid$.

At the same time participating in a raid will give following bonus:

- if casual: +3,
- if medium: +6,
- if hardcore: +9,

- if killer: +2,
- if achiever: +4,
- if explorer: +7,
- if socializer: +9.

Reaching a very low value in this field (<25) will make the player leave the game.

4   Results and Discussion

The simulation process described in the previous section runs for 300 times, to simulate an average video game year (300 days). At the end, every LS is assigned a value, corresponding to the average number of people that left guilds using that LS during raids. Every single simulation has been executed 50 times and the average for every LS calculated and compared with the others.

Figure 1 shows the data related to guild abandoning between various *game-time* types of agents. Analyzing the results of the simulation, the Dual Token ordered hybrid LS seems to be the LS with potential lower dissatisfaction for every type of *game-time* players. This result is in line with the results presented in [8].

Therefore, we can identify three major LSs groups, depending on their success rate. The first one is made up of LSs that clearly fail to make the player satisfied. We can consider not successful all LSs that base their core decision on a random value (rolling, dual token). The second group contains LSs that, at cost of some extra time needed to set up and use the model, give the players a fairer chance to obtain the loot wanted. This is generally the DKP system in its various applications. Lastly, the third group contains the LSs that are the most successful, as, in the case of the presented simulation, Dual Token ordered hybrid LS.

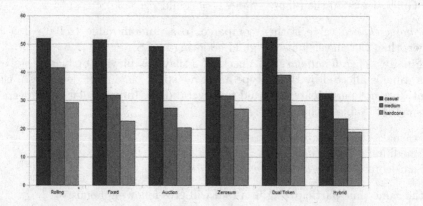

Fig. 1. Game-time type preferences population. The y axes define the average of players that leave a guild.

Generally we can say that a relational system (like the hybrid system), that takes into consideration both the loot already acquired and the time spent in the guild/game, could obtain a high general satisfaction from the average MMOG player. However it comes with the cost of harder and more complex implementation and maintenance.

The presented approach can be easily integrated with future proposed LSs and supplementary real data, and adapted to changes in general WoW settings. Moreover, the presented approach can contribute to influence the overall player well-being, by providing a fair and clear feedback to the time and efforts put in the game by the player, and, as a consequence, by maintaining a high level of engagement, and the will to continue to participate in the virtual world.

References

1. Taylor, T.L.: Play Between Worlds: Exploring Online Game Culture. MIT Press, Cambridge (2009)
2. Statista - The Statistic Portal. http://www.statista.com/statistics/276601/number-of-world-of-warcraft-subscribers-by-quarter/
3. MMOData blog. http://mmodata.blogspot.it/
4. Bartle, R.A.: Designing Virtual Worlds. New Riders Publishing, Indianapolis (2003)
5. Castronova, E.: Synthetic Worlds. University of Chicago Press, Chicago (2005). ISBN 0-226-09626-2
6. Maggiorini, D., Nigro, A., Ripamonti, L.A., Trubian, M.: Massive online games, loot distribution: an elusive problem. In: 5th International ICST Conference on Simulation Tools and Techniques, DISIO 2012, SIMUTools 2012, Desenzano, Italy (2012). 10.4108/icts.simutools.2012.247777
7. NetLogo. http://ccl.northwestern.edu/netlogo/
8. Maggiorini, D., Nigro, A., Ripamonti, L.A., Trubian, M.: The perfect lootingsystem: looking for a phoenix? In: IEEE Computational Intelligence and Games Conference (2012)
9. WoWWiki. http://www.wowwiki.com/Loot_system
10. Andrews, F.S.: The Guild Leader's Handbook. No Starch Press, San Francisco (2012)
11. Maggiorini, D., et al.: Loot Distribution in Massive Online Games: Foreseeing impacts on the players base. In: 2012 21st International Conference on Computer Communications and Networks (ICCCN). IEEE (2012)
12. Williams, D., Ducheneaut, N., Xiong, L., Zhang, Y., Yee, N., Nickell, E.: From tree house to barracks: the social life of guilds in world of warcraft. Games Cult. 1(4), 338–361 (2006)
13. Cole, H., Griffiths, M.D.: Social interactions in massively multiplayer online role-playing gamers. Cyber Psychol. Behav. 10(4), 575–583 (2007)
14. Ducheneaut, N., Yee, N., Nickell, E., Moore, R.J.: The life, death of online gaming communities: a look at guilds in world of warcraft. In: Proceedings of the SIGCHI (2007)
15. Ducheneaut, N., Yee, N., Nickell, E., Moore, R.J.: Building an MMO with mass appeal a look at gameplay in world of warcraft. Games Cult. 1(4), 281–317 (2006)
16. Griffiths, M.D., Davies, M.N.O., Chappell, D.: Demographic factors and playing variables in online computer gaming. Cyber Psychol. Behav. 7(4), 479–487 (2004)

17. Hours Played per week. http://www.nickyee.com/daedalus/archives/000758.php
18. Przybylski, A.K., Rigby, C.S., Ryan, R.M.: A motivational model of video game engagement. Rev. Gen. Psychol. **14**(2), 154 (2010)
19. Patil, A., Liu, J., Price, B., Sharara, H., Brdiczka, O.: Modeling destructive group dynamics in online gaming communities. In: International Conference Weblogs and Social Media, pp. 290–297 (2012)

Assessing the Emotional State of Job Applicants Through a Virtual Reality Simulation: A Psycho-Physiological Study

Daniela Villani[1(✉)], Chiara Rotasperti[1], Pietro Cipresso[1,2], Stefano Triberti[1], Claudia Carissoli[1], and Giuseppe Riva[1,2]

[1] Department of Psychology, Università Cattolica del Sacro Cuore, Milan, Italy
{daniela.villani,pietro.cipresso,stefano.triberti,
claudia.carissoli,giuseppe.riva}@unicatt.it
[2] ATNPLab, Istituto Auxologico Italiano, Milan, Italy

Abstract. Job interview is one of the most frequently used methods to assess candidates for employment and it often evokes feelings of anxiety and distress. The principal aim of this study is to use a VR simulation experience to assess the emotional state, and specifically anxiety, of job applicants. Two VR job simulations are proposed to twenty-five participants, before and after a five weeks training aimed to enhance their emotional skills. Results show differences in anxiety experienced by participants exposed to VR-simulated job interviews before and after the trainings and suggest adequacy of VR as an assessment tool sensitive to the changes in internal states of candidates.

Keywords: Virtual reality · Assessment · Anxiety · Emotional state · Psycho-physiological measures

1 Introduction

Around the world, job interview is one of the most frequently used methods to assess candidates for employment [1–3]. The job interview represents a critical moment for applicants: they expect interviews as part of a selection process [4] fundamental to job search success [5] and for this reason it often evokes feelings of anxiety and distress [6]. Anxiety is an inherent part of the interview process [7], and it could be related both to the fact that the interviewer is usually a stranger and talking with strangers could provoke anxiety [8] and to the lack of control perceived by the applicants [9]. A widely accepted explanation about the emergence of anxiety is related to the "test-taking anxiety". This view contains two principal components: performance anxiety, conceptualized as fear of failure, and behavioral anxiety that reflects the autonomic arousal due to the test-taking situation. Both these components were expected to be critical to job-interview situations, as job interviews could be considered as a type of test [10]. Anxiety can impair the individual's ability to retain information [11, 12] and thus determine serious implications for applicants [13]. For this reason, it is important to design structured situations

© ICST Institute for Computer Sciences, Social Informatics and Telecommunications Engineering 2017
K. Giokas et al. (Eds.): eHealth 2016, LNICST 181, pp. 119–126, 2017.
DOI: 10.1007/978-3-319-49655-9_16

helping applicants to reach a good performance and to reduce the risks of failure of their experience in a real job interview [14].

Today, thanks to the advances in technologies, Virtual Reality (VR) could represent a valid chance to overcome the limits related to the exposure in real life [15] and has been already applied in interventions aimed to reduce public speaking anxiety [16–19] VR is a human computer interaction in which users are active participants in a computer generated three-dimensional world [20] so convincing that it allows participants to have experiences that mimic those of real world. A simulated interactive environment available through VR can offer applicants an opportunity to practice and try out new skills without the worry of embarrassment or the risk of failure. This in turn can lead to improved job interview performance and, perhaps even more importantly, a sense of personal control or self-efficacy. Self-efficacy is defined as an individual's assessment of his or her ability to perform behaviors in specific situations [21] and this evaluation influences behavior. The first and most influential source of self-efficacy is past perform-ance accomplishments. Success experiences (e.g. being able to overcome an obstacle through effort and perseverance) generally enhance individuals' beliefs in personal competence [21]. Applied to applicants to job interview, self-efficacy theory suggests that the use of VR may provide them with a sense of mastery or self-efficacy and, in turn, result in improved perception of performance and satisfaction with performance.

Recently, Villani and colleagues [22] compared two different settings, an immersive VR job simulation and a real world simulation that was identical to its VR counterpart (same interviewer, same questions) but without technological mediation and without any social and cultural cues, and found that participants experienced higher level of presence during the virtual interview than in the real world simulation. This result supports the idea that the experience of presence is influenced by the ability of meaning attribution to the experience. In that case the design of the VR environment as a profes-sional setting enriched of social and cultural cues traditionally associated to the job interview context played a critical role.

Thus, VR can be used as an evaluation or a self-evaluation tool that provides infor-mation to the candidate about his/her emotional competence in coping with the event. This enables the candidate to decide whether he/she feels ready to face the situation or he/she believes that additional emotional skills must be developed to deal with the event successfully.

The principal aim of this study is to use a VR simulation experience to assess the emotional state, and specifically anxiety, of applicants. In particular, we proposed a VR job simulation experience enriched of social and cultural cues before and after a training aimed to enhance emotional skills of applicants. We expected to find differences between the two VR experiences related to applicants anxiety measured both with self-report and psycho-physiological measures. Specifically, we hypothesized a reduction of anxiety in VR experience measured after a training.

2 Method

2.1 Participants

Flyers were posted at Università Cattolica del Sacro Cuore and emails were sent to final years or graduated students of the same University to attract participants. We specified that we were interested in selecting people who had never had a job interview before. Twenty-five students, 9 males and 16 females, applied to participate and were included in the study. Participants' age ranged from 23 to 27 years. They were asked to imagine that they had applied for a desirable job and that they were undergoing a job interview.

2.2 Design

The VR job simulation was proposed two times during a face-to-face meeting with a psychologist, before and after a training aimed to enhance emotional skills of applicants. Participants were randomly assigned to two types of training: a more traditional one supported by a commercial book or a training supported by an ad hoc iBook developed using the iBooks Author tool from the Mac App store. Both trainings lasted five weeks and were focused on these issues: "prepare yourself for the job interview" (second and third weeks) included informative vs experiential materials about enhancing the aware-ness of candidate's profile and behavior aspects; "the job interview" (fourth and fifth weeks) included informative vs experiential materials about managing different inter-view types; "after the job interview" included informative vs experiential materials about dealing with the expected reply and evaluating the interview done in order to make better use of other occasions.

Within the VR job simulation the interview questions were general in nature, in order to allow participants to answer as if they were being interviewed for a job that they would like to have. The entire interview included eight questions and was split in half, yielding two sets of four questions (questions 1–4 vs. questions 5–8) each proposed in a random-ized order during the first or the second virtual simulation. The items were relatively short in length, based on concrete ideas, and included only straightforward language, to ensure that each item described only one idea [23]. Each VR job simulation lasted approximately 15 min.

2.3 Tools

The virtual environment was developed by using Xtranormal, a cost-free tool available online which allows non-expert users to easily modify the virtual scenes, in order to best suit the needs of recreating real world contexts and that has been adapted here for the specific goal.

For this experiment the environment was modeled on a typical manager's office and was meant to represent a place that would make the student feel at a job interview. Figure 1 (a and b) shows two screenshots of the VR environment.

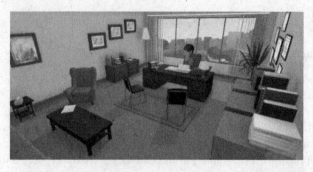

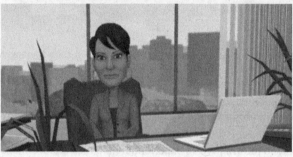

Fig. 1. The virtual office developed by using Xtranormal. Figure 1a shows the social and cultural cues (i.e. private office, furniture, books). Figure 1b shows the interviewer that is seated at a desk with laptop and applicant's Curriculum Vitae in front of her.

2.4 Measures

To identify the affective dimension of the participants, we proposed an integrated multi-modal assessment—combining subjective and objective measures.

The State Trait Anxiety Inventory [24, 25] is a self-report questionnaire that assesses both state and trait anxiety levels. We used the State Anxiety subscale (STAI-S), a 20-item measures in which participants rate their level of anxiety to each item on a 4-point Likert-type scale, to evaluate the "transitory emotional states". The State version was used as a manipulation check to measure anxiety levels at the end of each VR job simulation session.

The physiological signals were acquired using a ProComp Infiniti device from Thought Technology, including Biograph Infiniti 5.0.2 software to record and export all raw signals. According to the classic valence-arousal model [26, 27] we considered the two dimensions of physiological arousal and emotional valence for identifying affective states in participants during the experimental session. Following the guidelines of task force of the European Society of Cardiology and the North American Society of Pacing and Electrophysiology, typical Heart Rate Variability (HRV) temporal and spectral method indexes were used to evaluate the autonomic nervous system response [28, 29]. Specifically, we monitored the cardiovascular activity, by using two indexes such as Heart Rate (HR) and the ratio between low and high frequency components (LF/HF ratio) known as the sympathovagal balance index [30]. A baseline measure of the psychophysiological parameters was obtained with a 3-min registration in a steady state.

3   Results

Anxiety State Outcome. First of all, the level of anxiety experienced in both VR job simulations was investigated as measured by STAI State Pre-Post index compared by using a paired comparison T-test (first vs. second session). Results showed significant statistical differences ($t = 2.112$, df = 24, $p = .045$) between the two sessions. In the first session participants experienced a significant increase of anxiety state level, while in the second session they experienced a significant decrease of anxiety state level.

Physiological Outcome. The levels of physiological arousal and emotional valence calibrated on the baseline between the two VR sessions have been compared in order to verify differences in participants' affective states. After the noise reduction process we excluded some participants from the analyses. Results showed significant statistical differences both in HR ($t = 2.078$, df = 19, $p = .051$), and LF/HF ($t = 11.398$, df = 14, $p = .001$) between the two sessions. We found a significant reduction for both indexes.

Descriptive statistics of all measures are shown in Table 1.

Table 1. Descriptive statistics of the level of anxiety state change (STAI) and physiological indexes measured during VR job simulation sessions

	Session 1 M (SD)	Session 2 M (SD)
STAI Pre VR	35.92 (8.77)	36.96 (8.39)
STAIPost VR	36.72 (10.03)	34.20 (9.06)
HR	11.26 (8.30)	9.47 (6.70)
LF/HF	.94 (.21)	.24 (.29)

We also analyzed the differences between the trainings (paper book vs digital book) and we did not find differences between them.

4   Discussion and Conclusion

Results show differences in anxiety experienced by participants exposed to VR-simulated job interviews before and after the trainings, both measured with self-report and physiological signals. In addition to coming out in favor of the trainings' efficacy, this result implies an adequacy of VR for providing salient experiences to the participants. In other words, the results show that such experiences appear sensitive to the changes in internal states induced by trainings. Indeed, session 1 induced an increase in state anxiety such as the simulation had been experienced by the participants similarly to a real job interview. Consistently, after different trainings designed to empower participants' emotion regulation skills, the anxiety experienced during the virtual job interview was significantly reduced. This result does not seem attributable to the lack of novelty of the second virtual simulation, given that the group that had followed the Ibook training had more opportunities to try virtual job interview simulations.

Although the job interviews were simulated by means of VR, featuring cartoon-like characters and dialogues voiced by actors, the participants experienced them as immersive resources for meaningful role-playing. Indeed, the use of virtual environments and virtual characters has been found able to promote motivation for learning in role-playing [31]. Consistently, previous experiences have shown that such tools are useful to improve communicational and emotional skills, both in pathological and non-pathological contexts [32, 33]. In the present study, the coherence between self-report and physiological assessment leads us to consider that the VR simulation may be used both as an assessment experiential tool under laboratory setting, where traditionally the psychophysiological signals are used, and as a self-evaluation experiential tool by the candidates. Indeed, they reported to be aware of the change in the level of anxiety as measured by the questionnaire. This opens to the possibility of designing virtual environments for self-evaluation and self-empowerment, given that both immersive and non-immersive VR are more and more widespread resources, thanks to the emergence of commercial VR devices for home gaming and in the mobile technology industry [34].

Generally speaking, the main consequence the present study is that VR-based simulation of complex real-life experiences can be used to test the effectiveness of trainings for emotion regulation. In other words, effectiveness can be evaluated not only testing participants' emotional reactions to generalized, abstract stimuli, but also to controlled experiences that resemble (at least in virtual/simulative terms) the actual experiences they encounter in their own everyday life. Along with previous research [22] the present study suggests that VR-based simulations can be used as effective surrogates of complex real-life anxiety triggers, such as the job interview experience. Further research is needed to understand whether and how such a technology may be improved in its effectiveness resembling real life, and whether it can be applied to the empowerment of emotion regulation in multiple real-life problematic context [35].

References

1. Macan, T.: The employment interview: a review of current studies and directions for future research. Hum. Res. Manage. Rev. **19**(3), 203–218 (1981)
2. Ryan, A.N.N., et al.: An international look at selection practices: Nation and culture as explanations for variability in practice. Pers. Psychol. **52**(2), 359–392 (1999)
3. Wilk, S.L., Cappelli, P.: Understanding the determinants of employer use of selection methods. Pers. Psychol. **56**(1), 103–124 (2003)
4. Lievens, F., De Corte, W., Brysse, K.: Applicant perceptions of selection procedures: the role of selection information, belief in tests, and comparative anxiety. Int. J. Sel. Assess. **11**(1), 67–77 (2003)
5. Saks, A.M.: Multiple predictors and criteria of job search success. J. Vocat. Behav. **68**(3), 400–415 (2006)
6. Posthuma, R.A., Morgeson, F.P., Campion, M.A.: Beyond employment interview validity: A comprehensive narrative review of recent research and trends over time. Pers. Psychol. **55**(1), 1–81 (2002)

7. McCarthy, J., Goffin, R.: Measuring job interview anxiety: beyond weak knees and sweaty palms. Pers. Psychol. **57**(3), 607–637 (2004)
8. Ayres, J., et al.: Communication apprehension and employment interviews. Commun. Educ. **47**(1), 1–17 (1998)
9. Jones, D.B., Pinkney, J.W.: An exploratory assessment of the sources of job-interview anxiety in college students. J. Coll. Stud. Dev. **30**, 553–560 (1989)
10. Apa, A.P.A.: Standards for educational and psychological testing. American Psychological Association, Washington (1985)
11. Fiedler, K.: Emotional mood, cognitive style, and behavior regulation. In: Fiedler, K., Forgas, J.P. (eds.) Affect, Cognition and Social Behavior, pp. 100–119. Hogrefe, Gottingen (1988)
12. Luce, M.F., Bettman, J.R., Payne, J.W.: Choice processing in emotionally difficult decisions. J. Exp. Psychol. Learn. Mem. Cogn. **23**(2), 384 (1997)
13. Ayres, J., Crosby, S.: Two studies concerning the predictive validity of the personal report of communication apprehension in employment interviews. Commun. Res. Rep. **12**(2), 145–151 (1995)
14. Young, M.J., Behnke, R.R., Mann, Y.M.: Anxiety patterns in employment interviews. Commun. Rep. **17**(1), 49–57 (2004)
15. Riva, G.: Virtual reality in psychotherapy: review. Cyberpsychol. Behav. **8**(3), 220–230 (2005)
16. Anderson, P.L., et al.: Cognitive behavioral therapy for public speaking anxiety using virtual reality for exposure. Depression Anxiety **22**(3), 156–158 (2005)
17. Jo, H.J., et al.: The development of the virtual reality system for the treatment of the fears of public speaking. Stud. Health Technol. Inform. **81**, 209–211 (2001)
18. Pertaub, D.P., Slater, M., Barker, C.: An experiment on fear of public speaking in virtual reality. Stud. Health Technol. Inform. **81**, 372–378 (2001)
19. Slater, M., et al.: An experimental study on fear of public speaking using a virtual environment. CyberPsychol. Behav. **9**(5), 627–633 (2006)
20. Schultheis, M.T., Himelstein, J., Rizzo, A.A.: Virtual reality and neuropsychology: Upgrading the current tools. J. Head Trauma Rehabil. **17**(5), 378–394 (2002)
21. Bandura, A.: Self-efficacy: The Exercise of Control. Freeman, New York (2007)
22. Villani, D., et al.: May i experience more presence in doing the same thing in virtual reality than in reality? an answer from a simulated job interview. Interact. Comput. **24**(4), 265–272 (2012)
23. Spector, P.E.: Summated Rating Scale Construction: An Introduction. Sage, London (1992)
24. Spielberger, C.D., Gorsuch, R.L., Lushene, R.E.: State-trait Anxiety Inventory Manual. Consulting Psychologists Press, Palo Alto (1970)
25. Pedrabissi, L., Santinello, M.: Inventario per l'ansia di « Stato » e di « Tratto »: nuova versione italiana dello STAI Forma Y: Manuale, p. 44. Organizzazioni Speciali, Firenze (1989)
26. Lang, P.J.: The emotion probe: studies of motivation and attention. Am. Psychol. **50**(5), 372–385 (1995)
27. Russell, J.A.: Affective space is bipolar. J. Pers. Soc. Psychol. **37**(3), 345 (1979)
28. Camm, A., et al.: Heart rate variability. Standards of measurement, physiological interpretation, and clinical use. Eur. Heart J. **17**(3), 354–381 (1996)
29. Barbieri, R., Triedman, J.K., Saul, J.P.: Heart rate control and mechanical cardiopulmonary coupling to assess central volume: a systems analysis. Am. J. Physiol. Regul. Integr. Comp. Physiol. **283**(5), 1210–1220 (2002)
30. Cipresso, P., et al.: Computational psychometrics in communication and implications in decision making. Comput. Math. Methods Med. **2015**, 1–10 (2015)

31. Huang, H.-M., Rauch, U., Liaw, S.-S.: Investigating learners' attitudes toward virtual reality learning environments: Based on a constructivist approach. Comput. Educ. **55**(3), 1171–1182 (2010)
32. Sims, E.M.: Reusable, lifelike virtual humans for mentoring and role-playing. Comput. Educ. **49**(1), 75–92 (2007)
33. Park, K.-M., et al.: A virtual reality application in role-plays of social skills training for schizophrenia: a randomized, controlled trial. Psychiatry Res. **189**(2), 166–172 (2011)
34. Sharma, P.: Challenges with virtual reality on mobile devices. In: ACM SIGGRAPH Talks (2015)
35. Villani, D., Riva, G.: Does interactive media enhance the management of stress? suggestions from a controlled study. Cyberpsychol. Behav. Soc. Netw. **15**(1), 24–30 (2012)

Exergames on Line for Childhood Obesity: Using a Web Platform as an Ambulatory Program to Increase the Acceptance and Adherence to Physical Activity (PA)

Jessica Navarro[1], Patricia Escobar[1], Ausias Cebolla[1],
Juan Francisco Lisón[5], Julio Álvarez Pitti[2,4], Jaime Guixerres[2,3],
Cristina Botella[2,6], and Rosa María Baños[1,2(✉)]

[1] Department of Personality, Evaluation and Psychological Treatment,
Universitat de Valencia, Avda. Blasco Ibañez, 21, 46010 Valencia, Spain
{Jessica.Navarro,Ausias.Cebolla,Rosa.Banos}@uv.es,
paesva@gmail.com
[2] CIBER Fisiopatología Obesidad y Nutrición (CIBERObn),
Instituto Salud Carlos III, Santiago de Compostela, Spain
japnago@gmail.com, botella@uji.es
[3] Instituto Interuniversitario de Investigación en Bioingeniería y Tecnología
Orientada al Ser Humano, Polytechnic University of Valencia, I3BH/Labhuman,
Camino de Vera s/n, 46022 Valencia, Spain
jguixeres@lableni.com
[4] Child and Adolescent Cardiovascular Risk Unit, Pediatric Department,
Consorcio Hospital General Universitario de Valencia, Calle de la Casa
Misericordia, 12, 46014 Valencia, Spain
[5] Universidad CEU-Cardenal Herrera, Calle Luis Vives, 1,
46115 Valencia, Spain
juanfran@uchceu.es
[6] Department of Basic and Clinical Psychology and Psychobiology,
Universitat Jaume I, Avenida de Vicent Sos Baynat, s/n, 12071 Castello, Spain

Abstract. Many initiatives exist to promote physical activity (PA) in children but dropouts are a very common outcome. Information and Communication Technologies (ICTs) are considered as useful tools to promote adherence in PA. This study analyzes the acceptance and adherence of an Internet-based exergame (MOVE-IT) to promote PA compared to a non-technological ambulatory intervention (NTI). The role of clinicians support is also analyzed. Thirty one obese children (9–15 aged) were asked to do an exercise routine (3 times/week along 3 months), using a pamphlet (NTI) or MOVE-IT web. In addition, MOVE-IT participants were divided into two groups, with and without (S-EBW/NS-EBW) weekly support. Results showed no differences in adherence between conditions, but differences were found for acceptability and usability. MOVE-IT was considered more attractive and entertaining. Furthermore, S-EBW participants felt more comfortable and confident in the management of the program and informed greater intention to use it.

Keywords: Physical activity · Exergames · Adherence · Acceptance · Children · Obesity

© ICST Institute for Computer Sciences, Social Informatics and Telecommunications Engineering 2017
K. Giokas et al. (Eds.): eHealth 2016, LNICST 181, pp. 127–134, 2017.
DOI: 10.1007/978-3-319-49655-9_17

1 Introduction

According to the World Health Organization [1], childhood obesity is a serious and global public health problem and it is increasingly affecting many low and middle-income countries, especially in urban areas. In recent years the prevalence has increased at an alarming rate. As "The global strategy on diet, physical activity and health" [1] points out 42 million children were overweight worldwide. Evidence shows that obese and overweight children tend to remain obese in adulthood and they are more likely to develop at an earlier age, noncommunicable diseases such as diabetes and cardiovascular disease [2]. However, overweight, obesity and related diseases are largely preventable. Therefore, prevention of childhood obesity should be a priority.

Currently, overweight and obesity are more determined by environmental factors than by genetics ones [3] and physical inactivity and sedentary lifestyles are considered as crucial risks factors. For this reason, the promotion of physical activity (PA) among young people is considered as a priority for public health [4]. Many initiatives have been undertaken in order to promote PA in adults, children and adolescents. However, dropouts and failure of the proposed programs are a very common outcome [5]. Approximately 50% of individuals who start an exercise program abandon it in the first 6 months [6]. Therefore, the study of the variables that influence the acquisition and maintenance of PA becomes increasingly more relevant, especially in the adolescent stage where if achieved PA tends to keep to adulthood with health benefits [7]. Is needed to incorporate new ways to prescribe PA and Information and Communication Technologies (ICTs) are considered as useful tools to study the variables involved in the practice of PA and promote adhesion to these types of interventions and prescriptions.

Most interventions to promote PA have been applied in schools, especially for preventive purposes. However, interventions in this context are not able to respond specifically to the needs and peculiarities of overweight and obese children. Interventions implemented at hospital and clinical settings can be more easily adapted to the characteristics of these children providing a much more intensive and focused treatment. However, these interventions neither are exempt from difficulties such as cost and adherences. Lison et al. [8] compared the effect of a PA intervention for the treatment of childhood obesity in two contexts: hospital (face-to-face 3 times a week in sessions of 60 min) and ambulatory settings (pamphlet with PA instructions to be performed at home). Results of this study showed that both hospital and ambulatory interventions were effective and a reduction of BMI Z and waist circumference after 6 months. However, the ambulatory intervention was less expensive, allowed participant's greater flexibility, more privacy, more resources and involved parents and siblings.

In order to make more attractive the set of exercises, promote their availability at home, increase acceptance, adherence and expand the number of users who may receive the intervention, our group has designed an Internet-based exergame website (MOVE-IT) which replicates the exercise routine which has been shown to be effective [8]. The aim of this study is to analyze the acceptance and adherence of this Internet-based exergame (MOVE-IT) to promote PA in a sample of obese children, compared to a non-technological ambulatory intervention (NTI, a pamphlet). In addition, the role of clinicians support in acceptance and adherence of MOVE-IT is also explored and two groups with and without (S-EBW/NS-EBW) support of professionals are compared. It is expected to find higher scores in adherence and acceptance in those participants using MOVE-IT than those in NTI condition. Also, the participants in the supported exergame-based website (S-EBW) will obtain higher scores in adherence and acceptance compared to a non- supported web condition (NS-EBW).

2 Materials and Methods

2.1 Participants

Participants were recruited from the Unit Pediatric of the General Hospital of Valencia. The final sample was composed by 31 children (67.7% boys and 32.3% girls; 9–15 aged) with BMIz scores of the 2.12 (SD = 0, 41) in overweight and obesity treatment. Participants were randomly assigned in three conditions: 9 participants in NTI group, 10 participants in S-EBW group and 12 participants in NS-EBW group.

2.2 Instruments

The following questionnaires were designed ad hoc for this study:

(a) *Questionnaire about video games and physical activity:* It evaluates the use of video games (frequency, platform type, active video games, etc.) and sports habits (frequency, type and time of practice)

(b) *Questionnaire about acceptance and satisfaction with the intervention:* It was adapted to each of the 3 experimental conditions. It is composed by 11 questions evaluated by a Likert scale of 5 possible answers. The internal consistency was 0.812.

(c) *Questionnaire about usability of the intervention:* it was developed and adapted to each of the 3 experimental conditions. It was composed by 9 questions evaluated by a Likert scale of 5 possible answer. The internal consistency was 0.419.

(d) *Registration of use of "MOVE-IT":* Frequency of days and hours using the platform.

(e) *Physical activity intervention and "MOVE-IT":* It consists in a sheet which appears the days of the week and weekends of the intervention and participants note whether they have practiced exercise routine.

2.3 Procedure

Parent consent and child assent were obtained before data collection and intervention. After that, participants were assigned to each of the 3 experimental condition (NTI, S-EBW, NS-EBW) with 2 moments of assessment (pre and post intervention). The intervention lasted 3 months.

In all conditions participants were asked to make the set exercises at least 3 times a week. Similarly, the set of exercises increased the level of difficulty gradually and included resistance training and an aerobic activity. In the NTI condition participants received a pamphlet (paper with instructions and explanatory drawings). At the end, participants received a pencil-and- paper self-report and the date of the next session in 3 months. In both MOVE-IT conditions, participants had login and password to a web page "MOVE-IT" (http://moveit-etiobe.com/) which is self-administered and they had to repeat a set of exercises that avatar performed. In addition, participants received a CD with an explanation of the program and a demonstration of each exercise. Participants were asked to access "MOVE-IT" at least 3 times a week. In addition, the S-EBW condition (but not in the NS-EBW), participants received weekly emails with reminder and encouraging messages.

3 Results

3.1 Adherence to the Program

Regarding the adherence to the intervention 2 variables (frequency and regularity in the use of the program) were considered:

(a) *Comparison of MOVE-IT (S-EBW/NS-EBW) and (NTI).* Regarding the frequency of use of the program, one way ANOVA was conducted between the 2 conditions, and no differences were found between both conditions, $F(1,26) = 0.001 = 0.981$. In the NTI condition (M = 20.13, SD = 20.23) and in the S- EBW/NS-EBW (M = 19.9, SD = 23). As for the regularity in the use of the program, Chi square test was used and no differences were found between conditions X^2 (1) = 4, 178, p = 0, 056

(b) *Comparison of offering weekly support (S-EBW) or not (NS-EBW).* Regarding the frequency of use one way was conducted and no differences were found, F $(1,18) = 0.191 = 0.667$, between both conditions. As for the regularity in the use of the program, Chi square test was used and no differences were found between both conditions X^2 (1) = 0.069 p > 0.05.

3.2 Acceptability and Usability

(a) A.*Comparison of MOVE-IT (S-EBW/NS-EBW) and NTI.* One way ANOVA was conducted between the 2 conditions and significant differences were found in usability, acceptance and satisfaction, $F(1,28) = 4.375$, $p = .045$; $n = 0.125$. Participants in the MOVE-IT condition found it more entertaining than participants in the NTI condition (see Tables 1 and 2) Regarding the opinion of children on learning through intervention the participants in the MOVE-IT condition found it easier to learn the use of program than participants in NTI condition, F $(1,28) = 6.049$ p = 0.020; n = 0.168.

(b) *Comparison of offering weekly support (S-EBW) or not (NS-EBW).* One way ANOVA was conducted and significant differences were found in usability and acceptability. The participants in the S-EBW condition showed higher scores in usability and acceptability of the intervention (see Tables 3 and 4). Significant

Table 1. Descriptive statistics: Acceptance

	MOVE-IT	NTI
	M (SD)	M (SD)
Do you like to do it?	3,13 (1,16)	2,50 (0,84)
Do you prefer it?	2,83 (1,29)	2,00 (1,15)
Would you recommend it your friends?	3,22 (0,75)	3,20 (1,23)
Does it facilitate you to do PA?	3,09 (1,23)	3,20 (0,91)
Does it seem you entertaining?	3, 22 (1,11)	2,40 (0,84)
Does it seem you funny?	3,27 (1,12)	2,40 (1,07)
Does it hooked you?	2,31 (1,28)	2,20 (1,22)
Does it seem you difficult to use?	1,31 (0,77)	1,70 (0,82)
If you could continue to use it. Would you do it?	2,81 (1,18)	2,70 (1,16)
Do you think you have improved your fitness after using it?	2,77 (1,34)	2,60 (0,52)
Does it help you to be more physically active?	3,22 (1,23)	3,20 (1,13)

Table 2. Descriptive statistics: Usability

	MOVE-IT	NTI
	M (SD)	M (SD)
Did it take you a lot of time to learn how to use it?	1,54 (0,80)	1,70 (0,82)
Did it you seem difficult?	2,27 (1,48)	2,22 (0,83)
Did you like the design?	3,23 (1,19)	3,30 (1,49)
Did it seem complicated to use?	1,13 (0,64)	1,40 (0,96)
Would you like to use it more often?	2,90 (1,02)	3,00 (1,24)
Do you think other children quickly learn to use it?	3,90 (1,02)	2,90 (1,20)
Did you feel comfortable and confident with the management of the program?	3,40 (1,81)	3,20 (1,22)
Would you use it every day?	3,14 (1,06)	2,80 (1,03)
Did it seem you helpful?	3,75 (0,91)	3,50 (0,85)

differences between 2 conditions were found in comfort and confidence in the use of the program [$F_{(1, 19)} = 4, 104$ p = 0, 0178; n = 0, 238], intention of everyday use of the program [$F_{(1,18)} = 15, 474$ p = 0,001 n = 0,462] and the belief of improving their fitness after the intervention [$F_{(1, 19)} = 4,125$ p = 0,056; n = 0,179]. The participants in the S-EBW condition showed higher scores in comfort and confidence in the use of the program, in the intention of everyday use it and the belief of improving their fitness. In addition, the weekly support was evaluated by participants as a good communication means, easy to use and very useful to achieve the objectives of the intervention.

Table 3. Descriptive statistics: Acceptance

	NS-EBW	S-EBW
	M (SD)	M (SD)
Do you like to do it?	3,00 (1,18)	3,30 (1,19)
Do you prefer it?	2,60 (1,26)	3,12 (1,35)
Would you recommend it your friends?	3,27 (0,78)	3,18 (0,75)
Does it facilitate you to do PA?	3,09 (1,13)	3,09 (1,37)
Does it seem you entertaining?	3,45 (1,03)	3,00 (1,18)
Does it seem you funny?	3,45 (1,12)	3,00 (1,09)
Does it hooked you?	2,36 (1,36)	2,27 (1,27)
Does it seem you difficult to use?	1,18 (0,60)	1,45 (0,93)
If you could continue to use it. Would you do it?	3,00 (0,90)	2,63 (1,43)
Do you think you have improved your fitness after using it?	2,27 (0,90)	3,27 (1,56)
Does it help you to be more physically active?	3,18 (1,16)	3,27 (1,35)

Table 4. Descriptive statistics: Usability

	MOVE-IT	NTI
	M (SD)	M(SD)
Did it take you a lot of time to learn how to use it?	1,63 (0,92)	1,40 (0,69)
Did it you seem difficult?	2,18 (1,54)	2,40 (1,50)
Did you like the design?	3,73 (0,65)	2,70 (1,42)
Did it seem complicated to use?	1,27 (0,90)	1,00 (0,00)
Would you like to use it more often?	2,82 (0,98)	3,00 (1,10)
Do you think other children quickly learn to use it?	3,54 (0,93)	4,20 (1,01)
Did you feel comfortable and confident with the management of the program?	2,90 (1,04)	3,90 (1,14)
Would you use it every day?	2,50 (0,71)	3,73 (1,10)
Did it seem you helpful?	3,90 (0,74)	3,67 (0,88)
Did ICTs seem you helpful for PA?	2,8 (1,23)	3,7 (1,25)
Did MOVE-IT seem you easy to start?	2,5 (1,84)	4,30 (0,82)

4   Conclusions

The aim of this study was to analyze the acceptance and adherence to an Internet-based exergame (MOVE-IT) to promote PA in a sample of obese children and compared to a non-technological intervention. In addition, the role of the support on acceptance and adherence of Internet-based exergame was also explored and two groups with and without support (S-EBW/NS-EBW) were compared.

In relation to the adherence with the intervention the results did not support the hypothesis, as no significant differences between MOVE-IT and NTI were found. These results are in the line with those found in other study [9], which observed that children who used pencil and paper self-report showed more adherence in the intervention that children that used technological self-report. Participants in the pencil and paper condition filled out more records than participants in technological condition. However, when the complete records were taken into account, these differences disappeared because in the technological condition the records were more complete. Authors argued that in pencil and paper condition, participants could modify the information and in fact children reported that completed the self-report just before delivering. Therefore, the lack of differences could be due to a problem of reliability.

Regarding to the analyses of the acceptability and usability of the program, the results supported the hypothesis. The participants in MOVE-IT condition had higher scores than those in NTI condition. These results suggest that the web platform is more attractive and more entertaining than traditional interventions [9]. In this sense, the web platform could help to combat the major difficulties that professionals have encountered in the interventions such as lack of motivation, dropouts and failure. If children considerer the intervention more attractive and more entertaining is more likely that they continue the intervention.

Regarding the role of support in adherence with the intervention the results did not support the hypothesis, as no significant differences between both conditions (S-EBW/NS-EBW) were found. These results suggest that the weekly email support was not effective to promote adherence in the intervention and would be interesting to use other ways of support.

As for the acceptability and usability of the program comparing S-EBW/NS-EBW conditions, the results supported the hypothesis. The participants in the S-EBW condition felt more comfortable and confident in the management of the program than the participants in the NS-EBW condition. In addition, they informed greater intention to make daily use of the program and they expressed that their fitness improved. The weekly support was evaluated by participants as a good communication means, easy to use and very useful to achieve the objectives of the intervention. Therefore, although the weekly email support was not effective to promote adherence, was considered more acceptable and usable. These results suggest that the support provided in this intervention was assessed positively but it was insufficient and other ways of support should be explored.

Some limitations of the current study should be noted. The first one is the small sample size (N = 31). Another limitation was the absence of a control group treatment. For this reason, it is not possible to discriminate between the effects caused by PA program and other factors (regression to the mean, the natural evolution, etc.) Finally, the third limitation was the variables used to measure adherence to the program. In MOVE-IT condition the data was extracted directly from the web while in the NTI condition the data was extracted from the paper self-register with limitations of reliability and validity.

Despite of limitations, this study represents one of the first initiatives that assess an Internet-based exergame as a tool for ambulatory intervention in the field of childhood obesity. Our study found as the platform is more attractive and easier to use that the traditional pamphlet and it allows the collection of more reliable and valid data that the traditional self-register. With respect to the support, it has a positive impact in the acceptability and usability of the platform. However, we did not found significant influence in the adherence to the program, although it increased the scores in acceptability and usability.

For future implementation, the web platform is being introduced as a tool for the treatment of obesity and overweight in children. In fact, the MOVE-IT has been inserted into the ETIOBE system [10], a treatment program for childhood obesity in order to strengthen the specific component of PA in treatment program. Is necessary the development of this programs to give more importance to the PA in the control of body weight.

Acknowledgments. This work was supported by the Ministerio de Educación y Ciencia (Spain), Ministeio de Economía y competitividad (Spain) under grants "PROMOSAM" (PSI2014-56303-REDT) and CIBERON, an initiative of ISCIII (ISC III CB06 03/0052).

References

1. World Health Organization. http://www.who.int/es/
2. Sahoo, K., Sahoo, B., Choudhury, A.K., Sofi, N.Y., Kumar, R., Bhadoria, A.S.: Childhood obesity: causes and consequences. J. Family Med. Prim. Care **4**(2), 187–192 (2015)
3. Klesges, R.C., Klesges, L.M., Eck, L.H., Shelton, M.L.: A longitudinal analysis of accelerated weight gain in preschool children. Pediatrics **95**(1), 126–130 (1995)
4. Welk, G.J., Einsenman, J.C., Dollman, J.: Health-related physical activity in children and adolescents: a bio-behavioral perspective. In: Kirk, D., McDonald, D., O'Sullivan, M. (eds.) The Handbook at Physical Education, pp. 665–684. Sage, London (2006)
5. Lind, E., Welch, A.S., Ekkekakis, P.: Do 'mind over muscle' strategies work? Examining the effects of attentional association and dissociation on exertional, affective and physiological responses to exercise. Sports Med. **39**(9), 743–764 (2009)
6. Dishman, R.K., Buckworth, J.: Increasing physical activity: a quantitative synthesis. Med. Sci. Sports Exerc. **28**(6), 706–719 (1996)
7. Aedo, Á., Ávila, H.: Nuevo cuestionario para evaluar la autoeficacia hacia la actividad física en niños (2009)
8. Lisón, J.F., Real-Montes, J.M., Torró, I., Arguisuelas, M.D., Álvarez-Pitti, J., Martínez-Gramage, J., et al.: Exercise intervention in childhood obesity: a randomized controlled trial comparing hospital-versus home-based groups. Acad. Pediatr. **12**(4), 319–325 (2012)
9. Oliver, E., Banos, R.M., Cebolla, A., Lurbe, E., Alvarez-Pitti, J., Botella, C.: An electronic system (PDA) to record dietary and physical activity in obese adolescents; data about efficiency and feasibility. Nutr. Hosp. **28**(6), 1860–1866 (2013)
10. Banos, R.M., Cebolla, A., Botella, C., Garcia-Palacios, A., Oliver, E., Zaragoza, I., et al.: Improving childhood obesity treatment using new technologies: the ETIOBE system. Clin. Pract. Epidemiol. Ment. Health **7**, 62–66 (2011)

A VR-Based Serious Game to Regulate Joy in Adolescents: A Comparison of Different Devices

M. Dolores Vara[1], Rosa M. Baños[1,2(✉)], Paloma Rasal[1],
Alejandro Rodríguez[3], Beatriz Rey[3], Maja Wrzesien[4],
and Mariano Alcañiz[2,4]

[1] Department of Personality, Evaluation and Psychological Treatment,
University of Valencia, Avda. Blasco Ibañez, 21, 46010 Valencia, Spain
{m.dolores.vara,banos}@uv.es, paloma.rasal@gmail.com
[2] CIBER Fisiopatología Obesidad y Nutrición (CIBEROBN),
Instituto Carlos III, Santiago de Compostela, Spain
[3] Department of Graphic Engineering, Polytechnic University of Valencia,
I3BH/LabHuman, Camino de Vera s/n, 46022 Valencia, Spain
{alrodor,beareyso}@upv.es
[4] Instituto Interuniversitario de Investigación en Bioingeniería y Tecnología
Orientada al Ser Humano, Polytechnic University of Valencia, I3BH/LabHuman,
Camino de Vera s/n, 46022 Valencia, Spain
{mwrzesien,malcaniz}@labhuman.i3bh.es

Abstract. Adolescence is a crucial period to learn Emotional Regulation (ER) strategies to prevent future psychological problems. This work is aimed to test the efficacy of GameTeen System (GT-System), a serious game that teaches ER strategies to regulate joy (VAS scale) and perceived arousal (FAS scale) in a non-clinical sample of adolescents. We conducted a between-participants experiment in which participants (N = 63) played a joy induction game, and then an ER game using one of three types of devices (computer, smartphone, and RGB-D camera). Results revealed that GT-System was only effective in increase perceived arousal after the joy induction game and decrease after the ER game. Statistically significant differences were found between devices conditions after the joy induction game (more intense perceived arousal was reported by participants in RGB-D camera). This finding highlights that the type of device could be an important variable in the efficacy of serious game.

Keywords: Adolescents · Emotional regulation · Joy · Serious games · User interface

1 Introduction

Emotional dysregulation (ED) has been defined as "the difficulties in the intensity, frequency, and duration of emotional responses, as well as difficulties modulating emotional experiences in effective and adaptive ways" [1]. Adolescence is a crucial developmental period in where there are more typically problems of ED [2]. For this

© ICST Institute for Computer Sciences, Social Informatics and Telecommunications Engineering 2017
K. Giokas et al. (Eds.): eHealth 2016, LNICST 181, pp. 135–142, 2017.
DOI: 10.1007/978-3-319-49655-9_18

reason, learning Emotional Regulation (ER) strategies is considered an important component in the treatment of psychological disorders in childhood and adolescence [3].

Serious games have become a powerful tool to provide training in ER strategies to adolescents. For example, *RAGE-control* ("Regulate and Gain Emotional Control") [4], *ROC* ("Reach Out Central") [5], and *SPARX* ("Smart, Positive, Active, Realistic, X-factor thoughts") [6] have proved effective computers applications to teach ER strategies (i.e., relaxation techniques, cognitive behavior skills) in adolescents with emotional problems (i.e., aggressiveness, anxiety, depression).

Until now, few serious games teach ER strategies in non-clinical samples, and they have been more focused on adolescents with mental health problems. GameTeen System (GT-System) is a Virtual Reality (VR) system designed to train, evaluate, and monitor emotions and ER strategies that adolescents applied in their daily life [7]. Emotions are induced through a serious game, and subsequently participants have to learn and apply two ER strategies through other games focused on slow breathing and distraction. A previous study has shown that GameTeen games have been effective to increase and decrease frustration [7].

In order to study the user's experience in games, the "interface embodiment" is receiving special interest in the last years [8]. In this line, in a previous study we have analyzed the effect of the type of interface device (computer, smartphone, and RGB-D camera) on the efficacy of our GT-System to induce and reduce frustration [9]. The results showed differences among devices, and those participants who used the RGB-D camera (interacting with the full body), experienced less frustration after the induction game. We concluded that the participation of the body affected the users' emotional experience, and the type of device is a crucial variable in the efficacy of serious games.

In the present study, we explore the efficacy of GT-System to regulate a "positive" emotion (joy), and the influence of the type of user interface embodiment on users' emotional experience. The specific objectives are: 1) to validate the GT-System ("*joy induction game*") for teaching ER strategies ("*breathing strategy game*") in adolescents, and 2) to analyze the impact of user interface embodiment in the users' emotional responses. We expect that:

H1. The GT-System ("*joy induction game*" and "*breathing strategy game*") will be effective to induce and regulate joy and perceived arousal.

H2. Participants in the RGB-D camera condition will report more intense joy and perceived arousal than in the other two interface conditions (computer and smartphone).

2   Materials and Methods

2.1   Participants

The sample consisted of 63 volunteers (37 males) of a public High School (N = 51) and a Summer School (N = 12) aged from 10 to 16 years old (M = 13.62; SD = 1.27). Parent's informed consents were signed prior to their inclusion. Participants were randomly assigned to one of the three conditions: Computer (CC; N = 31), Smartphone (SC; N = 20) and RGB-D Camera (RCC; N = 12).

2.2 Instruments

The following quantitative measures were used:

- *Visual Analogue Scale* (VAS) [10]. It measures joy mood on a Likert scale from 1 (not at all) to 7 (completely).
- *Felt Arousal Scale* (FAS) [11]. It measures perceived arousal through a series of stylized drawings of faces on a Likert scale from 1 (very sleepy) to 5 (very alert).

2.3 Mood Induction and ER Procedure

- *Joy induction game:* It is a VR-based game, designed to induce positive mood (joy) in participants. The scene simulates an amusement park scene with many colorful balloons that appear in the sky continuously for 3 min. The objective is to prick the maximum possible number of balloons with different types of ammunition. Moreover, feedback messages (i.e., "You are achieving the goal") are displayed every 30 s during the game (see Fig. 1).
- *Breathing strategy game* [7]: It is a VR-based game, where users have to follow the movement of a virtual feather, which goes up and down during 45 s.

    For a more detailed description of the technical characteristics, see [9].

2.4 Procedure

Sample was recruited from the High School and Summer School. Researchers invited the students to participate in a virtual experience. The study was approved by the Internal Review Board at the University of Valencia. In order to randomly assign participants to one of the three conditions (CC, SC and RCC), the Random Allocation Software program was used. Participants fulfilled VAS and FAS scales before and after

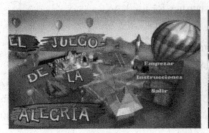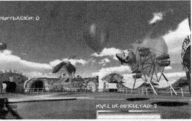

Fig. 1. Pictures of *joy induction game*.

the *joy induction game*. If joy scores exceeded 3 points or more on VAS and 2 or more on FAS, participants played the *breathing strategy game*. The experiment lasted about 20 min.

2.5   Statistical Data Analyses

In order to explore the efficacy of the GT-System and the influence of the type of different interface devices on the emotional experience, a repeated measures mixed ANOVA was performed, with the moment (pre-induction phase, induction phase, regulation phase) as within-factor and the group (CC, SC, and RCC) as between-factor. Analyses were performed using SPSS 22.0 (IBM) for Windows.

3   Results

3.1   Efficacy of the Mood Induction (*Joy Induction Game*) and ER (*Breathing Strategy Game*) Procedure

(a) Vas Scale (joy). A 3×3 ANOVA did not revealed a main effect for moment, indicating that the games were not effective in increasing and decreasing joy, $F(2, 120) = 2.18$, $p > .05$, $\eta_p^2 = .03$. No statistically significant differences were found between groups, $F(2, 60) = 2.27$, $p > .05$, $\eta_p^2 = .07$. Moreover, there was not a significant moment x group interaction effect, $F(4, 120) = .28$, $p > .05$, $\eta_p^2 = .01$ (see Table 1 and Fig. 2).

(b) FAS Scale. A 3×3 ANOVA revealed a main effect for moment, indicating that the games were effective in increasing and decreasing perceived arousal, $F(2,120) = 24.95$, $p < .001$, $\eta_p^2 = .29$. Statistically significant differences were found between groups, $F(2, 60) = 3.33$, $p < .05$, $\eta_p^2 = .1$. Moreover, there was a significant moment x group interaction effect, $F(4,120) = 2.86$, $p < .05$, $\eta_p^2 = .08$ (see Table 2 and Fig. 3). According to Cohen's (1988) indications, the effect size was moderate ($\eta_p^2 > .06$). Post-hoc analyses using Bonferroni correction indicated that the mean for perceived arousal differs depending on the moment and the group. After the induction

Table 1. Descriptive statistics for joy VAS.

Joy on the VAS scale						
	Pre-induction phase		Induction phase		Regulation phase	
	M (SD)	95% CI	M (SD)	95% CI	M (SD)	95% CI
Computer	5.03 (1.05)	4.61, 5.46	5.29 (1.19)	4.90, 5.68	5.16 (1.10)	4.75, 5.57
Smartphone	4.85 (1.19)	4.32, 5.38	5.05 (1.05)	4.56, 5.54	4.85 (1.22)	4.34, 5.36
RGB-D camera	5.03 (1.18)	4.65, 6.02	5.83 (.83)	5.20, 6.46	5.75 (1.05)	5.09, 6.40

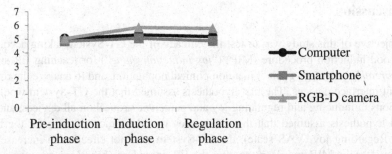

Fig. 2. Mean scores for joy on the VAS scale (out of 7) for different interface devices (computer, smartphone and RGB-D camera) in three experimental phases.

Table 2. Descriptive statistics for perceived arousal FAS scores.

Perceived arousal on the FAS scale						
	Pre-induction phase		Induction phase		Regulation phase	
	M (SD)	95% CI	M (SD)	95% CI	M (SD)	95% CI
Computer	2.06 (.85)	1.70, 2.43	2.54 (.96)	2.20, 2.90	1.94 (.81)	1.65, 2.22
Smartphone	2.55 (1.19)	2.09, 3	2.55 (1.05)	2.11, 2.99	1.55 (.76)	1.19, 1.91
RGB-D camera	2.83 (1.11)	2.24, 3.42	3.42 (.90)	2.85, 3.98	2.17 (.83)	1.70, 2.63

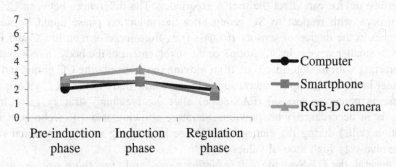

Fig. 3. Mean scores for perceived arousal on the FAS scale (out of 5) for different interface devices (computer, smartphone and RGB-D camera) in three experimental phases.

phase, perceived arousal increased significantly in the CC and RCC groups ($p < .05$) than the SC group. However, after the regulation phase, perceived arousal decreased significantly in all groups ($p < .05$).

4 Discussion

The objective of this study was to test the efficacy of the GT-System taking account a new mood induction procedure (MIP) ("*joy induction game*") for teaching ER strategies ("*breathing strategy game*") in a non-clinical population, and to analyze the role of different interface devices. The first hypothesis assumed that the GT-System would be efficacious in inducing and regulating joy and perceived arousal on all devices, and the second hypothesis assumed that these measures would be more intense for the RCC group. Regarding joy (VAS scale), the GT-System was not effective in increase this emotion after the MIP and decrease after the ER procedure (*breathing strategy game*) on all groups. Whereas for perceived arousal (FAS scale), results were different depending on the interface device. Only in the CC and RCC groups, perceived arousal increased significantly after the MIP. However, it decreased significantly in all groups after the ER procedure. Therefore, the first hypothesis was supported partially in terms of perceived arousal. Also the second hypothesis was supported partially for perceived arousal (it was more intense in the RCC group and also in the CC group after the MIP).

The fact that the GT-System has not been effective in inducing and regulating the target emotion (joy) could be explained by the high initial levels of joy (VAS scale) scores in the pre-induction phase on all groups. This result is not in line with previous studies that showed GT-System as an effective tool to regulate a negative emotion, frustration (the scores of frustration on the VAS scale were lower in the pre-induction phase on all groups) [7, 9].

Regarding perceived arousal, the results of the present study point out that the type of interface device can affect the user's experience. The differences between CC and RCC groups with respect to SC group after the induction phase could be due to differences in the degree of sensory richness (i.e., from larger screen in CC and RCC groups to smaller screens in SC group), or the involvement of the body (motor system) in interacting with the interface (i.e., from moving the mouse in the CC group, moving the finger in the SC group to interacting with the whole body in the RCC group). The decrease in perceived arousal (FAS scale) after the breathing strategy game in all groups is in accordance with previous literature showing that ER techniques (i.e., relaxation skills) during the games are effective in reducing intense emotional states that involve very high arousal values [4–6].

In general, the GT-System ("*joy induction game*" and "*breathing strategy game*") could be a useful tool to teach ER strategies in a non-clinical sample of adolescents, particularly in regulating perceived arousal. It allows them to develop the ability to identify and modify arousal during the games.

Adolescence is crucial period to learn to control and manage the emotions in adaptive way to avoid episodes of ED. The technologies could be an important channel to disseminate ER programs because they are so close to adolescents, who use them the most [12].

This research has some limitations. First, the sample size of the RCC group (N = 12) is smaller than the CC (N = 31) and SC (N = 20) groups. Second, the sample was composed of non-clinical adolescents, and so this study should be replicated in clinical patients (i.e., depression). Third, follow-ups would be necessary to corroborate that the short-term benefits obtained here, maintain over time.

In future studies, the sense of being in the game ("presence"), and physiological measures, such as heart rate or the galvanic skin response could be analyzed. In this sense, physiological measures could increase the potential of ER training through serious games, by providing biofeedback to the participants and therefore making them more aware of how the game is affecting their emotions and their physiological status.

Acknowledgments. This work was supported by the Ministerio de Educación y Ciencia (Spain), Project Game Teen (TIN2010-20187), and partially by Ministerio de Economía y Competitividad (Spain) under grants "PROMOSAM" (PSI2014-56303-REDT), "BODYTA" (Plan Nacional I+D+I 2013-2016 PSI2014-51928-R), and CIBEROBN, an initiative of ISCIII (ISC III CB06 03/0052).

References

1. Bloch, L., Moran, E.K., Kring, A.M.: On the need for conceptual and definitional clarity in emotion regulation research on psychopathology. In: Kring, A.M., Sloan, D.M. (eds.) Emotion Regulation and Psychopathology: A Transdiagnostic Approach to Etiology and Treatment, pp. 88–107. Guildford Press, New York (2010)
2. McLaughlin, K.A., Hatzenbuehler, M.L., Mennin, D.S., Nolen-Hoeksema, S.: Emotion dysregulation and adolescent psychopathology: a prospective study. Behav. Res. Ther. **49**, 544–554 (2011)
3. Gullone, E., Taffe, J.: The emotion regulation questionnaire for children and adolescents (ERQ-CA): a psychometric evaluation. Psychol. Assess. **24**, 409–417 (2012)
4. Kahn, J., Ducharme, P., Travers, B., Gonzalez-Heydrich, J.: RAGE control: regulate and gain emotional control. Stud. Health. Technol. Inf. **149**, 335–343 (2009)
5. Shandley, K., Austin, D., Klein, B., Kyrios, M.: An evaluation of 'Reach Out Central': an online gaming program for supporting the mental health of young people. Health Educ. Res. **25**, 563–574 (2010)
6. Merry, S.N., Stasiak, K., Shepherd, M., Frampton, C., Fleming, T., Lucassen, M.F.: The effectiveness of SPARX, a computerised self help intervention for adolescents seeking help for depression: randomised controlled non-inferiority trial. BMJ **344**, e2598 (2012)
7. Rodriguez, A., Rey, B., Vara, M.D., Wrzesien, M., Alcaniz, M., Baños, R.M., et al.: A VR-based serious game for studying emotional regulation in adolescents. IEEE Comput. Graph. Appl. **35**, 65–73 (2015)
8. Kim, S.Y., Prestopnik, N., Biocca, F.A.: Body in the interactive game: how interface embodiment affects physical activity and health behavior change. Comput. Hum. Behav. **7**, 376–384 (2014)
9. Vara, M.D., Baños, R.M., Rasal, P., Rodríguez, A., Rey, B., Wrzesien, M., et al.: A game for emotional regulation in adolescents: the (body) interface device matters. Comput. Hum. Behav. **4**, 267–273 (2016)
10. Stern, R.A., Arruda, J.E., Hooper, C.R., Wolfner, G.D., Morey, C.E.: Visual analogue mood scales to measure internal mood state in neurologically impaired patients: description and initial validity evidence. Aphasiology **11**, 59–71 (1997)

11. Hulley, A., Bentley, N., Clough, C., Fishlock, A., Morrell, E., O'Brien, J., Radmore, J.: Active and passive commuting to school: influences on affect in primary school children. Res. Q. Exerc. Sport **79**, 525–534 (2008)
12. Madden, M., Lenhart, A., Cortesi, S., Gasser, U., Duggan, M., Smith, A.: Teens, social media and privacy. Pew Internet and American Life Project, Washington, DC (2013)

Serious Games to Teach Nutrition Education to Children Between 9 to 12 Years Old. Pickit! and Cookit!

Alejandro Dominguez-Rodriguez[1], Elia Oliver[1,2], Ausias Cebolla[1,2],
Sussanna Albertini[3], Louis Ferrini[3], Ana Gonzalez-Segura[4], Enrique de la Cruz[4],
Karin Kronika[5], Tomas Nilsen[6], Cristina Botella[2,7], and Rosa Baños[1,2(✉)]

[1] University of Valencia, Valencia, Spain
{alejandro.dominguez,banos}@uv.es
[2] CIBER Obn, Madrid, Spain
elia.oliver.gasch@gmail.com, ausias.cebolla.marti@gmail.com
[3] FVA di Louis Ferrini and C, Rome, Italy
fvaweb@tiscali.it, info@fvaweb.it
[4] Everis, Valencia, Spain
{ana.gonzalez.segura,enrique.cruz.martinez}@everis.com
[5] BEST Institut für berufsbezogene Weiterbildung und Personaltraining GmbH,
Vienna, Austria
karin.kronika@best.at
[6] Rogaland School and Business Development Foundation, Stavanger, Norway
thomas@nilsen.com
[7] University Jaume I, Castellón de la Plana, Spain
botella@uji.es

Abstract. The current trend of increase in children obesity is worrying governments around the world and urgent actions are requested. The promotion of Nutrition Education in early stages has shown to be a factor to prevent the gain of weight in children. A tool that is gaining popularity in teaching contents to children are the Serious Games. The objective of this paper is to describe two Serious Games, Pickit! and Cookit! that has as objective to teach Nutrition Education to children between 9 to 12 years old. These games form part of the Modifying Eating and Attitudes through Learning platform, a pedagogical tool created for nutritionists and primary school teachers to transfer nutritional knowledge to children. These games contain relevant elements in the design of Serious Games as are avatars, levels and a system of points. It is expected that trough these games the children will increase their nutritional education knowledge.

Keywords: Nutritional education · Serious game · ICT platform · Children

1 Introduction

A healthy and balanced nutrition is important for the development of children. However, there is a current tendency of infants to eat in an unhealthy way, and to have a sedentary life, and this bring important health problems as obesity [1]. Currently, overweight and

© ICST Institute for Computer Sciences, Social Informatics and Telecommunications Engineering 2017
K. Giokas et al. (Eds.): eHealth 2016, LNICST 181, pp. 143–147, 2017.
DOI: 10.1007/978-3-319-49655-9_19

obesity affects millions of children around the world; according to the World Health Organization (WHO) in 2013 there were around 42 million with overweight or obesity [2].

Several attempts have been done in order to reduce or prevent this tendency. One of the most important is promoting Nutrition Education (NE) in children population [3]. NE is defined as "any combination of educational strategies, accompanied by environmental supports, designed to facilitate voluntary adoption of food choices and other food and nutrition- related behaviors conducive to health and well-being; NE is delivered through multiple venues and involves activities at the individual, community, and policy levels" (3, p 176-177). Also, it has been identified that the most recommended context to implement NE to children is through interventions in primary schools [4].

Regarding school-based interventions, Serious Games (SG´s) are one of the most innovative tools that have been designed to provide educational contents to children. Although there are several definitions of SG's, most researchers and developers agree that they are games used for purposes other than main entertainment, they inherit some of the game play characteristics from entertainment games and have focused on a principal goal as could be training or learning, with the objective of applying the learnt lessons in real-life work environments [5].

The MEAL (Modifying Eating and Attitudes through Learning) platform has been designed to implement a NE training for teachers and nutritionists in order to learn how to teach NE to children [6]. This platform is part of the MEAL project, an European Project funded under the Lifelong Learning Program (Project number: 543535-LLP-1-2013-1-ES-KA3-KA3MP). The platform contains two SG's, used as complementary tools to help the professionals to reinforce the lessons taught. The objective of this paper is to describe the SG's included in the platform MEAL, as long with their components, objectives, different levels and main characteristics.

2   Serious Games in MEAL Platform

The two SG's contained in the MEAL platform are: Pickit! and Cookit! They have been developed according to the characteristics of children on the range of age of 9 to 12 years old, and they contain basic elements that are considered relevant as a system of points, a ranking, and different levels of difficulty [7]. Also at the moment of designing these SG´s there were considered the main characteristics that according to the scientific literature should have the SG´s to motivate and excite the player, and therefore are perceived as acceptable and fun by those players. Among those characteristics we can find that the SG´s should has a clear system of competition with other players or the game itself, and goals to achieve inside the game, a clear system of rules of what is allowed and not to do inside the game, the option to perform choices, as could be to select or not an aliment, and establishment of challenges in order to overcome and make more fun the game [8], among others.

2.1 Pickit!

The first game that the children play as part of the MEAL program, is Pickit! http://www.mealproject.eu/ the game has been translated to 5 languages (English, Spanish, German, Norwegian, and Italian). This SG is aimed to teach to the children the composition of foods and their classification according to the food pyramid, as are whole grains, fruits and vegetables, milk and dairy products, fish, meat, oil, and sugared aliments (see Fig. 1). Pickit! includes a system of points where the child is rewarded when he/she performs a task requested by the game, and the player loose points when he/she does an action that is not requested. Also, this game was designed with a mechanism to use the time that the player takes to finish the game into adding or reducing points, meaning this that if the player finished the game in a short amount of time will be rewarded with extra points, and if the player takes a long period of time then he/she will lose points.

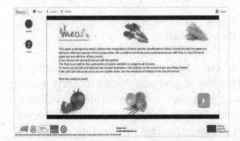 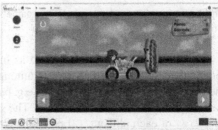

Fig. 1. Main screen with the instructions provided to the player in the SG Pickit!

Fig. 2. Example of junk food in the second level of Pickit!

At the beginning the player is requested to choose a character. There are two avatars available (boy and girl). In this SG the child controls a shopping cart and has the instruction of only selecting the aliments that are requested. For example, to pick only fruits or vegetables, and in this case if the child picks an aliment different the system reduces points and shows a message of error. Also as part of this game the child has to avoid picking junk food that appears in the game (see Fig. 2). Pickit! has 3 different levels, and provides a summary of the points achieved when the player finishes. In the first level the player is requested to pick only aliments that contain carbohydrates and vegetables. In the second level the instruction is to select only aliments that are fruits and dairy. In the third level the player is requested to pick only aliments with meat proteins. When the children finishes the game, the system provides a total score of the points gained and the total time that the player lasted to finish the 3 levels.

2.2 Cookit!

The second game included in the MEAL platform has the objective to teach to the players about the percentages of energy/calories, healthy and unhealthy levels for different ingredients and foods that are usually found at any home. This game has been also translated to 5 languages. At the beginning of the game, the player is asked to select a male or female avatar. Although during the game the player does not see an avatar as in Pickit! at the end of the game the selected character appears to provide a positive or negative feedback regarding the choices that the player made during the play (see Fig. 3).

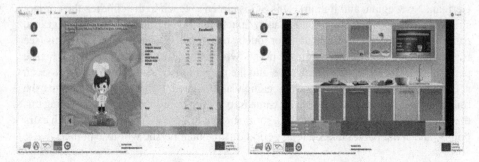

Fig. 3. Positive feedback provided by the game Cookit!

Fig. 4. Example of the indicator displayed in the SG Cookit!

In this game the children receive as instruction to compose a breakfast, meal or dinner; then, several aliments appear, among healthy (e.g. vegetables, fruits juice, whole meal bread, etc.) and unhealthy ones (e.g. bacon, chocolate, cakes, etc.) and the children could select as much as he/she wants. The game includes 3 general indicators: (1) level of energy of each aliment, (2) percentage of healthy elements of the aliment, and (3) percentage of unhealthy components of the aliment (see Fig. 4). The system also contains a general indicator to tell the sum of the total of energy, healthy and unhealthy elements according to the aliments selected. Regardless selecting the option to compose any of the 3 meals, the children will have to select one main dish and a secondary one, along with a beverage. At the end of the gameplay, the system provides a feedback regarding the decisions made by the player. This feedback will be positive (congratulations) if the child composes a healthy breakfast, meal or dinner, and it will be negative (warning) if the child selects a small amount of food or selects mostly hyper caloric food. Also this SG provides at the end a total score of the energy, healthy and unhealthy percentage of the total of the aliments selected.

3   Conclusions

These two SGs included in the MEAL platform have the objective to help teachers and nutritionists in their task of providing relevant NE to children population. This work is currently in progress and it is expected that these two SG´s will help the professionals to provide relevant contents of nutrition to children, and since they were designed considering the characteristics of effective SG´s it is expected that they will show high levels of acceptance as a teaching tool.

Also, it is expected that through these technological tools the children will learn concepts related with NE in a faster and funnier way. SG´s have been found to be a more enjoyable method for children to learn diverse subjects than traditional methods of learning, and also these games could help the educators to use a more flexible and less restrictive method of teaching [9].

Acknowledgements. MEAL ("Modifying eating attitudes and actions through learning") European Transversal Program LLP - PROGRAM KA3 (n°-LLP-1-2013-1-ES-KA3KA3MP). CIBERobn is an initiate of the ISCIII.

References

1. Wiles, N.J., Northstone, K., Emmett, P., Lewis, G.: 'Junk food' diet and childhood behavioural problems: Results from the ALSPAC cohort. Eur. J. Clin. Nutr. **63**(4), 491–498 (2009)
2. World Health Organization.: Facts and figures on childhood obesity (2014). http://www.who.int/end-childhood-obesity/facts/en/
3. Contento, I.R.: Nutrition education: linking research, theory, and practice. Asia. Pac. J. Clin. Nutr. **17**(1), 176–179 (2008)
4. Amini, M., Djazayery, A., Majdzadeh, R., Taghdisi, M., Jazayeri, S.: Effect of school-based interventions to control childhood obesity: a review of reviews. Int. J. Prev. Med. **6**(1), 68 (2015)
5. Wattanasoontorn, V., Boada, I., García, R., Sbert, M.: Serious games for health. Entertainment Comput. **12**(4), 231–247 (2013)
6. Oliver, E., Cebolla, A., Dominguez, A., Gonzalez-Segura, A., de la Cruz, E., Albertini, S., et al.: Meal Project: modifying eating attitudes and actions through learning. In: 9th International Technology, Education and Development Conference, March, 2–4, Madrid, Spain (2015). http://rogalandsbdf.com/n/wp-content/uploads/2015/06/MEAL-paper-for-conference.pdf
7. Kelly, H., Howell, K., Glinert, E., Holding, L., Swain, C., Burrowbridge, A., et al.: How to build serious games. Commun. ACM **50**(7), 44–49 (2007)
8. Charsky, D.: From edutainment to serious games: a change in the use of game characteristics. Games Cult. **5**(2), 177–198 (2010)
9. Girard, C., Ecalle, J., Magnan, A.: Serious games as new educational tools: how effective are they? a meta-analysis of recent studies. J. Comput. Assist. Learn. **29**(3), 207–219 (2013)

Ageing Positively with Digital Games

Daniela Villani[1]([⊠]), Silvia Serino[1,2], Stefano Triberti[1],
and Giuseppe Riva[1,2]

[1] Department of Psychology, Università Cattolica del Sacro Cuore,
Largo Gemelli 1, Milan, Italy
{daniela.villani,silvia.serino, stefano.triberti,
giuseppe.riva}@unicatt.it
[2] Applied Technology for Neuro-Psychology Lab,
IRCCS Istituto Auxologico Italiano, Milan, Italy

Abstract. Active ageing is the process of optimizing health, social participation and security in order to enhance the quality of life of older individuals. Building on the paradigm of Positive Technology, we argue that new advanced technologies may offer interesting solutions to enhance well-being in the elderly. Specifically, digital games deserve a special attention because recent studies show that the elderly are receptive towards the adoption of digital games and the number of older gamers is increasing. In the present contribution, we review the potential of digital games in enhancing positive emotions, engagement and social connectedness, and outline future challenges for research and guidelines for game designers interested in this peculiar field.

Keywords: Active ageing · Positive technology · Video games · Positive emotions · Engagement · Positive gaming

1 Introduction

It is well-known that one of the defining features of our society is that it is an "ageing society". By 2050, the ageing population (aged 65 and over) is projected to increase to 1.25 billion, accounting for 22% of the entire world's population [1]. Although the dramatic increase in life expectancy poses several critical challenges for health-care systems, since age-related diseases will consequently result in a dramatic increase in the use and costs of health services, there is a significant number of elderly individuals who wish to remain physically and cognitively healthy.

This shift in the definition of the ageing led institutions such as the World Health Organization to introduce concepts such as the so-called "active ageing" [2, 3], which may be defined as the process of optimizing health, social participation and security in order to enhance the quality of life of older individuals. Specifying the initial framework proposed by the World Health Organization [2], Walker [4, 5] explained the principles for building a strategy for structuring successful actions for active ageing and assigned a key role for well-being. Specifically, Walker [4, 5] emphasized that the "first principle" for all active ageing strategies should be the enhancement of individual and social well-being. It is interesting to note the also in considering elderly individuals,

© ICST Institute for Computer Sciences, Social Informatics and Telecommunications Engineering 2017
K. Giokas et al. (Eds.): eHealth 2016, LNICST 181, pp. 148–155, 2017.
DOI: 10.1007/978-3-319-49655-9_20

health is no more merely considered as the "absence of disease", but it is began to be conceived in a more holistic way, integrating also the social, cultural and psychological aspects. Indeed, the relationship between well-being and ageing is triggering considerable attention [6]. As recently highlighted by Steptoe and co-workers [6] in their Lancet paper: "As life expectancy increases and treatments for life-threatening disease become more effective, the issue of maintaining wellbeing at advanced ages is growing in importance" (p. 604).

The question is how to effectively promote well-being for an active and healthy ageing society. The incredible development of new advanced technologies may offer interesting solutions so that the full potential of active ageing will be achieved. In this direction, over the past decade, new disciplines have been developed for specifically exploiting the potentiality of technology for the elderly, such as the "gerontechnology", which refers to the "study of technology for ensuring good health, full social participation, and independent living throughout the entire life span" [7]. However, a theoretical perspective which may specifically guide the technological development emphasizing the promotion of well-being is that of Positive Technology [8–10]. Built on the conceptual framework of Positive Psychology [11–13], which can be defined as the scientific investigation of well-being to understand how exploiting human strengths and virtues to allow individuals, communities and societies to flourish, Positive Technology appears to be a promising approach to develop advanced technologies for both physical and mental health. More specifically, following the classification proposed by Seligman in analyzing the construct of well-being [14], it is possible to classify three different types of "positive technologies" [8–10] according to their roles in promoting different layers of well-being: (i) hedonic positive technologies: the use of advanced technologies to enhance positive emotions and to support enjoyable experiences ("the pleasant life"); (ii) eudaimonic positive technologies: the use of advanced technologies to support enriching, meaningful and self-actualizing experiences ("the engaged life"); and (iii) social/interpersonal positive technologies: the use of advanced technologies to connect individuals and groups improving social integration ("the meaningful life").

2 How to Promote Well-Being in Elderly: The Role of Positive Gaming

Focusing our attention on what Seligman called the "pleasant life" [14] (i.e., achieved through the continuous experiencing of pleasant experiences) which corresponds to the hedonic well-being [13], a growing body of evidence showed how positive emotions can play a crucial role in active and healthy ageing [15–18]. The application of advanced positive hedonic technologies may yield to more promising results since from the earliest stage of the recovery, focusing on the specific characteristics of different elderly individuals and specifically intended to promote well-being in terms of engaging pleasant experiences [19, 20].

A first prototype to enhance hedonic well-being of elderly individuals from the earliest stage of the recovery is given by Ohsuga and co-workers [21, 22], who developed the "Bedside Wellness System". The idea was to develop a system capable of reduce discomfort of elderly individuals caused by long period in bed by reproducing the sensation of walking immersed in enjoyable virtual reality environments (i.e., virtual forest).

A more recent and structured example on how to induce positive emotions using advanced technology for the elderly is offered by Banos and her co-workers [23]. They developed and tested two virtual environments as a part of the Butler System [24], i.e. an e-health platform designed to deliver health care to the elderly exploiting the potential of technology (mood monitoring and induction procedures, memory training, forum and chat, etc.). To specifically induce relaxation and joy, these two virtual environments reproduced a pleasant green park with a lake. Elderly participants were invited to freely navigate within them, recall positive autobiographical memories and learn mindfulness skills. For evaluating the efficacy of these two virtual environments in inducing positive affective states, 18 elderly individuals were asked to explore their interactive features in two different sessions. Findings showed a significant increase in relaxation and joy and a parallel significant decrease in anxiety and sadness [23].

Overall, these results confirmed the role of positive advanced technology, and in particular virtual reality, in promoting positive affect states and hence enhancing hedonic well-being for healthy elderly.

The situation appears still more promising if we consider the steady increase of older adults playing games between 2004 and 2011 (Entertainment Software Association, ESA [25]). In fact, among several leisure activities there are some that encourage mastery and achievement and provide an opportunity for people to develop and improve skills as well as achieving satisfaction and a sense of accomplishment [26]. This is the case of playing chess, learning a foreign language, playing a musical instrument and enjoy computer games. Recent studies have shown that the elderly are generally receptive towards the adoption of digital games [27] and that their attitudes become even more positive after computer game experiences showing the potential to positively affect their mental well-being [28]. Nap et al. [29] conducted two focus groups and a contextual inquiry with elderly to investigate seniors' motivation to play digital games and concluded that some of the main motivations to play games were fun and relaxation. Considering the elderly acceptance of technology and their availability of leisure time, the ageing population represents an important target that has to be considered by innovators and game designers, comparable if not better than younger consumers.

More than twenty years ago, Whitcomb [30] found that although only a limited number of games had been investigated at that time, it was possible to identify a range of benefits for older people from playing computer games. These included the recreational pleasures of satisfaction and accomplishment which positively influenced people's view of themselves and their abilities. More recently, Ijsselsteijn, Nap, de Kort and Poels [31] identified four potential areas in which games can enhance quality of life for older people. First, and perhaps most basically, is the use of digital games for relaxation and entertainment. Allaire and colleagues [32] recently compared Regular, Occasional, and non-gaming older adults and suggested that older adults who reported playing digital games score, on average, significantly better than non-digital game playing on measures assessing a number of domains of successful aging. Specifically, older adults who were classified as Regular and Occasional Gamers reported less depression and lower negative affect as well as higher well-being than their non-gaming counterparts. Importantly, the authors found also no significant differences among groups for positive affect, social functioning, and self-reported health. One possibility for these findings is that digital games serve as a source of entertainment which may lower negative affect and depression and increase well-being. Thus, gaming technology has significant potential to contribute positively to seniors' leisure time and to propose significant alternative to other well-established daily habits such as watching television.

Secondly, many elderly enjoy games as a means of socializing with others within and outside their social network. Digital gaming has become an increasingly social activity that provides a rich set of enjoyable topics of conversation, as well as a common activity that can serve as a way of decreasing social distance. For example, Al Mahmuda and colleagues [33] introduced the mobile phone game "Walk to Win" which aimed to encourage social engagement among the elderly. This is also the case of intergenerational programs that elderly people particularly appreciate [34]. This is related to a recent social trend involving games embedded in online social networks in particular [35]. Indeed, young gamers often invite their elderly relatives to play because of utilitarian reasons (e.g. gaining game resources thanks to multiple in-game friends visits). But then, the shared experience of the game provides new conversation material, fill the geographical distance, and constitutes a new affordance for relationship building. Recent studies showed that the interaction with the children's youth and enthusiasm functions as a source of emotional well-being for the elderly [36] sharing in the context of intergenerational gaming does foster connections and produce positive emotions for both generations [37]. Furthermore, elderly showed more positive attitudes toward younger people and increase life satisfaction [38].

Third, games can be played with the explicit motivation of sharpening one's mind. This area includes challenging mental activities, such as puzzles and quizzes, aimed to stimulate cognitive abilities such as memory and attention. Also recent randomized controlled trials demonstrated that video games designed to improve mental abilities, such as the so-called "brain training" games, can effectively improve cognitive abilities in the elderly [39]. The last area is represented by the possibilities of interacting that thanks to new technologies are both more natural in terms of affordances and engage the whole body. Keyani and colleagues [40] created the digital game "Dance Along" with the goal to promote social engagement combining exercises, dance and digital gaming for older people. The Sony EyeToy (using computer vision) and the Nintendo Wii (using position and acceleration sensing) are examples that allow for an embodied, physically active way of engaging with the game content. In such a context, digital games can be regarded as persuasive technologies that provide an additional incentive to engage in healthy behavior by engaging the user in a virtual fitness program, providing guidance and coaching that can be tailored to the individual [41].

What makes gaming a source of well-being? When performing a well-learned procedural activity people feel the experience of flow and engagement. Such experiences are intrinsically rewarding and positive, to the point they are commonly listed as reasons for approaching video games [42]. Flow can be defined as a positive experiential state occurring when the performer is totally connected to the performance, in a situation of balance between perceived personal skills and required challenges [43].

The experience of immersion in an activity reach a so intense level that one feels a sense of satisfaction and loses track of time. Essentially, flow can be seen as defining the conditions for positive, meaningful experience, and playing computer games provides an example of how this can be achieved using technology (e.g., [44, 45]) also with elderly population [46, 47]. This will open the chance to develop a new class of positive applications that may enhance well-being for the elderly not only by inducing positive emotions, but also by providing engaging, self-actualizing and social experiences.

3   How to Design Future Positive Technologies for Elderly? Future Challenges

There is a call from the research community for formulating digital games to meet the wellbeing and entertainment needs of elderly people. Although this area is growing, multi-user virtual environments and digital games have not yet been fully explored as potential positive technologies that can be utilized as a support tool in improving the affective state the older people. To reach this goal is important to recognize the need for specialized training and continuous support for the elderly who need to feel self-efficacy in using digital technologies and virtual worlds/games. A good design represents a strategic role to increase the degree to which a specific group of users are able to play a game and effectively accomplish tasks. Several aspect ranging from display selection, fonts, screen element organization, navigational elements, easiness of interaction, as well as rules and tutorials all play an important role in ensuring that games match the specific needs of the elderly, and ensure that the game environment is user-friendly, useful, simple and motivating [48, 49]. The elderly are frequently "casual" gamers [50], so that they prefer games with simple and positive narratives; thus gameplay should be adequately challenging but not devoted to the increasing of difficulty, and limited in time to allow players to have fun without excessive time investments.

To conclude, it is possible to identify digital game characteristics that may help in providing positive experiences to older gamers. As first, video games can feature pleasant environments and exploratory activities that foster relaxation and positive emotions. Secondly, game activities designed basing on measures of the players' ability may promote optimal experiences and engagement. Finally, game designers should exploit ways to enhance social aspects of gameplay, such as embedding the games within already-existing online social networks, in order to allow the gamers to experience new opportunities for social connectedness.

Acknowledgments. This study has been supported by Università Cattolica del Sacro Cuore of Milan (D3.2 Tecnologia Positiva e Healthy Aging - Positive Technology and Healthy Aging, 2014) and by Fondazione Cariplo (Research project Ageing and Healthy Living: A Human Centered Approach in Research and innovation as Source of Quality Life, 2014).

References

1. World Population Prospects: The 2004 revision highlights. Technical report, United Nations, New York City (2005)
2. WHO: Active ageing: a policy framework (2002)
3. WHO: Health for all: updated targets (1994)
4. Walker, A.: A strategy for active ageing. Int. Soc. Secur. Rev. **55**, 121–139 (2002)
5. Walker, A.: The emergence and application of active aging in Europe. J. Aging Soc. Policy **21**, 75–93 (2008)
6. Steptoe, A., Deaton, A., Stone, A.A.: Subjective wellbeing, health, and ageing. Lancet **385**, 640–648 (2015)
7. Harrington, T.L., Harrington, M.K.: Gerontechnology: Why and How. Herman Bouma Foundation for Gerontechnology & Shaker Publishing, Maastricht (2000)
8. Botella, C., Riva, G., Gaggioli, A., Wiederhold, B.K., Alcaniz, M., Banos, R.M.: The present and future of positive technologies. Cyberpsychol. Behav. Soc. Netw. **15**, 78–84 (2012)
9. Riva, G., Banos, R.M., Botella, C., Wiederhold, B.K., Gaggioli, A.: Positive technology: using interactive technologies to promote positive functioning. Cyberpsychol. Behav. Soc. Netw. **15**, 69–77 (2012)
10. Villani, D., Cipresso, P., Gaggioli, A., Riva, G.: Integrating Technology in Positive Psychology Practice. IGI Global, Hershey (2016)
11. Seligman, M.E.P., Csikszentmihalyi, M.: Positive Psychology: An Introduction. Springer, Berlin (2014)
12. Delle Fave, A., Massimini, F., Bassi, M.: Psychological Selection and Optimal Experience Across Cultures: Social Empowerment Through Personal Growth, vol. 2. Springer, Berlin (2011)
13. Ryan, R.M., Deci, E.L.: On happiness and human potentials: A review of research on hedonic and eudaimonic well-being. Ann. Rev. Psychol. **52**, 141–166 (2001)
14. Seligman, M.E.P.: Authentic Happiness: Using the New Positive Psychology to Realize Your Potential for Lasting Fulfillment. New York Free Press, New York (2002)
15. Newall, N.E.G., Chipperfield, J.G., Bailis, D.S., Stewart, T.L.: Consequences of loneliness on physical activity and mortality in older adults and the power of positive emotions. Health Psychol. **32**, 921–924 (2013)
16. Park-Lee, E., Fredman, L., Hochberg, M., Faulkner, K.: Positive affect and incidence of frailty in elderly women caregivers and noncaregivers: results of caregiver-study of osteoporotic fractures. J. Am. Geriatr. Soc. **57**, 627–633 (2009)
17. Fredman, L., Hawkes, W.G., Black, S., Bertrand, R.M., Magaziner, J.: Elderly patients with hip fracture with positive affect have better functional recovery over 2 years. J. Am. Geriatr. Soc. **54**, 1074–1081 (2006)
18. Meeks, S., Van Haitsma, K., Kostiwa, I., Murrell, S.A.: Positivity and well-being among community-residing elders and nursing home residents: What is the optimal affect balance? J. Gerontol. Ser. B Psychol. Sci. Soc. Sci. **67**(4), 460–467 (2012)
19. Riva, G., Marsan, P.A., Grassi, C.: Active Ageing and Healthy Living: A Human Centered Approach in Research and Innovation as Source of Quality of Life. IOS Press, Amsterdam (2014)
20. Riva, G., Villani, D., Cipresso, P., Repetto, C., Triberti, S., Di Lernia, D., Chirico, A., Serino, S., Gaggioli, A.: Positive and transformative technologies for active ageing. Stud. Health Technol. Inform. **220**, 308–315 (2016)

21. Ohsuga, M., Tatsuno, Y., Shimono, F., Hirasawa, K., Oyama, H., Okamura, H.: Bedside wellness - development of virtual forest rehabilitation system. In: Westwood, J.D., Hoffman, H.M., Stredney, D., Weghorst, S.J. (eds.) Medicine Meets Virtual Reality: Art, Science, Technology Healthcare (R) Evolution, vol. 50, p. 168. IOS Press, Amsterdam (1998)

22. Ohsuga, M., Tatsuno, Y., Shimono, F., Hirasawa, K., Oyama, H., Okamura, H.: Development of a bedside wellness system. CyberPsychol. Behav. **1**, 105–112 (1998)

23. Baños, R.M., Etchemendy, E., Castilla, D., Garcia-Palacios, A., Quero, S., Botella, C.: Positive mood induction procedures for virtual environments designed for elderly people. Interact. Comput. **24**, 131–138 (2012)

24. Botella, C., Etchemendy, E., Castilla, D., Baños, R.M., García-Palacios, A., Quero, S., Alcaniz, M., Lozano, J.A.: An e-health system for the elderly (Butler Project): a pilot study on acceptance and satisfaction. CyberPsychol. Behav. **12**, 255–262 (2009)

25. Entertainment Software Association: Essential facts about the computer and video game industry; 2010 sales, demographics, and usage data (2011)

26. Hultsch, D.F., Hertzog, C., Small, B.J., Dixon, R.A.: Use it or lose it: engaged lifestyle as a buffer of cognitive decline in aging? Psychol. Aging **14**, 245–263 (1999)

27. De Schutter, B.: Never too old to play: the appeal of digital games to an older audience. Game. Cult. **6**, 155–170 (2010)

28. Jung, Y., Li, K.J., Janissa, N.S., Gladys, W.L.C., Lee, K.M.: Games for a better life: effects of playing Wii games on the well-being of seniors in a long-term care facility. In: Proceedings of the Sixth Australasian Conference on Interactive Entertainment, p. 5. ACM Press (2009)

29. Nap, H.H., De Kort, Y.A.W., IJsselsteijn, W.A.: Senior gamers: preferences, motivations and needs. Gerontechnology **8**, 247–262 (2009)

30. Whitcomb, G.R.: Computer games for the elderly. In: Proceedings of the Conference on Computers and the Quality of Life, pp. 112–115

31. IJsselsteijn, W.A., Nap, H.H., de Kort, Y., Poels, K.: Digital game design for elderly users. In: Proceedings of the Future Play 2007, pp. 17–22. Institute for Human and Machine Cognition (IHMC), Pensacola (2007)

32. Allaire, J.C., McLaughlin, A.C., Trujillo, A., Whitlock, L.A., LaPorte, L., Gandy, M.: Successful aging through digital games: Socioemotional differences between older adult gamers and non-gamers. Comput. Hum. Behav. **29**, 1302–1306 (2013)

33. Al Mahmud, A., Mubin, O., Shahid, S., Martens, J.B.: Designing social games for children and older adults: two related case studies. Entertain. Comput. **1**, 147–156 (2010)

34. Kaplan, M., Hannon, P.: Intergenerational engagement in retirement communities: a case study of a community capacity-building model. J. Appl. Gerontol. **25**, 406–426 (2006)

35. Boudreau, K., Consalvo, M.: Families and social network games. Inf. Commun. Soc. **17**, 1118–1130 (2014)

36. Weintraub, A.P.C., Killian, T.S.: Intergenerational programming: older persons' perceptions of its impact. J. Appl. Gerontol. **26**, 370–384 (2007)

37. Osmanovic, S., Pecchioni, L.: Beyond entertainment motivations and outcomes of video game playing by older adults and their younger family members. Game. Cult. **11**, 130–149 (2016)

38. Meshel, D.S., MCGlynn, R.P.: Intergenerational contact, attitudes, and stereotypes of adolescents and older people. Educ. Gerontol. **30**, 457–479 (2004)

39. Nouchi, R., Taki, Y., Takeuchi, H., Hashizume, H., Akitsuki, Y., Shigemune, Y., Sekiguchi, A., Kotozaki, Y., Tsukiura, T., Yomogida, Y.: Brain training game improves executive functions and processing speed in the elderly: a randomized controlled trial. PLoS ONE **7**, e29676 (2012)

40. Keyani, P., Hsieh, G., Mutlu, B., Easterday, M., Forlizzi, J.: DanceAlong: supporting positive social exchange and exercise for the elderly through dance. In: CHI 2005 Extended Abstracts on Human Factors in Computing Systems, pp. 1541–1544. ACM (2005)

41. De Kort, Y.A.W., IJsselsteijn, W.A., Eggen, J.H., van den Hoven, E.A.W.H.: Persuasive gerontechnology. Gerontechnol. **4**, 123–127 (2005)

42. Hsu, C.L., Lu, H.P.: Why do people play on-line games? an extended TAM with social influences and flow experience. Inf. Manage. **41**, 853–868 (2004)

43. Csikszentmihalyi, M.: Flow the Psychology of Optimal Experience. Harper Row, New York (1990)

44. Sweetser, P., Wyeth, P.: GameFlow: a model for evaluating player enjoyment in games. Comput. Entertain. (CIE) **3**, 3:1–3:24 (2005)

45. Zhang, J., Fang, X., Chan, S.S., Zagal, J.: Measuring flow experience of computer game players. In: SOCRS 2011 Proceedings (2010)

46. McLaughlin, A., Gandy, M., Allaire, J., Whitlock, L.: Putting fun into video games for older adults. Ergon. Des. Q. Hum. Factors Appl. **20**, 13–22 (2012)

47. Astell, A.: Technology and fun for a happy old age. In: Sixsmith, A., Gutman, G. (eds.) Technologies for Active Aging, pp. 169–187. Springer, New York (2013)

48. Sauvé, L., Renaud, L., Kaufman, D., Duplàa, E.: Validation of the educational game for seniors: "live well, live healthy!". Procedia Soc. Behav. Sci. **176**, 674–682 (2015)

49. Marston, H.R.: Digital gaming perspectives of older adults. content vs. interaction. Educ. Gerontol. **39**, 194–208 (2013)

50. Juul, J.: A Casual Revolution. Reinventing Video Games and Their Players. MIT Press, Cambridge (2010)

Usability and Fun of the INTERACCT Client

Helmut Hlavacs[1]($\boxtimes$), Rebecca Wölfle[1], Konrad Peters[1], Daniel Martinek[1],
Jens Kuczwara[2], Fares Kayali[2], Andrea Reithofer[2], Ruth Mateus-Berr[2],
Barbara Brunmair[3], Zsuzsanna Lehner[3], and Anita Lawitschka[3]

[1] Research Group Entertainment Computing, University of Vienna, Vienna, Austria
{helmut.hlavacs,konrad.peters,daniel.martinek}@univie.ac.at,
rwoelfle@gmail.com
[2] Department Social Design, University of Applied Arts Vienna, Vienna, Austria
jens.kuczwara@gmail.com, fares@igw.tuwien.ac.at,
AndreaReithofer@gmx.at, ruth.mateus-berr@uni-ak.ac.at
[3] St. Anna Children's Cancer Research Institute, Vienna, Austria
barbara.brunmair@ccri.at, Susanne79@gmx.at, anita.lawitschka@stanna.at
http://entertain.univie.ac.at/~hlavacs/,
http://socialdesign.ac.at/team/ruth-mateus-berr/, http://science.ccri.at/

Abstract. We present the INTERACCT system, a smartphone app
and a Web page for fostering communication between young patients
in aftercare after a stem cell transplantation. In this phase of rehabilitation, daily communication between the patients and their clinicians is
key for detecting upcoming possibly deadly crises as early as possible.
The app consists of a communication part, a gaming part, a module for
daily medicine, and a daily story for further motivation. We describe the
system as well as an evaluation of the app with several healthy children.

1 Introduction

Allogeneic hematopoietic stem cell transplantation (HSCT) is a medical treatment in the field of hemato-oncology, proven to be a cure for many diseases
like leukaemia or red-cell disorders. Thanks to this life saving procedure, sur-
vival rates of more than 70% within the first two years after HSCT today
are possible. However, long-term survivors carry a high burden of morbidity,
including infections, treatment related organ toxicities, musculoskeletal disorders, endocrinopathies and immunological complications like graft versus host
disease (GVHD) [3]. They usually affect multiple organs and tissues, resulting in
multimorbidity and variable health developments [10]. In any case, early recognition is crucial, to initiate timely and sufficient treatment [8].

Currently, no adequate technological monitoring solutions are available, especially for young HSCT patients. The status-quo is a paper diary, where patients
track their health data and present it to their aftercare physician once they visit
the hospital, either during a scheduled visit or because the patient's condition
has worsened. Prior examples of electronic diary solutions have proven to provide
better integration into everyday routines.

© ICST Institute for Computer Sciences, Social Informatics and Telecommunications Engineering 2017
K. Giokas et al. (Eds.): eHealth 2016, LNICST 181, pp. 156–163, 2017.
DOI: 10.1007/978-3-319-49655-9_21

In the project INTERACCT[1] we have developed a communication system for daily health reports from children after stem cell transplantation to their clinicians. In order to foster longterm motivation to keep up communication, INTERACCT includes various motivational features such as a game system and daily stories.

2 Related Work

In project INTERACCT one of the core challenges is to sustain long term engagement by using games as motivators. For the purpose of this project, engagement is defined as the first and lowest-level stage of immersion as opposed to engrossment and total immersion [4].

Serious games with health relation were researched by Primack et al. [9], where various positive aspects like education in health matters, motivation during difficult episodes, enhancing treatment compliance as well as therapy support through physical exercises were covered.

Re-Mission and its successor *Re-Mission 2*[2] are serious games where the player is fighting cancer cells inside an infected body.

Aiming at education of their patients' disease and treatments, Gansohr et al. [5] present a multimetdia entertainment system with game elements. The patients are children and adolescents of differentiating age groups, therefore the design process described, which involved methods of user-centered design, was particularly important for INTERACCT.

Prior examples of electronic diary solutions have proven to provide better integration into everyday routines [1]. Furthermore it was shown that electronic health monitoring technology potentially eases the interaction between young patients and their parents [11].

Gronvall et al. [6] propose that health care technology focuses on participative and collaborative approaches to doctor-patient communication.

A system for smart phones or tablets to support children with cancer to keep up with the curriculum of their school classes is presented by Barbosa et al. [2].

3 The INTERACCT Project

INTERACCT is an acronym standing for Integrating Entertainment and Reaction Assessment into Child Cancer Therapy, and denotes an Austrian research project funded nationally be the Austrian Research Promotion Agency FFG. Partners are the Research Group Entertainment Computing of the University of Vienna, the University of Applied Arts Vienna, Department Social Design, Arts as Urban Innovation, the St. Anna Children Cancer Research Institute and outpatient clinic, and the IT service provider T-Systems.

---

[1] http://interacct.at/.
[2] http://www.re-mission2.org/ (accessed May 7th 2015).

The St. Anna outpatient clinic takes care of children after a stem cell transplantation (which essentially wipes out the child's immune system and replaces it with a new one), who are sent home after some months to recover. Often, these children have to stay home all day for a period of between one and two years, being isolated from their friends and school mates, since the danger if contracting life threatening diseases is imminent. In this volatile phase, compliance to treatment is paramount, as is regular communication with the clinicians in order to quickly identify upcoming crises.

Therefore facilitating the communication process of the patient informing the physician about actual health data is key to a successful recovery. In the project INTERACCT we have developed a communication tool for children and adolescents for reporting their health status to their clinicians on a daily basis. The tool is basically a smartphone app that facilitates a module for entering health related data, a gaming system for keeping up fun and motivation, a medical system informing the patients about their daily medicine to be taken, and a daily story for keeping up spirits, taken from our story database comforting stories.

In order to design an appealing interface and gaming system we followed a participatory design process, conducting a three-stage methodological approach towards evaluating gaming preferences of children. These involved mainly exploratory design sessions, a quantitative survey and a proxy design approach based on drawing [7].

3.1   The Clinician Interface

INTERACCT provides a Web interface to involved cinicians who can assign patient profiles to their patients. For example, a kidney profile would involve all relevant parameters for monitoring patients with problematic kidneys. Such parameters would then include daily communication of the amount of water drunk, pain at the kidney, nausea, how often the patient urinated, etc. However, such profiles can be adapted and for each patient, parameters can be excluded or added as the clinicians see fit.

Communicated parameters can then be selected and shown stacked onto each other as time-value diagrams. This way, clinicians can visually correlate problematic episodes and therefore identify crises. Figure 1 shows such a stacking.

3.2   The INTERACCT Client

The INTERACCT app consists of various submodules designed for communication and motivation of young patients. The overview over the possible data categories that can be communicated are shown in Fig. 2. Only those categories that have been selected by the clinician will appear in the app.

One such category is how much water the child has drunk. This can be done every time a glass of water has been drunk, or in the evening to enter the total amount of drunk water (Fig. 3). Another category is pain. Here children can select the region of their body they feel pain at (Fig. 4). Other categories

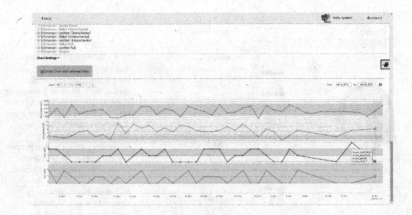

Fig. 1. Clinician Web interface

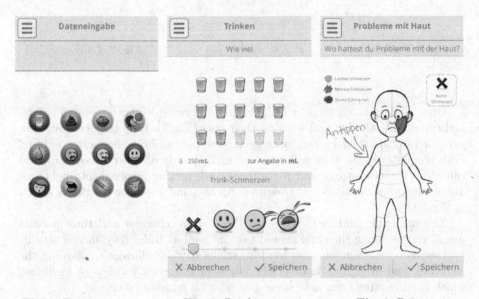

Fig. 2. Data entry.   **Fig. 3.** Drinking.   **Fig. 4.** Pain.

include defecation, mental wellbeing, physical activity, eating, pain in the mouth, nausea, throwing up, fever, and sleeping. When designing the data entries, care was taken to make the design child friendly and as non-verbal as possible, since our medical partner St. Anna Children's Hospital treats many children with non-German background.

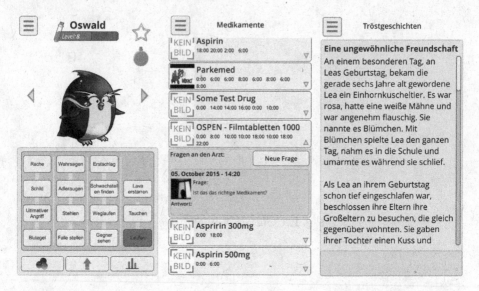

Fig. 5. Pet lab.   **Fig. 6.** Medication.   **Fig. 7.** Daily story.

Once all data has been provided, children are rewarded with research points, and can go into the lab and work on their pets (Fig. 5). Here they can buy new pets, or upgrade their current ones by buying new abilities like better fighting skills etc. Afterwards, they will find new islands daily on their island map, and can go to the newest one and roam the island, getting involved into fights, or discovering magic potions and treasures. An in-game screenshot of this is shown in Fig. 10.

The medicine module is shown in Fig. 6. Here children and their parents see all the medicine the child should take, as well as when they should take it. Furthermore, children can also send questions to their clinicians regarding the medicine, and even take fotos of the labels of unknown versions of medicine, which is more often than note some generic with unusual labels.

Furthermore, every day the app offers a new comforting story taken from our story database, which currently holds over 250 stories written by healthy children for ill children (Fig. 7).[3]

4   Evaluation

We asked 5 girls and 4 boys in the ages between 12 and 15 to participate in an experiment in order to collect their opinions in the INTERACCT client, here

---

[3] http://www.interacct.at/troestgeschichten/.

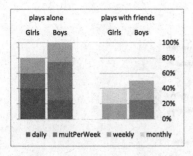

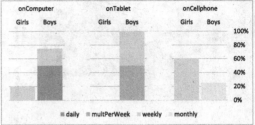

Fig. 8. Playing alone or with friends.   **Fig. 9.** Preferred platform.

testing for understandability of the process and accuracy of the exercise detection system.

The process was as follows: we first explained the purpose of the system, and showed the various parts of the app: data entry, pet laboratory, island gaming system, medicine module, and daily story. Then we gave them around 15 min for each of these parts to use them, play with them, and collect experiences. After about an hour we handed out the questionnaires and collected their opinions about the app.

The questionnaire has three parts. We first asked about their experiences and habits on playing computer games on various platforms. Figure 8 shows the distributions of the children on whether they prefer to play alone, or with friends, and Fig. 9 shows the distribution of preferred gaming platforms. Values are given for girls and boys separately. It can be seen that girls seem to prefer smaller smart phones, whereas boys prefer larger screens like tablets and PCs.

Figure 11 shows the results from the app questionnaire regarding the usability of the overall app. The green bars denote the more positive scores yes/fairly, while the orange bars show the no/marginally answers. Neutral answers have been omitted. The upper part of the diagram shows the categories where a positive answer is favourable, while the lower part shows the opposite. It can be seen that the results are quite satisfying and positive. Overall, using the app was regarded to be quite easy and unchallenging, which is of course important since the target audience consists mostly of very ill children with reduced cognitive skills.

Figure 12 shows the engagement felt in the game system. Here children reported again that the game is quiet easy and unchallenging, again something that we designed intentionally for ill children to be used. Generally the children felt anticipation for the app, which they regarded as being fun and useful.

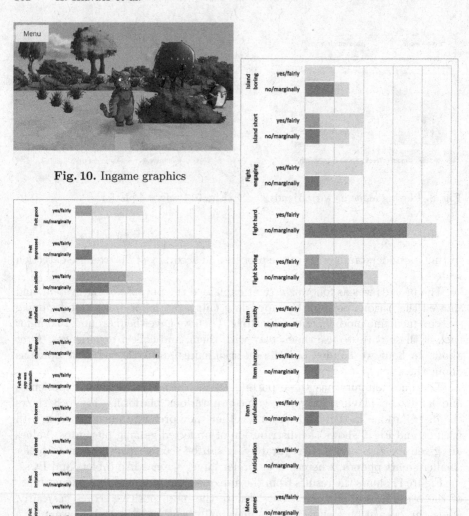

Fig. 10. Ingame graphics

Fig. 11. Usability of app. (Color figure online)

Fig. 12. Game engagement.

5 Conclusion

In the presented communication system INTERACCT we found good results in our evaluation with the intended age categories, but in our case only healthy children. While the design of the app and the game system per se was rated quite positive, healthy children are underchallenged by our game system, which has been designed for ill children with possibly severe cognitive and motoric restrictions. For example, the fight system is round based, there are generally no time-based challenges demanding fast moves.

However, since INTERACCT is more a game container rather than only one particular game, we intend to create a larger variety of games to be found on the islands, presenting more challenges for different skill sets.

References

1. Aarhus, R., Ballegaard, S.A., Hansen, T.R.: The ediary: bridging home and hospital through healthcare technology. In: Wagner, I., Tellioğlu, H., Balka, E., Simone, C., Ciolfi, L. (eds.) ECSCW 2009, pp. 63–83. Springer, London (2009)
2. Barbosa, D., Bassani, P., Mossmann, J., Schneider, G.T., Reategui, E., Branco, M., Meyrer, L., Nunes, M.: Mobile learning and games: experiences with mobile games development for children and teenagers undergoing oncological treatment (2014)
3. Bhatia, S., Davies, S.M., Baker, K.S., Pulsipher, M.A., Hansen, J.A.: Nci, NHLBI first international consensus conference on late effects after pediatric hematopoietic cell transplantation: Etiology and pathogenesis of late effects after HCT performed in childhood-methodologic challenges. Biol. Blood Marrow Transplant. **17**(10), 1428–1435 (2011)
4. Brown, E., Cairns, P.: A grounded investigation of game immersion. In: CHI 2004 Extended Abstracts on Human Factors in Computing Systems, pp. 1297–1300. ACM (2004)
5. Gansohr, C., Emmerich, K., Masuch, M., Basu, O., Grigull, L.: Creating age-specific interactive environments about medical treatments for children and adolescent patients diagnosed with cancer. In: Göbel, S., Wiemeyer, J. (eds.) Game-Days 2014. LNCS, vol. 8395, pp. 141–152. Springer, Heidelberg (2014). doi:10.1007/978-3-319-05972-3_15
6. Gronvall, E., Verdezoto, N., Bagalkot, N., Sokoler, T.: Concordance: a critical participatory alternative in healthcare IT. Aarhus Ser. Hum. Centered Comput. **1**, 21–24 (2015)
7. Kayali, F., Silbernagl, M., Peters, K., Mateus-Berr, R., Reithofer, A., Martinek, D., Lawitschka, A., Hlavacs, H.: Design considerations for a serious game for children after hematopoietic stem cell transplantation. Spec. Issue Fun. Engaging Comput. Technol. Health Entertainment Comput. **15**, 57–73 (2016)
8. Kedia, S., Acharya, P.S., Mohammad, F., Nguyen, H., Asti, D.: Infectious complications of hematopoietic stem cell transplantation. J. Stem Cell Res. Ther. **3**(002), 10–4172 (2013)
9. Primack, B.A., Carroll, M.V., McNamara, M., Klem, M.L., King, B., Rich, M., Chan, C.W., Nayak, S.: Role of video games in improving health-related outcomes. Am. J. Prev. Med. **42**(6), 630–638 (2012)
10. Tamari, R., Castro-Malaspina, H.: Allogeneic haematopoietic stem cell transplantation for primary myelofibrosis and myelofibrosis evolved from other myeloproliferative neoplasms. Curr. Opin. Hematol. **22**(2), 184–190 (2015)
11. Toscos, T., Connelly, K., Rogers, Y.: Best intentions: health monitoring technology and children. In: SIGCHI Conference on Human Factors in Computing Systems, pp. 1431–1440. ACM (2012)

Gamification of a System for Real Time Monitoring of Posture

Alberto Cavallo, Alessio Robaldo, Flavio Ansovini,
Ivan Carmosino[✉], and Alessandro De Gloria

University of Genoa – EliosLab, via Opera Pia 11A, Genoa, Italy
Cavallo.Alberto.ca@gmail.com,
Robaldo.Alessio@gmail.com,
{Flavio.Ansovini,Alessandro.DeGloria}@unige.it,
Ivan.Carmosino@elios.unige.it

Abstract. In this paper the gamification of a system for monitoring bad postural behavior is presented. The system is designed having children as main target users. Bad posture is a known cause of possible severe disorders in childhood and, in the worst-case scenario, may entail permanent spinal deviations. The developed system consists of two main components: a device equipped with inertial sensors (accelerometer, magnetometer and gyroscope), which are able to measure the patient's spinal curvature, and a Game Engine plugin (Unity3D and Udk) that provides the reading of the device data and through which the game programmer can link the posture information to a game variable such as: life count, number of enemies, energy and so on. If the player is in a bad posture, he gets negative feedback during the game, which affects the value of the associated variable.

Keywords: Posture · Inertial measurement unit · Serious game for health · Game engine plugin

1 Introduction

Bad posture attitude is one of the main causes of backache which can easily degenerate into more severe disorders, especially in childhood. Giving a feedback about the posture maintained during a class, for example, we can reduce the amount of ache complained by students [1].

In general, completing and wrapping a product (e.g., a medical device in the present case) in the form of a game (usually called serious game) is expected to sensitively improve its attractiveness, especially if it is aimed at children [2]. And serious games for improving people wellness are becoming very popular [3].

The structure of this document is as follows: Sect. 2 introduces the main features for a method for recognizing bad postures and shows the related state of the art. Section 3 presents the project, describing both the hardware elements and the developed algorithms. In Sect. 4 the advantages deriving from including some typical aspects of gamification. are discussed and a related plug-in is described. Section 5 provides the conclusions and illustrates future work.

© ICST Institute for Computer Sciences, Social Informatics and Telecommunications Engineering 2017
K. Giokas et al. (Eds.): eHealth 2016, LNICST 181, pp. 164–168, 2017.
DOI: 10.1007/978-3-319-49655-9_22

2   Postural Attitudes Monitoring and State of the Art

In order to develop our project, a device able to monitor postural habits suitable for an everyday life environment (e.g. in a school or in an office) is needed; the latter should be non-invasive, not restricting nor altering the user's motion in any way. Nowadays, a lot of systems have already been proposed but no one has at the same time all three features we want develop. The main techniques for analyzing human posture use camera and optoelecronics sensor; they has a high precision, but their employing is restricted to a controlled environment [5]. Another method of analysis realizes the procedure using an electromagnetic tracking system, but the presence of metallic objects during the measurements can alter the results. The last system examined is based on potentiometric goniometers, but it restricts the patient's movements (Fig. 2).

3   The System

On the basis of the previous considerations, we decided to implement a system based on inertial sensors composed by a three-axis gyroscope, a three-axis magnetometer and a three-axis accelerometer. These sensors measure the orientation of a rigid body in the space in terms of its Euler angles with respect to a fixed system of reference. Accelerometers and gyroscopes are already been used for monitoring the spine position of a human being [4–7].

However, our system makes use of a further component (a magnetometer) in order to avoid the drift problem, typically caused by gyroscopes.

Our system may be divided in two separate parts, the former being devoted to measure the patient posture and the latter analyzing the data and allowing the user interaction. The two elements are able to communicate each other by means of a Bluetooth connection (Fig. 1).

The device equipped with sensors is composed by an ST iNemo module [8]. This module contains different kind of sensors, including inertial sensors we need. It has also a microprocessor able to filter sensors data and compute Euler angles.

The analyses of the user's posture is realized using two devices, built as we have descripted previously, placed in different spots of the user's spinal column. One of them, called master, provide the data transmission via Bluetooth, in addition to its measuring task, The second Inertial Measurement Unit (IMU), called slave, can only obtain and elaborate data from the sensors, and send them to the master using a wired connection.

The system architecture is designed to quickly change the number of IMUs employed, improving the measurement precision. The graphic user interface (GUI) is designed to run on an Android device. The device connects with the sensors through the Bluetooth protocol and it can update the GUI according to the received data, so the user can see a view of his position in real time. The mobile device is able to warn the user while he's keeping an incorrect posture in three different ways: a graphical one (Fig. 3), an acoustic one, and a haptic one. The data about a session can be stored within a database, allowing the user to analyze them at a later time.

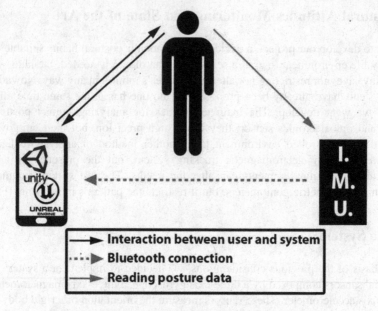

Fig. 1. System components relation

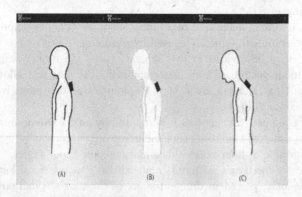

Fig. 2. Graphic User Interface: (a) Correct curve; (b) Medium curve; (c) Wrong curve.

Finally, the master IMU have to send data to a Unity3D plugin, which will be describe more in detail in the next section.

4   Improve Postural Habits with a Social Game

An aspect that has been considered in studying our system is the great achievement that social games have obtained in the last few years. A lot of studies show that the possibility of sharing results in a community makes a system more engaging [9–11].

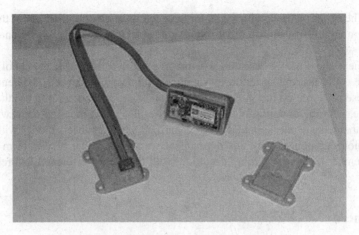

Fig. 3. The system hardware prototype.

This is an aspect applicable to every kind of goals reached by the user, who is nowadays accustomed to share his life events through social networks.

In the light of the above argument, we decided to develop an Inertial Measurement Unit (IMU) connection plugin designed for the two most popular game engines which are widespread within both the indie developers' community as well as big companies: Unity3D and Udk.

The plugin encapsulate the posture sensor and thus sends a value representing the correctness of the player's posture to the game which uses this information in a way that the game designer deems suited. As an example, the player's bad posture may be set to cause the game life bar to decrease more rapidly even in the absence of negative game events, such as the presence of enemies. The game designer may also, or alternatively, decide to correlate the plugin's signal to the enemies' generation, thus entailing a more difficult game experience when the player's posture is not correct.

Taking the player's posture into account, the value sent by the plugin is an accumulator which is:

- incremented by one every minute spent in a correct position
- unchanged every minute spent in a partially incorrect posture
- decremented by one every minute spent in a bad posture

If directly associated with a variable used for computing the overall game's score, the value delivered by the plugin could be also used to give game points to the players.

5   Conclusions

Preliminary experiments conducted in lab have shown the validity of the approach, both for the precision in measuring the posture and for the feedback given to the user.

In order to verify the real impact of our device, we have developed a social game exploiting a plugin, that delivers to the game the posture assessment provided by the device. The experiments conducted so far have left us quite optimistic about the results our system could give but, the real impact on social games is still to be analyzed in depth.

The next steps of our research will involve a partnership with a school through which we could test the system on a significant number of subjects. The general idea we propose is to split up the students in two groups: the first one should use the system as a game, with the opportunity of sharing the results and comparing them with other gamers; the second one should use only the real time feedback mode, without the gamification component. For this experiment we expect better results from the students' member of the first group, according with the theory explained beforehand.

References

1. Robbins, M., Johnson, I.P., Cunliffe, C.: Encouraging good posture in school children in using computers. Clin. Chiropractic **12**, 35–44 (2009)
2. 10 stats on the growth of gamification. http://www.gameifications.com/learning/10-numeri-sulla-gamification-nelleducazione/
3. Health a fitness news. http://seriousgamessociety.org/index.php/2014-07-11-14-15-51/explore/137-health-a-fitness-news
4. Wong, W.Y., Wong, M.S.: Trunk posture monitoring with inertial sensors. Eur. Spine J. **17**, 743–753 (2008)
5. Lee, R.Y.W., Laprade, J., Fung, E.H.K.: A real-time gyroscopic system for three-dimensional measurement of lumbar spine motion. Med. Eng. Phys. **25**, 817–824 (2003)
6. Lou, E., Raso, J., Hill, D., Durdle, N., Moreau, M.: Spine-straight device for the treatment of kyphosis. Stud. Health Technol. Inf. **91**, 401–404 (2002)
7. Nevins, R.J., Durdle, N.G., Raso, V.J.: A posture monitoring system using accelerometers. In: Electrical and Computer Engineering, pp. 1087–1092 (2002)
8. INEMO_M1 official documentation. www.st.com/web/en/catalog/sense_power/FM89/SC1448/PF253162
9. University of Pennsylvania Annenberg School for Communication, Social networks can motivate people to exercise more: Compared to motivational messaging, the social influence of online peers proved more effective in improving exercise habits (2007). www.sciencedaily.com/releases/2015/10/151007110738.htm
10. Simoes, J., Redondo, R.D., Vilas, A.F.: A social gamification framework for a K-6 learning platform. Comput. Hum. Behav. **29**, 345–353 (2013)
11. Hamari, J., Koivisto, J.: Social motivation to use gamification: an empirical study of gamifying exercise. In: ECIS 2013, Paper 105 Completed Research (2013)

Positive Technologies for Promoting Emotion Regulation Abilities in Adolescents

Esther Judith Schek[1]([✉]), Fabrizia Mantovani[1], Olivia Realdon[1],
Joao Dias[2], Ana Paiva[2], Sarit Schramm-Yavin[3],
and Ruth Pat-Horenczyk[3,4]

[1] Department of Human Sciences for Education, CESCOM-Centre for Studies in
Communication Sciences, University of Milano-Bicocca, Milan, Italy
e.schek@campus.unimib.it
[2] INESC-ID, Instituto Superior Técnico, Universidade de Lisboa,
Lisbon, Portugal
[3] The Israel Center for the Treatment of Psychotrauma, Herzog Hospital,
Jerusalem, Israel
[4] Paul Baerwald School of Social Work and Social Welfare,
Hebrew University of Jerusalem, Jerusalem, Israel

Abstract. In recent years there is a growing interest in the use of emerging advanced technologies in supporting well-being and health promotion. Although few existing programs employ innovative technologies to foster social and emotional learning in adolescence, they do not specifically focus on emotion regulation skills. Further, research in this domain has primarily tested the efficacy of these trainings with one type of measurement technique at a time, although most recent theories highlight that emotions are multi-dimensional and multi-component processes. With the above in mind and to overcome these limitations, we developed a technology-enhanced protocol for the enhancement of emotion regulation, based on evidenced based program, the Building Emotion and Affect Regulation, age-adjusted and combined with virtual characters and wearable physiological sensors. The objective of this paper is to present an overview of the design and development process of this innovative protocol: EmoRegulators.

Keywords: Positive technology · Emotion regulation · Adolescents

1 Introduction

Emotion regulation (ER) refers to a set of processes involved in the initiation, maintenance and modification of emotion [1]. ER strategies are especially important during adolescence, when the transition from middle school to high school requires adolescents to develop new skills and to cope with new situations, and deficits in this area might result in psychosocial and behavioral problems [2]. Research has shown that students with well-developed social skills and emotional awareness are more motivated to engage in studies and to collaborate with peers and are better able to manage stress [3].

© ICST Institute for Computer Sciences, Social Informatics and Telecommunications Engineering 2017
K. Giokas et al. (Eds.): eHealth 2016, LNICST 181, pp. 169–174, 2017.
DOI: 10.1007/978-3-319-49655-9_23

Today's students are called "digital natives": they are in their natural habitat when using technological interfaces [4], so that technology-enhanced interventions can be an attractive alternative for them compared to traditional ones. Although training programs that employ innovative technologies to foster social and emotional learning have been developed (e.g., Playmancer [5], eCircus [6], and Interstress [7]), they either are not targeted specifically to adolescents or focus on social and/or emotional issues, rather than on the specific aim of building ER skills. Moreover, the adoption of emerging advanced technologies in supporting well-being and health promotion has been recently highlighted within the Positive Technology paradigm, identifying the pathways of personal experience through which technology can build strengths and resilience in individuals, organizations and society [8]. Based on these premises, we propose an innovative technology-enhanced protocol aimed at enhancing ER abilities in adolescents. In the current paper we will present an overview of the process of the development and of the research design for testing its efficacy.

2 Adaptation of the BEAR Training to a Technology-Enhanced Protocol

Among existing interventions for children and youth, a recent program for strengthening the abilities of emotion regulation has shown preliminary promising results [9]: The Building Emotion and Affect Regulation (BEAR). The BEAR program is a group intervention geared for enhancing ER capacities in children (aged 7–12) and it was developed by the Israel Centre for the Treatment of Psychotrauma (ICTP) and implemented in Singapore, Israel and in the US. It is based on a number of theoretical and clinical sources [10–12], and it incorporates various components from several evidence-based interventions. The BEAR is an eight-session protocol. Each session focuses on a different domain of regulation, including physical, cognitive, emotion and social regulation and it includes the following themes: Becoming a Group; Resources; Physical Regulation; Cognitive and Emotional Regulation; Cognitive Behavioral Regulation; Interpersonal Regulation; and Social Support. The intervention is structured around the following core components, which are repeated in each of the session: Mindfulness exercises; Psycho-education; Experiential exercises; Narrative approach; and opening and closing rituals.

The design and development of the technology-enhanced version was carried out in different phases and involved three universities: the University of Milano-Bicocca (UNIMIB), the Hebrew University of Jerusalem (HUJI) and the University of Lisbon (IST-UL). A User-Centred Design was adopted and 4 schools and 2 youth organizations in Italy were involved. First, 5 focus groups were conducted with students aged 13–17. 3 main areas were analyzed: (a) stress experienced by adolescents in their day-to-day activities; (b) their physical awareness of stress effects and their coping abilities; (c) their expectations about a technology-enhanced training protocol. Then, during the development phase, 3 different graphic design versions were directly evaluated by 30 high-school students (15 male) and on the basis of the results, the cartoon style version was selected. Finally different usability tests were conducted, to evaluate the total time required to complete the protocol and to have their opinions and suggestions about the interface of the training, the animation of the avatars and the biosensors adopted. The development of the training evolved step by step in response to the main findings. All sessions and exercises were adapted and adjusted for the relevant age group, and further changes and adaptations were made based on the youth experiences.

3   Definition of the Functional Requirements of EmoRegulators

Once the training was adapted, the various functional requirements were chosen and integrated:

Computational model: The computational model adopted is FAtiMA [13, 14].

FAtiMA (Fearnot AffectTIve Mind Architecture) is an Agent Architecture with planning capabilities designed to use emotions and personality to influence the agent's behaviour. The architecture was recently extended with interpersonal emotion regulation capabilities [15] and this was the main reason why FAtiMA was selected. In fact, our long-term goal is to create a virtual facilitator that is able to perceive the user's emotional state and help him cope with negative emotions that may arise from the use of the application. In the initial prototype version, we've only used the emotional reactive capabilities, fixing the appraisal process so that the emotions generated are always the same.

Software: Unity 3D was used as the development environment due to the existence of a large set of community-developed assets that can be used to extend Unity's functionalities, and due to the already existing integration of FAtiMA Agent Architecture with Unity 3D.

Avatars: Daz 3D software was chosen for avatars. A cartoon graphic design was selected to avoid the uncanny valley problem [16], a well-known problem in games, 3D animation and robotics. Two cartoon style characters were used from the 3D library: Jason and Jasmine (See Fig. 1), for male and female user. Jasmine was also used for the assistant avatar modifying some physical characteristics, with the Genesis platform.

Biosensors: Bioplux sensors (See Fig. 2), a wearable device, non-invasive, able to connect in wireless, was used to obtain psycho-physiological data of HR, muscle activity and EDA. In addition, the physiological value of heart rate measured by the device was always displayed on the monitor, giving an immediate feedback to the user and, at the same time, obtaining an objective data of the effectiveness of the training.

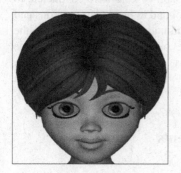

Fig. 1. Facial female 3D avatar

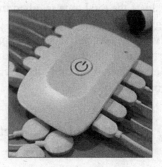

Fig. 2. Bioplux sensors

4 Conclusion and Next Steps

As mentioned, according to the PT approach, technology can increase emotional, psychological and social well-being [17] and with this vision in mind we've proposed an innovative technology-enhanced protocol aimed at enhancing ER abilities in adolescents. The main strength of this innovative tool is the combination of different advanced technologies: gamification aspects, virtual characters and wearable physiological sensors. In fact, it is widely recognized that stress detection technologies can help people better understand and relieve stress by increasing their awareness of heightened levels of stress that would otherwise go undetected [18]. Further, in the last couple of years, gamification has been a trending topic and a subject to much hype as a means of supporting user engagement and enhancing positive patterns in service use [19]. A limitation of this first prototype development was that no VR biofeedback was associated to the HR, although it has been shown to be more effective in inducing relaxation than simple audio and visual cues [20]. We took this choice since we wanted to test only the training itself, avoiding any other kind of variable that could influence the final result.

A pilot study is currently ongoing to explore the impact of Emoregulators, focusing on the feasibility and benefits of the innovative tool. We are testing in particular one specific session of the BEAR, physical regulation, developed in 3 different versions: (a) Written instructions at pc & 3D user's avatar doing exercises; (b) Instructions given by a 3D avatar-assistant & 3D user's avatar doing exercises; (c) Traditional adapted BEAR.

As said, in a future pilot version the Emotional Intelligent Component of FAtiMA will be added, so that avatars will become agents able to understand emotions of the user and able to behave accordingly. Further, we would like to integrate it with biofeedback, as an effective means of strengthening regulation abilities in youth.

References

1. Gross, J.J.: Emotion regulation: taking stock and moving forward. Emotion **13**, 359–365 (2013)
2. Saarni, C.: The social context of emotional development. In: Lewis, M., Haviland-Jones, J.M. (eds.) Handbook of Emotions, 2nd edn, pp. 306–322. The Guilford Press, New York (2000)
3. Cherniss, C., Extein, M., Goleman, D., Weissberg, R.P.: Emotional intelligence: what does the research really indicate? Educ. Psychol. **41**, 239–245 (2006)
4. Prensky, M.: Digital Game-Based Learning. McGraw-Hill, London (2001)
5. Ben Moussa, M., Magnenat-Thalmann, N.: Applying affect recognition in serious games: the playmancer project. In: Proceedings of the 2nd International Workshop on Motion in Games, MIG 2009, pp. 53–62 (2009)
6. Lim, M.Y., Leichtenstern, K., Kriegel, M., Enz, S., Aylettt, R., Vannini, N., Hall, L., Rizzo, P.: Technology-enhanced role-play for social and emotional learning context-Intercultural empathy. Entertainment Comput. **2**, 223–231 (2011)
7. Riva, G., Raspelli, S., Pallavicini, F., Grassi, A., Algeri, D., Wiederhold, B.K., Giaggioli, A.: Interreality in the management of psychological stress: a clinical scenario. Stud. Health Technol. Inf. **154**, 20–25 (2010)
8. Riva, G.: Personal experience in positive psychology may offer a new focus for a growing discipline. Am. Psychol. **67**, 574–575 (2012)
9. Pat-Horenczyk, R., Sim Wei Shi, C., Schramm-Yavin, S., Bar-Halpern, M., Tan, L.J.: BEAR - building emotion and affect regulation (BEAR): preliminary evidence from an open trial in children's residential group homes in Singapore. Child Youth Care Forum **44**, 175–190 (2014)
10. Ford, J.D., Russo, E.: A trauma-focused, present-centered, emotional self-regulation approach to integrated treatment for post-traumatic stress and addiction: trauma affect regulation: guidelines for education and therapy (TARGET). Am. J. Psychother. **60**, 335–355 (2006)
11. Lahad, M.: BASIC Ph: the story of coping resources. In: Lahad, M., Cohen, A. (eds.) Community Stress Prevention, pp. 117–145. Community Stress Prevention Center, Kiryat Shmona (1993)
12. Pat-Horenczyk, R., Berger, R., Kaplinsky, N., Baum, N.: The journey to resilence: coping with ongoing stressful situations. Protocol for guidance counselors (adolescent's version) (2004)
13. Dias, J., Paiva, A.: Feeling and reasoning: a computational model for emotional characters. In: Bento, C., Cardoso, A., Dias, G. (eds.) EPIA 2005. LNCS (LNAI), vol. 3808, pp. 127–140. Springer, Heidelberg (2005). doi:10.1007/11595014_13
14. Dias, J., Mascarenhas, S., Paiva, A.: FAtiMA modular: towards an agent architecture with a generic appraisal framework. In: Bosse, T., Broekens, J., Dias, J., van der Zwaan, J. (eds.) Emotion Modeling. LNCS (LNAI), vol. 8750, pp. 44–56. Springer, Heidelberg (2014). doi:10.1007/978-3-319-12973-0_3
15. Dias J., Paiva A.: I want to be your friend: establishing relations with emotionally intelligent agents. In: Proceedings of Autonomous Agents and Multi-Agent Systems Conference (AAMAS) (2013)
16. Tinwell, A.: The Uncanny Valley in Games and Animation. CRC Press, Boca Raton (2014)
17. Serino, S., Cipresso, P., Gaggioli, A., Riva, G.: The potential of pervasive sensors and computing for positive technology. In: Mukhopadhyay, S.C., Postolache, O.A. (eds.) Pervasive and Mobile Sensing and Computing for Healthcare: Smart Sensors, Measurement and Instrumentation. Springer, New York (2013)

18. Dishman, R.K., Nakamura, Y., Garcia, M.E., Thompson, R.W., Dunn, A.L., Blair, S.N.: Heart rate variability, trait anxiety, and perceived stress among physically fit men and women. Int. J. Psychophysiol. **37**, 121–133 (2000)
19. Hamari, J., Lehdonvirta, V.: Game design as marketing: how game mechanics create demand for virtual goods. Int. J. Bus. Sci. Appl. Manag. **5**, 14–29 (2010)
20. Gaggioli, A., Pallavicini, F., Morganti, L., Serino, S., Scaratti, C., Briguglio, M., Tartarisco, G.: Experiential virtual scenarios with real-time monitoring (interreality) for the management of psychological stress: a block randomized controlled trial. J. Med. Internet Res, **16**, e167 (2014)

Technology for Well-Being at School. App iNclusion by CeDisMa: A Support for Teachers to Teach Inclusively, for Students to Really Learn

Maria Concetta Carruba[✉]

Department of Pedagogy (Education), Università Cattolica Del Sacro Cuore,
Largo Gemelli N. 1, 20123 Milan, Italy
MariaConcetta.Carruba@unicatt.it

Abstract. The iNclusion App by CeDisMa (available in iTunes Store: https://itunes.apple.com/it/app/inclusion/id1093478813?mt=8) is an innovative research tool that allows to integrate quantitative data with qualitative analysis. This application invites teachers to reflect upon motivation and technology. Answering to the questions included in the App, teachers will collect information about their students' approach to learning, including students with special needs or learning disabilities; motivation and classroom management; the effects of best practices on classroom management in the teaching-learning process.

Keywords: Well-being · School · Technology · Inclusion · App · iNclusion

1 Introduction

Based on the research project "Motivation and Pedagogy: a study of the relationship between social inclusion and class management" (it is a study by Ilaria Folci teacher and researcher at Catholic University of Sacred Heart, in Milan), the Study and Research Centre on Disability and Social Marginality (CeDisMa, Centro Studi e Ricerche sulla disabilità e la marginalità, http://centridiricerca.unicatt.it/cedisma, directed by Luidi d'Alonzo) has developed an application for teachers in cooperation with Marketing Media Network (a business structure in Milan that promote ICT solutions for school, expert and corporation, http://www.mmn.it). CeDisMa's main interest areas are: developing knowledge on education, leaning, teaching and training professionals in the field of special education needs. The Centre primarily deals with education, special needs and social inclusion. It cooperates with local administrations on projects financed by the EU Structural Funds for equal opportunities. It currently organizes post-graduate courses on care, education and training based on European programs. Marketing Media Network (MMN) promotes ICT solution for business and technical support in education processes (also through Apple's partnership). The project has grown out of a multidisciplinary team (CeDisMa's teachers and researchers together with MMN's ICT experts) whose joint efforts made their idea far more complete and valuable [14] This tool will help to analyze and understand how a

© ICST Institute for Computer Sciences, Social Informatics and Telecommunications Engineering 2017
K. Giokas et al. (Eds.): eHealth 2016, LNICST 181, pp. 175–182, 2017.
DOI: 10.1007/978-3-319-49655-9_24

student's well-being influences motivation in learning. Several variables must be taken into account in the teaching-learning process. Motivation, defined as proactive acting in order to reach set targets, is definitively one of them. Scientific studies in this field are based on the assumption that the dynamics of motivation are determined by multiple social, cognitive and emotional factors such as:

- Self-concept;
- Perception of competence;
- Locus of control effects;
- The goals that the student aims at achieving;

Evertson and Weinstein's considerations [8] are particularly interesting in these regards as they underline the positive consequences of motivated acting in the personal development of a sense of responsibility and self-regulation when being in the class, studying, dealing with classmates and, in general, towards the educational and learning processes.

1.1 Motivation and Pedagogy: Best Practices for Inclusion and Classroom Management

Nowadays, studies on motivation are based upon the awareness that its underlying dynamics result from the influence of several factors – social, cognitive and emotional – such as self-concept, perception of competence, locus of control effects and the goals that the student aims at achieving (see Deci and Ryan, who listed the three needs that determine the individual's approach to motivation: competence, affection and autonomy; see also Harter, who relates self-concept with motivation, asserting that the latter is influenced by the self-concept that the individual has, according to age and other contextual aspects). These causes are strictly connected with elements of the social environment and they are mediated by pedagogical and educational practices. On the basis of these studies, it is necessary to consider that "motivational orientation that better takes into account the fact that motivational behavior is not a mere consequence of a 'need' or 'push', it is instead a pattern or result of many cognitive and emotional factors, which influence the start and the continuation of the effort towards an objective" [1]. Therefore, it plays a fundamental role in how individuals set their own goals. The choice of goals is directly linked to the individuals' inclination to achieve success or avoid failure, and to their beliefs on the value of the results, which are good indicators of positive behaviors [7].

These considerations are very important, especially when challenging students are concerned. Finding academic goals that the students themselves perceive as achievable motivates them towards this target.

In this framework, teachers play a fundamental role because through specific teaching techniques, they can support a proactive learning behavior and improve learning success. Classes–environments in which each student's individual needs coexist - should be managed in an inclusive manner, to support each student without losing the focus on the whole group. The class social and relational mood affects the learning process, which is itself linked to all of the entities involved in the educational process: teachers, students, family, specialists and the whole school network.

Establishing an adequate environment, both as a physical space and as a collection of material, human and symbolic resources, influences the quality of the students' performance and allows teachers to value and respect each student's potential. Teachers work in a class and must therefore be aware that they are operating in a group dimension. The students didn't choose to belong to the group itself, but they are forced to accept it and be an active part of it [4].

The tools for effective teaching are defined as "the pillars of class management" [6] that current studies have identified as necessary to positively influence students. A good class management lies in the teacher's ability to show his/her students the right educational path, to promote a proactive attitude to learning, to meet the students' personal needs and, while supporting and keeping a profitable learning environment [5]. Therefore, it is clear that some of these teaching factors influence the individuals' motivational needs, fostering or inhibiting school performances. We are referring specifically to:

- Approaching studying with enthusiasm and fluency;
- Managing more activities simultaneously [5];
- Diversifying to be committed [5].

These factors are strictly connected with elements of the social context and they are mediated by daily teaching and educational practices.

Teachers play a fundamental role because they play a key role in a successful education and decrease the risk of failure through specific teaching strategies.

2   iNclusion App: Research Summary

In the field of education, the well-being of students is a necessary condition to make them feel included, accepted, part of the class and therefore ready to learn. iNclusion App is a technological tool for Italian teachers to analyze how the classroom management can support students' motivation. It is based on a qualitative questionnaire which will be filled in by primary, middle and secondary school teachers (in Italy) to find out how often they implement educational actions. These actions include:

- Letting teachers' beliefs about students' motivation and learning abilities emerge;
- Pushing teachers to implement some teaching strategies in order to increase students' motivation and learning levels;
- Analyzing the effect of teaching-related class management factors on students' personal motivation to learn, and their consequences on the whole class.

The App allows the collection of data through a specific Apple platform, Research Kit (http://www.apple.com/it/researchkit/). Teachers can use the application with IOS devices and respond to the survey anonymously. The data will be analyzed by CeDisMa's research team. The App is 13.1 MB, it's the first version, it's in Italian and it is available in the App Store in the category "Education". To use the App you need IOS 8.4 or following.

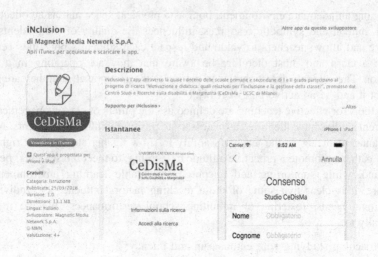

(https://itunes.apple.com/it/app/inclusion/id1093478813?mt=8)

How teachers can use the App:

- they login to the format and agree to transfer their data to the platform;
- they read a short presentation about CeDisMa research center and the aim of the study;
- they enter the teacher's questionnaire;

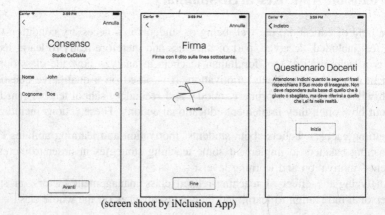

(screen shoot by iNclusion App)

- they answer the questions (60 question about classroom management, students in the class, teacher and student needs - special needs included).

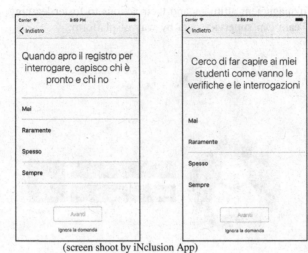

(screen shoot by iNclusion App)

The questionnaire will also drive teachers to reflect on the importance of students' motivation. A motivated student is a student that feels well in the class.

Good class management creates a positive work environment and therefore plays an important role in implementing a more functional "context" for learning, as a social and physical reality. The data collected will make it possible to analyze and "measure" the relationship between class management, students' motivation and the subsequent impact on their learning. The platform will allow the research team to provide a qualitative data analysis. Technology is no longer just a way of processing statistics and data, but it's an invaluable support for research. Teachers will find it useful to analyze their own class management skills and to share procedures, good practices and needs.

3   Research Kit: A Platform to Collect Data as Technical Tool for Research

Research Kit (http://researchkit.org) is an open source framework introduced by Apple that allows researchers and developers to create powerful apps for medical research. Easily create visual consent flows, real-time dynamic active tasks, and surveys using a variety of customizable modules that you can build upon and share with the community. And since Research Kit works seamlessly with Health Kit, researchers can access even more relevant data for their studies — like daily step counts, calorie use, and heart rate. The Research Kit platform will be used to collect data in order to create a database (or information repository). Up to now, similar repositories have only been available in the medical field.

In this study, access to the platform is granted through a dedicated application ("iNclusion") that will allow teachers to fill in the questionnaire, and researchers to process the data in real time. The easy-to-use application will allow teachers to reflect on their class management attitudes and their actions to foster learning.

CeDisMa Team can supervise data by way of platform:

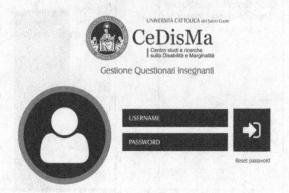

The researchers login into the platform and can have a general view about the users' feedback:

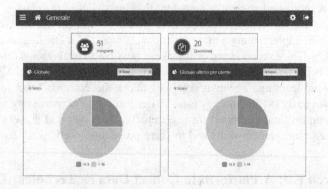

The researchers can view all questionnaires and survey response.

The Research Kit platform makes it possible to obtain more quantitative data and the questionnaire allows the Research Centre on Disability and Social Marginality to study how teachers teach and manage their classroom. The more the data, the more reliable is the study itself. As Apple confirmed at the platform launch, the Research Kit will allow researchers to focus more on their studies rather than losing too much time in adding and storing data. We can login to the platform to view, analyze and export the data collected. Since the App was launched on March 25th, 2016, the amount of available data is still limited.

4   iNclusion App: A Support for Teachers to Teach Inclusively, for Students to Really Learn

iNclusion App can promote:

– Actions and interventions to encourage well-being, supported by technology
– Technologies to support students' engagement in learning processes;
– Technologies to enhance the social well-being.

The App stresses the importance of creating a collaborative and profitable environment in order to enhance learn in the classroom. To do so, relationships (teachers-students, students- students, students- teachers) are unavoidable. Teachers can be a "good guide" [10] in the classroom but only if they are able to involve their students in the teaching-learning process, making them feel like actors, not like passive passersby. Technology, if used by good teachers, can act as a support to teach inclusively and can help students to learn more [3].

The questions of the questionnaire invite teachers to observe their classroom from a new prospective and manage it in the best way possible to allow progress.

Each single class needs to be considered as a community having its own special needs, points of view as well as its very own approach to learning. When teachers teach on the basis of the Universal design for learning, they can be inclusive [9]. When teachers teach with different approaches, planning their lessons keeping into account their classes' special needs, they promote the well-being of their own students. Thanks to the iNclusion App, teachers can think over their own strategies to improve the learning environment in the name of inclusion of all their students. The first tool they need to use to do so is of course observation.

During the teaching-learning process, teachers can observe but they are also active in this process. Therefore they need a tool to enable them to lead the most impartial analysis possible, even though they are part of the process itself and not mere observers.

iNclusion App can be a support for teachers to observe the learning process, and to manage their classes in a rational way.

During the collection of data, teachers can focus on:

– classroom management [11];
– relationships in the teaching-learning process [12];
– students' behaviour in the classroom [2];
– best practices to teach [15].

iNclusion App can support teachers to teach and manage the classroom in order to create a positive atmosphere in the classroom.

Well-being in classroom is possible if:

– students have a good relationship to each other and also to teachers;
– teachers are able to teach inclusively and to support students to avoid failure;
– teacher's classroom management supports the learning process and the establishment of relationships;
– teachers promote motivation to learn.

Teaching and learning should bring joy. Every child deserves a champion, an adult who will never give up on them, who understands the power of connection, and insists that they become the best that they can possibly be [13].

Thanks to a simple app, teachers will be able to think over important subjects such as inclusion and motivation. If students feel actively part of a lesson, they can learn better and more effectively. This can be possible if teachers are able select their methodology according to the single individuals they're teaching to. At moment data collected isn't too much, but the App is available from April 2016 and collection data started from 29 April 2016. However, feedback received (at moment) can support CeDisMa's thesis about the App' utility. During the data collection is also possible receive information about the critical element connected to the use and the efficacy of the App. iNclusion allows teacher to take part in the research, making their point and their need clear. Teachers are no more simple passive spectators or data readers, they have a chance to become proactive participants in research.

References

1. Booth, T., Ainscow, M.: Index for Inclusion: Developing Learning and Participation in Schools. CSIE, Bristol (2002). Revisited edition
2. Camaioni, L.: La teoria della mente. Laterza, Bari-Roma (2003)
3. Carruba, M.C.: Tecnologia e Disabilità. Pedagogia Speciale e Tecnologia per Un'inclusione Possibile. Pensa Multimedia, Lecce (2014)
4. Carruba, M.C.: Tecnologie per l'inclusione e la promozione del benessere a scuola. TD J **23** (3), 190–192 (2015)
5. d'Alonzo, L.: Come Fare per Gestire la Classe Nella Pratica Quotidiana. Giunti Scuola, Firenze (2012)
6. d'Alonzo, L.: La Gestione Della Classe. Modelli di Ricerca e Implicazioni per la Pratica. La Scuola, Brescia (2004)
7. Eccles, J.S., Wigfield, A.: Motivational beliefs, values and goals. Annu. Rev. Psychol. **53**(1), 109–132 (2002)
8. Evertson, C.M., Weinstein, C.S. (eds.): Handbook of Classroom Management: Research, Practice, and Contemporary Issues, pp. 1041–1062. Routledge Taylor & Francis Group, New York (2006)
9. Gargiulo, R.M., Metcalf, D.: Teaching in Today's Inclusive Classrooms: a Universal Design for learning. CENGAGE, Boston (2015)
10. Hopkins, D.: A Teachers Guide to Classroom Research. Open University Press, Berkshire, England; and Kounin, J.S, Discipline and Group Management in Classrooms, Krieger, Huntingont (1977)
11. Kanizsa, S.: Il Lavoro Educativo: l'importanza Della Relazione Nel Processo di Insegnamento-apprendimento. Bruno Mondadori, Milano (2007)
12. Pianta, R.C.: La relazione bamino-insegnante. TR. IT, Raffaello Cortina Editore, Milano (2001)
13. Pierson, R.: Every child needs a champion, [video]. In: TED Conference (2013). Retrieved https://www.ted.com/talks/rita_pierson_every_kid_needs_a_champion?language=it
14. Sing-Kong, L.: Toward a better future: education and training for economic development in Singapore, p. 187. The World Bank, Washington D.C. (2008)
15. Stone, R.: Best Practices for Teaching Social Studies: What Award-winning Classroom Teachers Do. Corwin Press, New York (2015)

Interacting with Videogames in Adolescence: Effects of Graphic Visualization on Perceived Presence and Visuospatial Competences

Luca Milani[✉], Stefano Ambrosioni, and Paola Di Blasio

Centre for Research on Developmental and Educational Dynamics (C.Ri.d.e.e.), Department of Psychology, Catholic University of Milan, Largo Gemelli 1, 20123 Milan, Italy
{luca.milani,paola.diblasio}@unicatt.it,
stefano.ambrosioni@hotmail.it

Abstract. The study here described had the aim of studying the effects of the interaction with videogames characterized by different modalities of graphic visualization (two-dimensional vs. three-dimensional) on presence and visuo-spatial competences. Participants were 129 adolescents (74 M and 55 F) aged 14–18 years old (mean of age = 16.11; SD = 1.31), recruited in a high school in Northern Italy. Participants were instructed to use for a week on their home PC a specific videogame and were divided in five experimental conditions: 2D Tetris, 3D Tetris, 2D Adventure, 3D Adventure, control. Videogames provided to participants were chosen so to have a continuum in terms of complexity of graphics, complexity of interaction possibilities and degree of immersivity. At the end of the week of playing with the given videogame, participants were administered specific checklists for measuring the degree of presence experimented during the interaction with the videogame and their visuo-spatial performance. This results show that there is a strong and direct correlation between the degree of complexity, immersivity and cognitive demands of videogames and the level of presence conveyed. Results also show that some of the visuo-spatial abilities are progressively and positively improved as the complexity of the graphic environment increases.

Keywords: Presence · Videogames · Visuo-spatial abilities · Graphic visualization · Immersivity

1 Introduction

Presence can be defined as a medium-related function, i.e. the perceptive illusion of *non-mediation*, in a context of mediated environment [1]. This effect is due to a cognitive disappearance of the medium from the conscious subjective experience [2].

The term "presence" in its present meaning was subject of scientific debate from 1992, when Sheridan [3] used it instead of "telepresence" as a result of the first experimental studies in the field of virtual reality applied to remote control of equipment. Differently from the early Nineties, nowadays most of virtual reality technology is used to generate environments to foster participation in socio-cognitive activities via

© ICST Institute for Computer Sciences, Social Informatics and Telecommunications Engineering 2017
K. Giokas et al. (Eds.): eHealth 2016, LNICST 181, pp. 183–189, 2017.
DOI: 10.1007/978-3-319-49655-9_25

interaction with a computer. The common ground is that the participant ceases to think about himself as interacting with a computer and starts to directly interact with the virtual environment. The virtual environment allows the participant to project his cognitive, perceptive and motor abilities in a simulated environment, and the feeling of presence is the consequence of a seamless and successful performing of an action in that environment [4, 5].

The similarity between the feedback to an action in the virtual environment and the real feedback to the same action in the real world is crucial in fostering a sense of presence. From a perceptual and cognitive point of view, the subject implicitly evaluates the contents of virtual environments in terms of opportunities and affordances: as the formers increase, the sense of presence is more likely to occur. The result of the increase in the sense of presence is a sort of paradoxical "invisibility" of the medium [6] and a sense of inseparability between the self and the virtual environment [7]. Presence has also a clear effect on emotions, in a "circular" path of mutual influence [8].

More recently, one of the most intriguing applications of virtual reality is the world of videogaming: modern videogames often can boast among the most sophisticated and complex virtual environments in the consumer market. The illusion of being in a synthesized virtual environment is maximised in the top productions, both from an aural and a visual point of view [9]. Modern videogames are generally characterized by very complex virtual environments in which the players can interact in many ways, and conceived to let the player have the impression that there are no boundaries and no limits to their exploration (e.g. the so-called "free roaming games").

Videogames are also one of the most widespread forms of entertainment among children and adolescents, and often represent the first mean of approach with the information technologies for the new generations. In the developmental psychology literature, videogames have been linked with potential negative effects such as increased aggression due to violent contents [10], addiction [11] and seizures [12]. The literature has also clearly pointed out that videogame play can exert significant positive effects in terms of cognitive processes, such as visuospatial abilities [13], problem-solving skills and inductive reasoning [14].

Given these findings, it appears of interest to link the study of presence to the strong literature on the effects of videogame use. A few researches studied the degree of graphical complexity of videogames in relation with the sense of presence. Ivory and Kalyanaraman [15] found that the improvement in terms of graphics between mid-1990s and 2003 games led to stronger sensations of presence in their participants. Bracken and Skalski [16] found similar results: undergraduates that played a high definition (HD) version of a modern videogame felt a stronger sense of presence than controls who played a standard definition (SD) version of the same videogame.

1.1 Aims of the Research

Moving from these results, the present study has the aim of deepening the knowledge about the effect of visualization on both the sense of presence conveyed by videogames and the visuo-spatial competences. Given the paradigmatic shift seen in the last 20 years in the videogame industry (i.e. the introduction of complex and real-time three-dimensional graphics), assessing the effects of the different types of visualization it is of some importance. This holds even truer when thinking about the learning potential embedded in videogames: choosing the "right" balance between immersion, presence and conveying of contents to be learned could be crucial in order to design videogames for learning purposes.

2   Materials and Methods

2.1   Participants

Participants were 129 students, aged 14–18 (mean = 16.11; SD = 1.31), recruited in a high school in Northern Italy. 74 (57.4%) participants were male and 55 (42.6%) female. No gender differences in terms of mean age were found at t test for independent samples (t = .88 ns).

2.2   Procedure

The research was approved by school managers and was proposed to students during curricular activities in their classrooms. Parents of the participants signed a written consent to allow their children to take part in the study. Participants were randomly assigned to five experimental conditions: 2D Tetris, 3D Tetris, 2D Adventure, 3D Adventure and control condition. No age differences were found between the five experimental conditions at ANOVA (F = .01 ns).

Participants were tested for visuospatial abilities with five subscales of the "Kit of Factor Referenced Cognitive Tests" [17], before they were given a CD-ROM containing a specific videogame (described below) and were asked to play with the provided videogame for a week on their home PCs. Participants were overtly asked to refrain from using other videogames during the week.

Videogames provided to participants were chosen so to have a continuum in terms of complexity of graphics, complexity of interaction possibilities and degree of immersivity, starting from 2D Tetris (the simplest) to 3D Adventure (the most complex):

- 2D Tetris: two-dimensional version of the classic Pazhitnov's 1984 puzzle game.
- 3D Tetris: three-dimensional version of Tetris, with a rotation of shapes in the three axes instead of one.
- 2D Adventure: for both the adventure conditions, the game "The Secret of Monkey Island" was chosen. Being an adventure videogame, the player need to solve puzzles in order to progress with the plot. The player interacts with the videogame via a two-dimensional interface, controlling a character and pointing with the mouse over various objects and characters and performing on them a fixed set of actions.
- 3D Adventure: participants assigned to this condition played with the fourth episode of the "Monkey Island" series. This episode shares the same adventure structure of the first episode but is displayed via a real time three-dimensional environment. The

player controls the character and performs actions via a combination of mouse and keyboard inputs.

The videogames were chosen in order to avoid any possible violent content and for their ease of play. Thus, there were two distinct features of variation in experimental conditions:

1. depth of interaction: Tetris provided limited interactive affordances, giving the repetitiveness of action, whereas the Adventure provided more complex problem-solving puzzles and a degree of free exploration;
2. visualization: 2D isometric representation of shapes and environments vs. 3D real time reconstruction of shapes and landscapes.

At the end of the week of training with the videogame, participants were re-assessed for visuo-spatial abilities and were administered the Italian version of the ITC-SOPI questionnaire [18] in order to assess the degree of presence experimented during the videogame play. Questionnaires were administered the day after the end of the one-week training with videogames, in order to make sure they had still a vivid recall of their gaming activity. Participants were also asked to state their previous experience with videogames in terms of mean of hours per week spent videogaming.

2.3 Measures

Visuo-spatial abilities were assessed prior and after the training with videogames by using five subscales of "Kit of Factor Referenced Cognitive Tests" [17]. The subscales administered were:

- Matrix of points (CF-3).
- Recognition of identical figures (P-3).
- Reconstruction of images (CS-1).
- Rotation of figures (S-1).
- Rotation of cubes (S-2).

Cronbach's alpha was .88.

In order to assess the degree of presence experimented by using the videogames provided, participants were administered a specific measure, the ITC-SOPI by Lessiter et al. [18]. The instrument specifically focuses upon the subjective experience when interacting with a medium, is comprised of 42 items on a 5-point likert scale.

The instrument provides four subscales, each measuring a distinct feature of presence:

- SP (physical space): measures the feeling of being physically placed in a virtual environment. This is related also to a personal evaluation of the sense of "being there".
- ENGAGE (engagement): measures the degree of subjective psychological engagement in the virtual experience.
- ECO (ecological validity): this subscale measures the overall appeal and believability of the environment and its content, and to perceive them as lifelike and real.

- NEG (negative effects): this subscale refers to potentially negative feedbacks from the interaction with the medium, such as dizziness, headaches, nausea.

Cronbach's Alpha of the ITC-SOPI was .97.

3 Results

We performed a MANOVA to compare the visuo-spatial performance before and after the experience with videogames, and the degree of presence conveyed by the different experimental condition. In order to precisely pinpoint the specific contribution of the experimental conditions on both visuospatial abilities and presence, we splitted the two facets of the experimental condition and inserted them as fixed factors: "visualization" (i.e. 2D vs. 3D), and "interaction" (i.e. high interaction, Adventure vs. low interaction, Tetris). To control for prior experience with videogames, we inserted the hours per week of videogames use as covariate. We found two significant main effects: one of visualization (Wilks' $\Lambda = .315$, $F = 7.74$, $p < .001$, multivariate $\eta2 = .685$) and one of interaction (Wilks' $\Lambda = .135$, $F = 22.76$, $p < .001$, multivariate $\eta2 = .865$). Interestingly, we found no significance for the combined effect visualization * interaction. As can be seen from Table 1 (only significant scores reported), follow-up ANOVAs indicate a clear and significant trend among the main facets of experimental conditions (interaction and visualization) as regards presence: the degree of presence steadily increased from the least immersive and interactive condition (2D Tetris) to the most immersive and interactive condition (3D Adventure). The experimental condition also has an effect on some of the visuospatial competences: CF-3 and S-1 subscales showed a clear increase from pre- to post-test, and the more complex and immersive the environment, the more increment was found. These results hold true regardless habitual experience with videogames (weekly hours were controlled as covariates).

Table 1. Differences between experimental conditions in terms of presence and visuo-spatial abilities.

Experimental condition mean scores					Variable	F	η	p
2D Tetris	3D Tetris	2D Adv.	3D Adv.	Control				
1.80	2.11	2.62	3.23	–	SP	76.38	.761	.001
2.59	2.86	3.54	3.83	–	ENGAGEMENT	44.66	.650	.001
1.47	2.18	2.35	3.02	–	ECO	80.07	.769	.001
1.50	1.35	1.54	1.59	–	NEG	2.82	.105	.05
20.26	21.42	20.23	22.11	20.47	CF-3 (pre-test)	2.72	.036	ns.
23.73	23.89	23.66	27.05	22.78	CF-3 (post-test)	4.10	.054	.05
43.36	44.36	38.71	48.00	40.96	S-1 (pre-test)	3.18	.042	ns.
47.73	49.36	44.42	53.61	45.54	S-1 (post-test)	4.08	.054	.05

4   Discussion

The aims of the research were to verify if the graphic visualization of the videogame could be related to the degree of presence experimented by the player and to an increase in visuospatial competences. Data show that participants who played the three-dimensional versions of the games felt a higher degree of presence than participants who played the two-dimensional versions.

Of more interest is that – regardless of graphic complexity – participants who played the adventure obtained higher scores in terms of presence than participants who played the puzzle game. This clearly calls into play the level of cognitive challenge and cognitive complexity of tasks as a key factor in the fostering of presence. Put in other words, the level of graphic complexity is only a part of the picture: it seems that the level of challenge in terms of cognitive skills is just as important as the formal properties of the graphics.

Nonetheless, the level of realism in terms of virtual environments is also a key factor, at least for the impression of being physically placed in a virtual environment. The more detailed and lifelike the graphics are, the more the subject gains the feeling of "being there". In our sample, this is clearly shown by the ICT-SOPI "SP" subscale: mean scores of the 3D Adventure experimental condition almost double those of 2D Tetris condition and are roughly the 20% higher than even the 2D Adventure condition. Regarding the "ENGAGE" subscale we can detect the same trend: players enjoyed the more detailed and vivid experience of both the Adventure experimental conditions over the more simple and less interactive gameplay of Tetris. If we consider the "ECO" subscale, data suggest that players felt the Adventure environments as more ecologically credible than the Tetris ones. This comes quite obvious since both Tetris are puzzle games whose objectives are not to recreate a fictional world. Finally, regarding the "NEG" subscale, none of the experimental conditions conveyed substantial uneasiness in the participants. Only the 3D Adventure causes a marginal discomfort, probably due to the difficulty to detect the "hotspots" (the areas where the player could interact with objects) in the environment. No instances of motion sickness were reported by participants.

Also, our results show that the level of presence and complexity of the videogame could have some effects also on the increase of visuo-spatial abilities. Our participants shown better performances in the task of completing matrices of points (CF-3) and mentally rotate shapes (S-1) after the training with videogames. The more complex the environment of the game (i.e. 3D Adventure), the more increase was found.

These results as a whole have significant spin-offs in terms of implications for educational software development. If we think at the growing educational potentiality of videogames in formal and informal education, being able to identify the optimal level of presence of an educational videogame could be crucial for adjusting the level of interaction to the appropriate learning goals.

On a second instance, assuming that the habitual experience with videogames is irrelevant in terms of presence could encourage to produce learning games without having to worry much about the steepness of the learning curve. Put in other words: provided the game is challenging both in terms of appearance and content, the cognitive feedback will be the roughly same regardless of the videogaming habits of the user.

References

1. Riva, G., Waterworth, J.A.: Presence and the Self: A cognitive neuroscience approach, Presence-Connect. 3 (2003). http://www8.informatik.umu.se/~jwworth/Riva-Waterworth.htm
2. Banos, R.M., Botella, C., Alcaniz, M., Liano, B.A., Guerrero, B., Rey, B.: Immersion and emotion: their impact on the sense of presence. Cyberpsychol. Behav. 7, 734–740 (2004)
3. Sheridan, T.B.: Musings on telepresence and virtual presence. Presence: Teleoper. Virtual Environ. 1, 120–126 (1992)
4. Draper, J.V., Kaber, D.B., Usher, J.M.: Speculations on the value of telepresence. Cyberpsychol. Behav. 2, 349–362 (1999)
5. Riva, G., Waterworth, J., Murray, D. (eds.): Interacting with Presence: HCI and the Sense of Presence in Computer-mediated Environments. Walter de Gruyter GmbH & Co KG, Berlin (2014)
6. Schuemie, M.J., Van der Straaten, P., Krijn, M., Van der Mast, C.A.P.G.: Research on presence in VR: a survey. Cyberpsychol. Behav. 4, 183–201 (2001)
7. Usoh, M., Alberto, C., Slater, M.: Presence: experiments in the psychology of virtual environments (1996). http://citeseer.nj.nec.com/did/61357
8. Riva, G., Mantovani, F., Capideville, C.S., Preziosa, A., Morganti, F., Villani, D., Alcañiz, M.: Affective interactions using virtual reality: the link between presence and emotions. CyberPsychol. Behav. 10(1), 45–56 (2007)
9. Riva, G., Davide, F., IJsselsteijn, W.A.: Being there: concepts, effects and measurements of user presence in synthetic environments. In: Riva, G., Davide, F. (eds.) Emerging Communication: Studies on New Technologies and Practices in Communication. Ios Press, Amstredam (2003)
10. Milani, L., Camisasca, E., Caravita, S.C., Ionio, C., Miragoli, S., Di Blasio, P.: Violent video games and children's aggressive behaviors. SAGE Open 5(3) (2015). Doi: 10.1177/2158244015599428
11. Petry, N.M., Rehbein, F., Gentile, D.A., Lemmens, J.S., Rumpf, H.J., Mößle, T., Auriacombe, M.: An international consensus for assessing internet gaming disorder using the new DSM-5 approach. Addiction 109(9), 1399–1406 (2014)
12. Ferrie, C.D., De Marco, P., Grunewald, R.A., Giannakodimos, S., Panayotopoulos, C.P.: Video game induced seizures. Neurol. Neurosurg. Psychiatry 57, 925–931 (1994)
13. Feng, J., Spence, I., Pratt, J.: Playing an action video game reduces gender differences in spatial cognition. Psychol. Sci. 18(10), 850–855 (2007)
14. Bartolomeo, A.: Il videogioco: uno strumento per "pensare". In: Bartolomeo, A., Caravita, S. (eds.) Il Bambino e i Videogiochi. Carlo Amore, Roma (2004)
15. Ivory, J.D., Kalyanaraman, S.: The effects of technological advancement and violent content in video games on players' feelings of presence, involvement, physiological arousal, and aggression. J. Commun. 57, 532–555 (2007)
16. Bracken, C.C., Skalski, P.: Telepresence and video games: the impact of image quality. PsychNology J. 7, 101–112 (2009)
17. Ekstrom, R., French, J., Harman, H., Dermen, D.: Kit of factor referenced cognitive tests. Educational Testing Service, Princeton (1976)
18. Lessiter, J., Freeman, J., Keogh, E., Davidoff, J.: A cross-media presence questionnaire: the ITC-sense of presence inventory. Presence: Teleoper. Virtual Environ. 10, 282–297 (2009)

HealthWear 2016

Use Moving Average Filter to Reduce Noises in Wearable PPG During Continuous Monitoring

Yan Chen, Dan Li$^{(\boxtimes)}$, Yanhai Li, Xiaoyuan Ma, and Jianming Wei

Shanghai Advanced Research Institute, Chinese Academy of Sciences,
No.99 Haike Road, Pudong, Shanghai, China
{cheny,lid,liyh,maxy,wjm}@sari.ac.cn

Abstract. In order to improve the accuracy of heart rate extracted from wearable photoplethysmography (PPG) signal, a new processing method based on moving average filtering is proposed. There are two cascaded moving average filters. The first filter is designed to remove baseline wandering as preprocessing. The second filter whose window size is adjusted according to the additional accelerometer signal is used to remove motion artifacts. During continuous monitoring, the parameters of these two filters change adaptively in accordance with a batch processing method. The results show that the proposed method can reconstruct a better waveform and improve the signal quality for calculating the beats per minute (BPM). Referenced with the vital sign monitoring instrument VS800 of Mindray company, the detecting accuracy of the proposed method is 7%–10% higher than adaptive filtering.

Keywords: Heart rate · PPG · Moving average

1 Introduction

With the wide application of wearable devices in the field of health care, the technology of heart rate detection based on PPG is developing rapidly. Wearable PPG technology, consisting of light emitting diode (LED) and photoelectric detector, provide a simple, low cost and noninvasive heart rate detection method [1]. Alternative measurement sites commonly include finger [2], wrist [3] and ear [4]. However, poor reliability and accuracy of heart rate detection bring problems to the practical application. It is mainly because of the motion artifact which is a noise aliasing in the clean PPG signal. In most cases, motion artifacts falls within the same frequency band as the physiological signal of interest [5]. Exercises, especially strenuous exercises (e.g., high leg lifting, quick running, etc.), damage the waveform seriously and affect the measurement of PPG's periodicity, which eventually lead to the error of heart rate.

Sweeny K.T., et al. [6] make a detailed analysis of current artifact removal techniques including adaptive filtering, wiener filtering, bayes filtering and blind source separation. An on-line and automatic processing technique is necessary for wearable devices. Han, H. and Kim J. [7] propose a least mean square based active noise cancellation method applied to accelerometer data to reduce periodical artifacts and

K. Giokas et al. (Eds.): eHealth 2016, LNICST 181, pp. 193–203, 2017.
DOI: 10.1007/978-3-319-49655-9_26

recover pulse from PPGs efficiently. Gibbs P.T., Wood L.B., and Asada H.H. [8] motivate a recursive least squares active noise cancellation technique using the MEMS accelerometer reading as an input for a FIR or Laguerre model. Lee B., et al. [9] use kalman smoother with simultaneous accelerometry to reduce motion artifacts from PPG signal. These filters calculate and update corresponding coefficients by sampling point. There is high time complexity in these algorithms and most of them are not able to remove burst noises during continuous monitoring perfectly.

We consider the ear is the best measurement site as there is no movable joints. We integrate LED, photoelectric sensor and accelerometer sensor into an earphone. In this paper, from the principle of PPG, we propose a simple model of the in-ear PPG signal and analyze different noise sources. Then we design two kind of moving average filters to reduce different noises from the actual PPG signal. This paper also puts forward a batch processing method to adjust the parameters of the filters as the heartbeat and motion state keep changing during continuos monitoring.

2 Analysis

2.1 Principle of PPG

Part of the incident light will be absorbed by vascular tissue, and the transmitted light intensity follows Lambert-Beer's law [10] which is the theoretical basis of understanding PPG:

$$I = I_0 \cdot exp(-KCL) \tag{1}$$

In formula (1), I_0 represents incident light intensity, K is the absorption coefficient which is only related to the physical properties of substances and wavelength of the incident light, C denotes the density, L is the optical path. While our light intensity in-ear photoelectric detector receives is:

$$I = I_1 + I_2 \cdot exp(-KCL) \tag{2}$$

I_1 is the part of light reflected directly. I_2 is the light irradiation to skin, muscle and blood vessel. Ideally, the acquired result only changes with the vascular pulsation caused by heart beats, so PPG waveform is an alternating component (AC) superimposed on a direct-current component (DC). Actually, respiratory, nervous sympathetic activity and body temperature changes can cause a slow change of the baseline [11]. The muscle will be squeezed during motion state which will also affect the optical path. The actual light intensity is:

$$\begin{aligned} I &= I_1 + \Delta I + I_2 \cdot exp[-KC(L + \Delta L)] \\ &= I_1 + \Delta I + I_2 \cdot exp(-KCL) \cdot [exp(-\Delta L) - 1 + 1] \end{aligned} \tag{3}$$

Where ΔI represents the change of baseline which is called baseline wandering, ΔL represents the change of optical path caused by vascular pulsation and muscle squeeze. As ΔL is extremely little, our PPG signal can be shown as:

$$S = S_0 + \Delta S - S_1 \cdot \Delta L_1 - S_2 \cdot \Delta L_2 \tag{4}$$

Where S_0 is the baseline signal, ΔS is the baseline wandering signal, $S_1 \cdot \Delta L_1$ is the desired signal, and $S_2 \cdot \Delta L_2$ is the motion artifact signal. In order to study the change of motion artifacts signal, we add an accelerometer sensor into the sensing unit.

2.2 Actual PPG Signal

Before proceeding further discussion, it is necessary to check the actual signal waveform. Figure 1 shows a period of actually acquired signal including three axis accelerometer signals and photoelectric signal. The sampling rates are both 62.5 Hz. In order, the motion state is standing, running and standing. From the beginning to the end, the photoelectric signal waveform has a gentle wandering which is called baseline wandering noise. During the running state, the morphology of PPG signal is corrupted seriously as motion artifacts noise exits.

Through Fourier analysis, according to the amplitude spectrum figure, we find that the frequency of motion artifacts is similar to accelerometer signals which is pointed out by Zhang Z.L. [12]. As x axis is the major factor in this case, we only show its amplitude spectrum figure. In Fig. 2, the green arrows pointing at about 2 Hz are motion artifacts, the black arrow nearby 0 Hz represents the baseline wandering and the red arrow neighbouring 1 Hz is the frequency of hear rate we desired. Of course, motion artifacts noise has different forms in different motion states. This rhythmic motion artifact most severely affects the heart rate detection, as it destroys the periodicity and morphology of the PPG signal. In other cases, random irregular motions leading the PPG signal shake suddenly and randomly will also affect the estimated period.

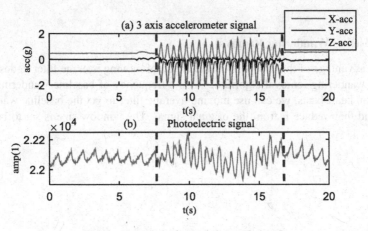

Fig. 1. A period of actual detected signal.

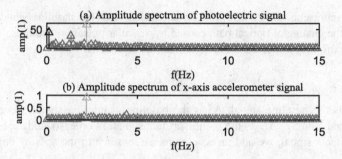

Fig. 2. Fourier analysis of the photoelectric signal and accelerometer signal of Fig. 1 in the running state. (Color figure online)

3 Algorithm

It is known that moving average filter with narrow window has a smoothing effect on the signal and the moving average filter with wide window can get the general trend of a signal. That means we can reduce abrupt motion artifacts noise and get the baseline signal in the actual PPG signal through moving average filtering. Now some previous works present that moving average filter is very useful to remove high-frequency noise and intermittent motion artifact. It can reduce effects of mutations on the PPG signal waveform [13]. However, it is difficult to remove a large amplitude motion artifact, and the higher the filter order, the worse the quality of the waveform [14]. We take advantage of the most simple moving average filter:

$$y[n] = \frac{1}{N} \sum_{i=0}^{N-1} (x[n-i]), n = N, N+1, \ldots, L \tag{5}$$

Where N is the widow size and L is the data length. We design two filters to reduce noises in the original signal utilizing the different characteristics of moving average filtering.

3.1 Baseline Wandering Removal

We take advantage of the low-pass characteristic of moving average filter to design the baseline wandering removal algorithm. As the frequency of baseline wandering is far lower than heart beats, we can use moving average filter to get the baseline wandering signal and then reduce it from the original signal. The window size is set to be:

$$N_{BW\_} = \frac{N_S \cdot 60}{BPM} \tag{6}$$

In formula (7), N_S is the number of sampling points per second. The output signal with base wandering removal $S_{BW\_}$ is acquired as following steps:

Step 1. Get a temperate baseline wandering signal BW_{tmp} from the original signal S using moving average filter (MAF) with window size $N_{BW\_}$:

$$BW_{tmp} = MAF(S, N_{BW\_}) \tag{7}$$

Step 2. To compensate for the lost data and get the complete baseline wandering signal BW:

$$\begin{cases} BW[1:P] = BW_{tmp}[1:P] + BW_{tmp}[1] - BW_{tmp}[P+1] \\ BW[P+1:Q] = BW_{tmp} \\ BW[Q+1:L] = BW_{tmp}[Q - N_{BW\_}:Q-P] + BW_{tmp}[Q-P] \\ \qquad\qquad - BW_{tmp}[Q - N_{BW\_} - 1] \end{cases} \tag{8}$$

where $P = \begin{cases} \frac{N_{BW\_} - 1}{2}, N_{BW}\_ is\ odd \\ \frac{N_{BW\_}}{2}, N_{BW}\_ is\ even \end{cases}$, and $Q = L - N_{BW\_} + P + 1$.

Step 3. Subtract the baseline wandering signal from the original signal:

$$S_{BW\_} = S - BW \tag{9}$$

3.2 Motion Artifact Removal

After removal of baseline wandering, we need to remove the motion artifacts. As moving average filter has a perfect inhibition of the signal near the cut-off frequency, we can reduce rhythmic motion artifacts by moving average filter with window size $N_{MA\_}$. $N_{MA\_}$ is the cycle of motion artifacts in discrete domain. If the motion artifact is irregular, then $N_{MA\_}$ can be set as a constant to smooth the signal. The motion artifact removal algorithm is described specifically as following:

Step 1. From the normalized auto correlation function (NACF) [15] of accelerometer signal, determine whether there is rhythmic motion artifact or not. If the peak value of NACF is larger than the setting threshold, the rhythmic motion artifact exits and set the peak point as $N_{MA\_}$. If the peak value is lower than the setting threshold, $N_{MA\_}$ is set to be a constant.

Step 2. Get a temperate signal Y_{tmp} without motion artifacts using MAF with window size of $N_{MA\_}$:

$$Y_{tmp} = MAF(S_{BW\_}, N_{MA\_}) \tag{10}$$

Step 3. Estimate the period T of Y_{tmp} in the discrete domain by average magnitude difference function (AMDF) [16]. And the result of BPM detection is $BPM = N_s \cdot 60/T$.

Step 4. To compensate for the lost data and get the complete signal with amplitude suppressed Y.

$$\begin{cases} Y[1:\mu] = Y_{tmp}[T-\mu:T-1] \\ Y[\mu+1:\tau] = Y_{tmp} \\ Y[\tau+1:L] = Y_{tmp}[\tau-\mu-T+2:L-\mu-T+1] \end{cases} \quad (11)$$

Where $\mu = \begin{cases} \frac{N_{MA\_}-1}{2}, N_{MA\_} \text{ is odd} \\ \frac{N_{MA\_}}{2}, N_{MA\_} \text{ is even} \end{cases}$, $\tau = L - N_{MA\_} + \mu + 1$.

Step 5. To compensate for the amplitude attenuation and get the reconstructed signal S_R:

$$S_R = Y/A(x) \quad (12)$$

Where $A(x) = x^3 - 2x^2 + 1, x = \frac{N_{MA}}{T}$. $A(x)$ is acquired by curve fitting from the amplitude-frequency curve of moving average filter.

3.3 Dynamic Monitoring

Because of continuous changes of motion state and heartbeat in the long-time monitoring, the coefficients of moving average filters need to be changed relatively in order to remove motion artifacts more effectively and improve the accuracy of BPM detection. The flow chart of the whole algorithm is shown as Fig. 3 where $MAF_{BW\_}$ is the baseline wandering removal algorithm and $MAF_{MA\_}$ is the motion artifact removal algorithm. We call this method as batch processing method. We select 3–4 s data as a batch and set $N_{BW\_}$ in the next batch to be T in the current batch (except initialization in the first batch). We assume heart beats cannot change suddenly in 3–4 s.

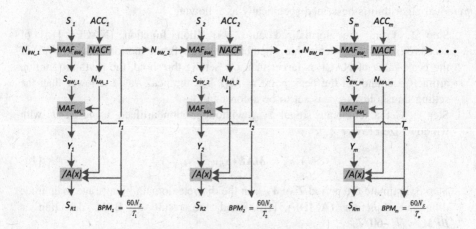

Fig. 3. Batch processing method of dynamic monitoring.

4   Results

Firstly, we collect the photoelectric signal and accelerometer signal in different rhythmic motion states those will affect in-ear PPG signal to improve the artifacts existence criterion. Figure 4 simply shows the data under 6 common condition in daily life. The tester wears the heart rate detecting earphone and makes the corresponding action according to the instruction in order. The earphone can transport data out by bluetooth connecting. As long as there is rhythmic motion artifact in the PPG signal, the accelerometer signal has the similar rhythm. Conversely, we cannot determine whether the rhythmic motion artifact exits or not when the accelerometer has a rhythmic. So in the Step.1 of motion artifact removal algorithm, the sum amplitude of 3-axis accelerometer should be taken into consideration. We set two thresholds when we estimate the coefficient $N_{MA\_}$. $N_{MA\_}$ is set to be the period of accelerometer signal only when the sum amplitude of all three axis is larger than the first threshold and the peak value of NACF is larger than the second threshold. During continuous monitoring, when the point of NACF is less than the previous T, $N_{MA\_}$ is set to be the period of accelerometer signal. In other cases, $N_{MA\_}$ is set to be a constant. Table 1 shows the accelerometer data analysis under the 6 common states. After a lot of experiments, in this paper our first threshold is 3 g, the second is 0.5 and the constant is 7 (about 9 Hz).

Secondly, we select the worst signal acquired in the high leg lifting case to verify the effectiveness of base wandering removal algorithm $MAF_{BW\_}$ and motion artifact removal algorithm $MAF_{MA\_}$. As shown in Fig. 5, we intercept 500 points of the data acquired during rapid leg lifting. In Fig. 5(b), $N_{BW\_}$ is assigned to be 63 as sampling rate is 62.5 Hz and heart rate is commonly 1 Hz. We calculate the amplitude of the baseline BW. BW is reduced from 439.92 to 23.83. As the sum amplitude of 3-axis accelerometer signal is larger than 3 g and from the NACF of y-axis accelerometer signal as shown in Fig. 6(a) we set $N_{MA\_}$ to be 11. Then from the AMDF of the

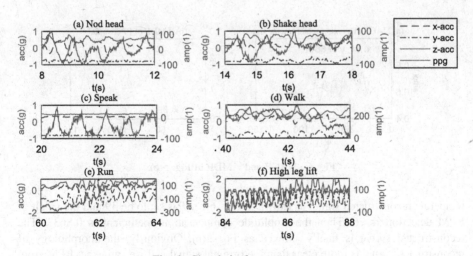

Fig. 4. Signals in 6 common cases.

Table 1. Accelerometer data analysis in 6 common cases.

Cases	AMP ACC/g			SUM of ACC/g	NACF of MAX[X,Y,Z]	
	X	Y	Z		Point	Value
Nod	1.0469	0.2969	0.4844	1.8282	44	0.5793
Shake	0.6094	0.3906	0.7813	1.7813	67	0.5632
Speak	0.1875	0.0781	0.0938	0.3594	92	0.1581
Walk	0.6875	0.7031	0.5938	1.9844	36	0.6513
Run	*1.1719*	*1.8281*	*1.4688*	*4.4688*	*17*	*0.5291*
High Leg lift	*1.5781*	*2.1875*	*1.1563*	*4.9219*	*11*	*0.6298*

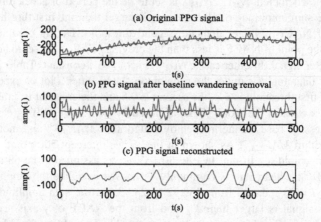

Fig. 5. Result of baseline wandering removal and motion artifact removal.

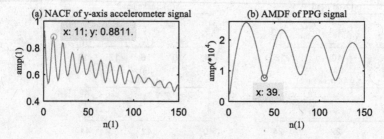

Fig. 6. NACF and AMDF in Fig. 5(c).

temperate reconstructed signal as shown in Fig. 6(b), T is set to be 39 and the result of BPM detection is 96. Then the amplitude compensation coefficient is 0.8633. The reconstructed signal is finally showed as Fig. 5(c). Obviously, the morphology of reconstructed signal is more clear than the original signal and we can exact BPM from it accurately.

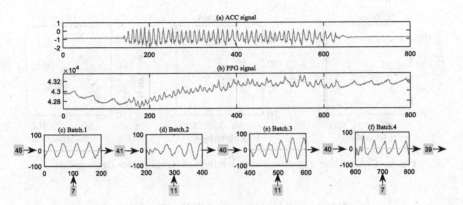

Fig. 7. Result of dynamic monitoring.

Thirdly, we select 200 points data as a batch and the batch processing result is shown in Fig. 7, where x label is discrete sequence, y label is amplitude. The right arrow represents $N_{BW\_}$ from the current batch to the next. The up arrow represents $N_{MA\_}$ determined from the current accelerometer signal. However, the motion artifacts cannot exactly start at the beginning of one batch and finish at the end of one batch, so in Fig. 7(d) and (f) there are a little distortion in the signals. The distortion will not affect the accuracy of BPM estimation.

Finally, we make a comparative experiment between the proposed algorithm and adaptive filtering referenced with a medical instrument VS800, which is a vital sign monitoring product of Mindray company. We record the time and BPM on the display screen of VS800 by video. Tester wears our device with his finger clipped by the VS800's probe and does some daily life actions during 10 min. We collect our device's data to a computer whose time is synchronized with the VS800 and process the signal by different algorithms simutaneously. NLMS is shown as formula (13):

$$\begin{cases} y = H \cdot \omega^T \\ e = x - y \\ H = H + \frac{\alpha}{\beta + \omega \cdot \omega^T} \cdot e \cdot \omega \end{cases} \tag{13}$$

RLS recursion equations can is obtained as formula (14):

$$\begin{cases} g = \left(\frac{P \cdot \omega^T}{\delta + \omega \cdot P \cdot \omega^T} \right)^T \\ y = H \cdot \omega^T \\ e = x - y \\ H = H + g \cdot e \\ P = \frac{1}{\delta}(P - g \cdot \omega^T \cdot P) \end{cases} \tag{14}$$

The result of the BPM detected is shown in Fig. 8 whose y label is detecting BPM and x label is reference BPM. The red crosses are out of the interval ±5 bpm and blue cycles are in the interval. The detecting accuracy of the proposed method is the highest and 7%–10% higher than adaptive filtering. The statistical analysis of the result is

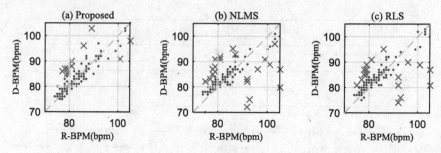

Fig. 8. Comparative experiment with a reference signal (Color figure online)

Table 2. Statistical analysis of the result in Fig. 8.

Algorithm	Accuracy/%	MSE	SROCC	PROCC	PLCC
Proposed	*91.67*	*5.2091*	*0.8659*	*0.7318*	*0.8851*
NLMS	80.83	6.3608	0.7103	0.5918	0.6368
RLS	84.17	5.6436	0.7253	0.6066	0.7085

shown in Table 2. SROCC is spearman rank order correlation coefficient. KROCC is kendall rank order correlation coefficient. PLCC is pearson linear correlation coefficient. The statistical result indicates that the BPM detected by the proposed algorithm is more accurate and has a stronger correlation to the reference BPM.

5   Conclusion

In this paper, with additional accelerometer, we propose algorithms based on moving average filtering which effectively remove noises of base wandering and motion artifacts in ear PPG signal. During continuous monitoring, the coefficients of filters adaptively change through a batch processing method. We can reconstruct better waveform from the corrupted original signal and improve the accuracy of BPM detection.

References

1. Tamura, T., et al.: Wearable photoplethysmographic sensors—past and present. Electronics **3**(2), 282–302 (2014)
2. Millasseau, S.C., et al.: Contour analysis of the photoplethysmographic pulse measured at the finger. J. Hypertens. **24**(8), 1449–1456 (2006)
3. Lee, Y., et al.: Development of a wristwatch-type PPG array sensor module. In: 2011 IEEE International Conference on Consumer Electronics-Berlin (ICCE-Berlin) (2011)
4. Budidha, K., Kyriacou, P.A.: The human ear canal: investigation of its suitability for monitoring photoplethysmographs and arterial oxygen saturation. Physiol. Meas. **35**(2), 111–128 (2014)

5. Ming-Zher, P., Swenson, N.C., Picard, R.W.: Motion-tolerant magnetic earring sensor and wireless earpiece for wearable photoplethysmography. IEEE Trans. Inf. Technol. Biomed. **14**(3), 786–794 (2010). A Publication of the IEEE Engineering in Medicine & Biology Society

6. Sweeney, K.T., et al.: Artifact removal in physiological signals-practices and possibilities. IEEE Trans. Inf Technol. Biomed. **16**(3), 488–500 (2012). A Publication of the IEEE Engineering in Medicine & Biology Society

7. Han, H., Kim, J.: Artifacts in wearable photoplethysmographs during daily life motions and their reduction with least mean square based active noise cancellation method. Comput. Biol. Med. **42**(4), 387–393 (2011)

8. Gibbs, P.T., Wood, L.B., Asada, H.H.: Active motion artifact cancellation for wearable health monitoring sensors using collocated MEMS accelerometers. In: Proceedings of SPIE - The International Society for Optical Engineering, vol. 5765, pp. 811–819 (2005)

9. Lee, B., et al.: Improved elimination of motion artifacts from a photoplethysmographic signal using a Kalman smoother with simultaneous accelerometry. Physiol. Meas. **31**(12), 1585–1603 (2010)

10. Shi Ping, Y.H.: Principles of photoplethysmography and its applications in physiological measurements. J. Biomed. Eng. **30**(4), 899–904 (2013)

11. Allen, J.: Photoplethysmography and its application in clinical physiological measurement. Physiol. Meas. **28**(3), R1–39 (2007)

12. Zhang, Z.: Photoplethysmography-based heart rate monitoring in physical activities via joint sparse spectrum reconstruction. IEEE Trans. Biomed. Eng. **62**(8), 1902–1910 (2015)

13. Lee, J.: Motion artifacts reduction from PPG using cyclic moving average filter. Technol. Health Care Official J. Eur. Soc. Eng. Med. **22**(3), 409–417 (2014)

14. Lee, H.W., et al.: The periodic moving average filter for removing motion artifacts from PPG signals. Int. J. Control Autom. Syst. **5**(6), 701–706 (2007)

15. Yousefi, R., Nourani, M., Panahi, I.: Adaptive cancellation of motion artifact in wearable biosensors. In: Conference: International Conference of the IEEE Engineering in Medicine & Biology Society IEEE Engineering in Medicine & Biology Society Conference (2012)

16. Hui, L., Dai, B.Q., Wei, L.: A pitch detection algorithm based on AMDF and ACF. In: IEEE International Conference on Acoustics (2006)

Effective Prognosis Using Wireless Multi-sensors for Remote Healthcare Service

Rahul Krishnan Pathinarupothi[1(✉)] and Ekanath Rangan[2]

[1] Amrita Center for Wireless Networks and Applications,
Amrita School of Engineering, Amrita Vishwa Vidyapeetham, Amritapuri, India
rahulkrishnan@am.amrita.edu
[2] School of Medicine, Amrita Institute of Medical Sciences,
Amrita Vishwa Vidyapeetham, Kochi, India

Abstract. Remote healthcare delivery is one of the most promising solutions to tackle global trends in falling health care access and quality of service. A wireless network of sensors, IoT devices, and cloud is presented here. New innovative algorithms for effective prognosis are designed and developed based on motifs and profile matrices. The system consisting of the sensor network and algorithms together enable delivering remote healthcare services.

Keywords: Body sensor network · Sensor data summarization · Consensus abnormal motif

1 Introduction

Telemedicine and remote health monitoring are gaining attention in ensuring better access to quality healthcare services for the growing population. The use of body sensors for vitals monitoring has gained large scale acceptance with the high proliferation of smartphones. The physiological parameters such as blood pressure (BP), blood glucose, oxygen saturation (SpO2), electrocardiogram (ECG) etc. are monitored, processed and send from the smartphone for further analysis to doctors in remote hospitals, where they can suggest interventions. Though such innovations are of great benefit to patients, it increases the load on the doctors, technicians and nurses. To obtain a fast and accurate summarization of huge amount of sensor data is still an open challenge. Some of the earlier works on data summarization [1,2] focused on quantizing continuous time series data into most frequently occurring patterns that they call motif. There has been recent work [3] where sensor data summarization has been used to identify abnormal activities from prior experience database for monitoring people in old age homes. However, the challenge of identifying abnormal motifs has not been explored much for multi-sensor time series data.

Working in collaboration with medical practitioners we have developed a novel express data summarization technique specifically designed for large scale sensor based healthcare monitoring applications. This is achieved by identifying

© ICST Institute for Computer Sciences, Social Informatics and Telecommunications Engineering 2017
K. Giokas et al. (Eds.): eHealth 2016, LNICST 181, pp. 204–207, 2017.
DOI: 10.1007/978-3-319-49655-9_27

what we call *Consensus Abnormality Motif* (CAM) that represents the most frequent deviations from the normal values. In the following sections, we present a formal model and evaluation of this summarization technique.

2   Multi-sensor Architecture

We consider N physiological sensors attached to a patient as shown in Fig. 1. The data is first quantized into K finite severity levels by the severity quantizer. Each sensor value is quantized as A_n++, A_n+, A_n, A_n-, A_n--, etc., where n represents the sensor type while the symbols + and - represents above-normal and sub-normal severity levels in comparison to the normal value. For instance, A represents normal range of values, A+++ represents higher than normal, while A— suggests subnormal level. It may be noted that the number of severity levels, K, depends upon the type of sensors too. It might be easier to visualize this as a matrix where the columns represent time-ordered tuple of quantized sensor values (A_1^t+, A_1^{t+1}, A_1^{t+2} etc.) and rows represent values from different sensors during the same time. This matrix is passed to the multiplexer to form a multi-sensor matrix (MSM) in which temporally related values from different sensors are sequentially arranged, while preserving the synchronous ordering of sensors. For example, the first two rows in the MSM represents the quantized values for time t and t+1 as: A_1^t+, A_2^t,..., A_n^t-- and $A_1^{t+1}+$, A_2^{t+1},..., $A_n^{t+1}--$. The output of the MUX is fed to the Physician Assist Filter (PAF) which helps in CAM discovery and analysis. The PAF-CAM engine has three functionalities, namely: PAF-CAM pre-processing, PAF-CAM discovery and PAF-CAM alerting engine. These form the basic building blocks for the smart summarization technique that we describe next.

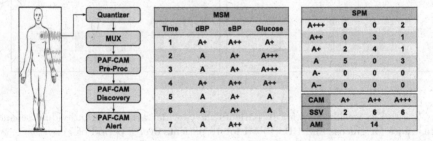

Fig. 1. Smart Summarization and analytics architecture based on PAF-CAM technique.

3   Smart Summarization

In the first part of the PAF-CAM pipeline, i.e., the pre-processing engine, each column of MSM is analysed to calculate the weighted-frequency of occurrence of each symbol and is used to derive the Severity Profile Matrix (SPM). Suppose a predefined weight w_n^k is assigned for the kth severity level of nth sensor, and the frequency of occurrence of a symbol A_n^t is f_n^k, then the $(k,n)^{th}$ element of SPM would be $w_n^k * f_n^k$. After forming the SPM, PAF-CAM discovery engine calculates the Consensus Abnormal Motif, which is a collection of symbols that summarizes the severity level of the nth sensor data over a time duration of D. The CAM is calculated by comparing the weighted-frequencies in the SPM along a column and then assigning the corresponding CAM as the symbol having the highest value. In effect, CAM also removes fluctuations in the sensor signals since the CAM is dominated by the highest frequency component parameterized by the severity. This makes CAM an error resilient summarization technique thereby providing the doctors with reliable and relevant data. The next module in the PAF-CAM pipeline is the alerting engine that calculates a Sensor Severity Value (SSV) which is the highest $w_n^k * f_n^k$ value for the nth sensor. The SSV represents the summarized severity level of a given sensor data over a time duration D. Furthermore, we calculate an Alert Measure Index (AMI), which is an aggregate score that represents the combined severity of all sensors and is used to classify the patients severity level. Based on AMI, the PAF-CAM alerting engine alerts the doctors and caregivers if the values are above a preset threshold.

$$AMI = \sum_{i=1}^{n} max(w_i^k * f_i^k) \tag{1}$$

In the following section, we describe how we have used this method to identify patients requiring urgent attention in remote healthcare monitoring.

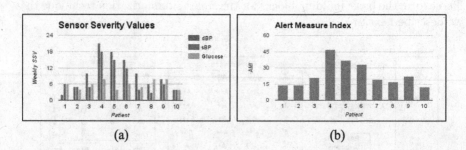

(a)   (b)

Fig. 2. (a) The weekly SSV for 10 patients shows wide variation in individual sensor data values for glucose and BP. (b) MI for 10 patients over a period of 7 days.

4   Evaluation and Results

We obtained the vitals data of ten patients from an anonymized patient database that included systolic blood pressure (sBP), diastolic blood pressure (dBP) and blood glucose levels over a seven day monitoring period. Each day of data consists of one reading for sBP, dBP and fasting glucose. Here, variables N = 3 and D = 7 days were used. We assumed k = 6; with A+++, A++, A+, A (normal), A- and

A–. For each sensor, the individual range for each symbol was decided based on known levels of severity. For the calculation of SPM, the weights w_n^k used were: A+++ (3), A++ (2), A+ (1), A (0), A- (1), A– (2). The zero weighted normal values ensure that only abnormalities are detected from the SPM. After deriving the SPM, the corresponding CAM, SSV and AMI were calculated. Figure 2 (a) shows the weekly SSV for all the patients. The normal value would be zero and hence a deviation from the baseline shows higher severity. Figure 2 (b) shows the AMI for all the ten patients. It can also be observed that the effect of individual SSVs are very evident in the overall AMI. We can infer from these results that patient 4 shows unusually high severity level while 5, 6 are in the higher range. Most of the other patients in this study showed higher than normal AMI, though it is at least two times less severe than patients 4, 5 and 6. This technique of classifying patients based on their severity level would prove highly useful for doctors, nurses and technicians, who would otherwise have to identify the most severe signs of a patient by going through a huge amount of data. Though these are early results from PAF-CAM technique, we believe that the simplicity and usability of this can be extended to many other areas of prognosis too.

5 Conclusion

We have presented initial work towards the development of a fast, effective and usable prognosis support technique using consensus abnormal motifs. The physician assist filters help in summarization of large amount of sensor data into insightful prognosis-supporting reports that can reduce the work load on doctors. In the near future, we intend to use the PAF-CAM algorithm to identify CAMs for known disease conditions to help in CAM matching. We also believe that the area of medical data summarization will gain further momentum as we head towards large scale deployment of remote monitoring systems.

References

1. Chiu, B., Keogh, E., Lonardi, S.: Probabilistic discovery of time series motifs. In: Proceedings of the Ninth ACM SIGKDD International Conference on Knowledge Discovery and Data Mining, pp. 493–498. ACM (2003)
2. Lonardi, J., Patel, P.: Finding motifs in time series. In: Proceedings of the 2nd Workshop on Temporal Data Mining, pp. 53–68 (2002)
3. Hajihashemi, Z., Popescu, M.: Early illness recognition using frequent motif discovery. In: Proceedings of Annual International Conference of the IEEE Engineering in Medicine and Biology Society, pp. 3699–3702. IEEE (2015)

Qualitative Study of Surgeons Using a Wearable Personal Assistant in Surgeries and Ward Rounds

Shahram Jalaliniya[✉] and Thomas Pederson

IT University of Copenhagen, Copenhagen, Denmark
{jsha,tped}@itu.dk

Abstract. In this paper, we report on the utility of a wearable personal assistant (WPA) for orthopedic surgeons in hospitals. A prototype of the WPA was developed on the Google Glass platform for supporting surgeons in three different scenarios: (1) touch-less interaction with medical images in surgery room, (2) tele-presence colleague consultation during surgeries, and (3) mobile access to the Electronic Patient Records (EPR) during ward rounds. We evaluated the system in a simulation facility of a hospital with two real orthopedic surgeons. The results of our study showed that while the WPA can be a viable solution for touch-less interaction with medical images and remote collaborations during surgeries, using the WPA in the ward rounds can have a negative impact on social interaction between surgeons and patients.

Keywords: Wearable Personal Assistant · Google Glass · Hospital work

1 Introduction

Mobility is one of the main characteristics of work in hospitals. Due to the spatial distribution of departments, wards, and offices in clinical settings, clinicians need to move between different departments all the time. Aside from the considerable time that clinicians waste on moving in hospitals, having access to the right information in different situations is a big challenge. The majority of previous work on providing remote access to the patient information have used mobile devices (e.g. PDAs and smartphones). However, most mobile devices do not support interaction on the move, which means the users need to stop, pick up their device, and direct their attention away from the task at hand [1]. This way of interaction often requires the user's full attention and occupies at least one hand which most of the time interferes with the task at hand. Furthermore, interaction with the dominant touchscreen-based mobile devices does not comply with sterility restrictions in hospitals. Emerging new generation of eyewear computers e.g. Google Glass that provide various hands-free input modalities (e.g. head motion and voice commands), raises the question as to whether this new platform can address some of the challenges of interaction on the move.

© ICST Institute for Computer Sciences, Social Informatics and Telecommunications Engineering 2017
K. Giokas et al. (Eds.): eHealth 2016, LNICST 181, pp. 208–219, 2017.
DOI: 10.1007/978-3-319-49655-9_28

What are the potential advantages and limitations of using such devices in hospitals? To answer these questions, we implemented and evaluated a wearable personal assistant (WPA) for orthopedic surgeons based on a previous study on design of wearable personal assistants for surgeons [2]. Our WPA supports three specific tasks throughout a workday of surgeons: (1) touch-less interaction with medical images, (2) tele-presence during surgeries, and (3) mobile access to the Electronic Patient Records (EPR) during ward rounds.

2   Related Work

2.1   Early Wearable Assistants for Clinicians

The first generation of wearable computers for hospital work domain [3–7] comprised a head mounted display (HMD), a microphone and earphone for vocal interaction, a compact processing unit connected to a wireless network, and other peripherals such as wrist-mounted keyboards, trackball mice, and etc. RNPSS [3] was one of the first wearable systems for clinicians. The main goal of this system was to decrease the medical errors of nurses. A similar project [6] was done to support nurses in home care tasks. Supporting physicians in ward rounds was another application for the early wearable assistants [4]. The ward round system supported hand gesture interaction using inertial sensors [4] and conductive textile sensor [8]. These initial prototypes of wearable assistant for clinicians increased hopes for using wearable computers in practice, but due to the technical, social, and usability challenges [9] those system never took off.

2.2   Using Google Glass in Healthcare

In [10], an expert surgeon provided guidance to a local surgeon over distance. The guidance was provided through vocal communication and the image of the remote surgeon's hand was superimposed on the live view of the surgical site on the Google Glass HMD. This study showed some problems with battery life, audio and image quality, and difference between camera view and the surgeon view. In another study [11], Google Glass was used to retrieve similar medical cases by sending a picture and relevant keywords to a remote server. In this paper, similar technical issues were reported such as limited battery life, unstable WIFI connection, lack of auto-focus functionality, which decreases the quality of the pictures. Muensterer et al. [12] showed the utility of the Google Glass for hands-free photo and video recordings, hands-free calls, looking up billing codes, and searching for unfamiliar medical terms in a hospital. The feasibility of using Google Glass for monitoring patient's vital signs in the surgeon's eye was investigated by Vorraber et al. [13]. Their study showed that using Google Glass decreases head and neck movements of the surgeon and increases the surgeon's focus on the operation. They reported over-heating problems of the Google Glass in addition to the other technical issues. While previous work has focused on the technical feasibility of using Google Glass in healthcare scenarios, our focus here is on human-computer interaction challenges emerging from using the device as a wearable assistant in hospitals.

In the work presented in this paper we investigate the ecological validity of the WPA design explained in more detail elsewhere [2] by asking real orthopedic surgeons use the WPA in a clinical simulation.

3   Method

Since deploying the WPA in a real clinical setting needs legal approval, we evaluated the WPA in a clinical simulation facility. Such simulations is common and have been proven efficient in the medical work domain [14]. Our simulation facility includes different hospital departments from patient wards to surgery rooms. We set up the facility for the above-mentioned three scenarios. The touch-less interaction and tele-presence scenarios were played out in the surgery room (see Fig. 1b), and for the mobile access to the EPR scenario we set up a patient room with two beds (see Fig. 1a).

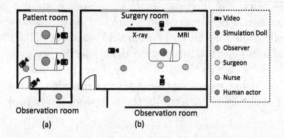

Fig. 1. (a) The simulation setup for the ward round scenario. The room is equipped with hidden cameras, microphones, and an observation room behind a one-way mirror. (b) The simulation surgery room for touch-less interaction and tele-presence scenarios is equipped with surgical equipments, a simulation doll connected to a monitor displaying simulated vital signs, and two large screens for displaying X-rays and Magnetic Resonance Images (MRIs).

3.1   Participants

During a full day simulation, two orthopedic surgeons, a senior nurse, and two human actors (to play the role of patients) participated in the study. Since surgeons are extremely busy and hard to recruit for such studies we could manage to find only two surgeons. This is a big limitation for finding statistical significance; therefore, we only rely on qualitative findings from interviews and observations. The entire simulation was recorded using video cameras, note taking, photographing, and observations behind a one-way mirror. After welcoming the participants, a brief introduction was delivered on the purpose of the study and the scenarios. Both surgeons performed all three scenarios. Before starting each scenario, the surgeons were briefly trained on how to use the WPA.

Each training session took about 30 min. After each scenario, the surgeons were asked to complete a structured questionnaire polling their experiences completing the task and using the system. The result of questionnaires is represented in Fig. 3. Immediately after the questionnaire the surgeons were interviewed to get deeper insights into their experience of using the WPA.

3.2   Scenario-Based Evaluation

We took a scenario-based approach in evaluation of the WPA. The scenarios were defined based on a previous study [2]. Scenarios included: (1) Touch-less interaction, (2) Tele-presence, and (3) Mobile access to the EPR in ward rounds. These three scenarios are part of a bigger scenario which starts with a patient getting an orthopedic surgery. Before the surgery, the surgeon needs to review the medical images of the patient. The WPA helps the surgeon find relevant medical images and adjust the view through touch-less modalities. During the surgery, the surgeon needs another experienced surgeon's opinion about the surgery. The WPA helps the local surgeon to have a tele-presence session with the remote colleague. After surgery, the patient is moved to the ward, and the surgeon visits the patient in the ward. The WPA enables the surgeon to see the patient electronic records on the go and review the new medical images after the surgery.

3.3   Preparing Data for the Study

Since all three scenarios are related to each other, for this study we needed real medical cases. We selected two cases with the help of our medical partner. We anonymized the data and assigned unreal names to the selected cases. Two human actors from university staff played the role of the patients during the ward round scenario. We also used real pictures of the surgical site taken during real surgeries. The pictures were printed and attached to the simulation doll to create a more realistic view (see Fig. 2-a).

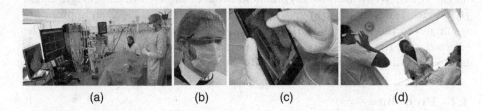

    (a)   (b)   (c)   (d)

Fig. 2. (a) A surgeon uses the WPA for touch-less interaction with X-rays and MRIs. (b) The local surgeon sees the visual guidance on the HMD in real-time. (c) A remote surgeon uses a tablet device to provide guidance to the local surgeon. (d) A surgeon uses the WPA to browse EPR and X-rays in the ward round scenario.

4   Scenario 1: Touchless Interaction

In the surgery room, the surgical team including a surgeon and a nurse, are about to start the surgery. Before starting the surgery, the surgeon looks at X-rays and MRIs. But his/her hands are sterile and s/he cannot touch the mouse or keyboard. Therefore, the surgeon uses the WPA for browsing X-rays and MRIs on two different screens in the operation room through voice commands and head movements. The surgeon might need to zoom in, rotate, or navigate through the medical images until s/he finds a good view. The surgeon can also take a snapshot of the screens and see the content on the HMD.

4.1   Apparatus

We used Google Glass to implement the WPA since Google Glass provides at least two touch-less input modalities: voice commands and head movements. Moreover, the unobtrusive form factor of the Google Glass and covering small part of the users field of view makes the Google Glass the best available option for applications where having a good view over the real-world is crucial. We developed a simple image browser for displaying the X-rays in the surgery room. To visualize MRIs and X-ray scans, we modified Invesalius software that is an open-source medical imaging system[1].

All three systems were connected to a dedicated local WIFI network. We used UDP protocol for communication between Google Glass and other two medical systems. The WPA app on the Glass accepts both voice commands and head movements for interaction. Voice modality is used for discrete commands such as activating/deactivating the interaction, switching between X-rays, zooming in/out X-rays, changing the views in MRIs between (sagittal, coronal, and axial). While head motion is used for continuous commands such as adjusting the position of the X-rays on the screen. In the latter case, we used the user's head similar to a mouse where the vertical and horizontal head movements are translated into the vertical and horizontal movements of the pointer displayed on the HMD. We defined some command areas in the GUI of the Google Glass. By moving and keeping the pointer in each area, the WPA sends an appropriate command to the X-ray and MRI systems. As soon as the pointer exits from the selected area the WPA stops sending commands. Table 1 shows the modalities used for sending commands to the WPA.

4.2   Procedure

After briefing the participants and setting up the surgery room, the surgeons started the scenario one after another. First the nurse gave a brief explanation about the patient to the surgeon. Then the surgeon activated the stationary X-ray system through the WPA to find an X-ray and adjust the scale and position of it on the large display. To find a good view the surgeon used either voice

---

[1] http://svn.softwarepublico.gov.br/trac/invesalius/.

Table 1. Input modalities for each module of the WPA

System module	Commands to the WPA	Voice	Head	Touch
Touchless interaction	Wake up the Glass		×	
	(De)activate the X-ray/MRI system	×		
	Switching X-rays (next/previous)	×		
	Positioning X-rays on the screen		×	
	Changing MRI views	×		
	Change the depth of the MRI views		×	
	Take snapshot of X-rays/MRI views	×		
Tele-precense	Wake up the Glass		×	
	(De)activate the tele-precense system	×		
	Take a picture	×		
	Select a picture for sharing	×		
	Call a clinician	×		
	End call	×		
EPR	Wake up the Glass		×	×
	(De)activate the EPR system	×		×
	Select a patient record	×		×
	Switch X-rays	×		×
	Zoom in/out X-rays	×		×
	Rotate X-rays	×		×
	Navigate through X-rays		×	
	Browse EPR pages	×		×

commands or head movements as shown in Table 1. After finding the appropriate view, the surgeon took a snapshot of the stationary X-ray which made it come up on the HMD. This snapshot helps the surgeon to examine the X-ray image during the surgery without having to change the head orientation towards the large display. Each surgeon repeated the scenario for both patients. Since the second patient had also some MRIs, in the second surgery, the surgeons used the WPA for interaction with both X-rays and MRI systems. To interact with the MRI system, the surgeon needed to activate three different views (sagittal, coronal, axial) through voice commands and adjust an appropriate depth view.

4.3   Results

Interview: We asked surgeons about the pros and cons of the WPA for touchless interaction compared to the current indirect interaction (asking a nurse to control a computer mouse as proxies for surgeons). Participant 1 (P1) indicated the higher speed of interaction using the WPA; however, he believes that it might take more time for older surgeons to learn how to use the WPA. P2 thinks the direct interaction through the WPA can be a big advantage and saves time of surgeons in the surgery room because sometimes it is very hard to explain to a nurse the view that the surgeon is looking for. However, interaction with X-rays by head movements is not easy since the user needs to look through the HMD to see the pointer and at the same time look at the X-rays or MRIs on the large screens which demands frequently switching between the HMD and the large screens.

We also asked whether they prefer voice commands or head movements for interaction with X-rays and MRIs. P1 thinks the voice commands are more convenient for interaction with X-rays where the user usually needs to provide a few commands while in the MRI case the head movements can be more beneficial since finding the right depth view among a lot of slices can be frustrating by voice commands. P2 prefers voice commands since interaction through head movements was challenging for him due to the need for switching frequently between the HMD and the large screens.

The last question was about the snapshot function. Both P1 and P2 indicated that the snapshot functionality can be extremely useful when the surgeon needs a reference X-ray or MRI to monitor the state of the surgical site during the surgery. In such cases, the surgeon needs to frequently turn his/her head towards the screen. To have a snapshot of such reference images in the HMD, saves surgeons' time and energy for the surgery.

Observations: Both surgeons quickly learned how to use the voice commands for interaction through the WPA; however, P1 felt more comfortable with head-based interaction compared to P2. When P2 wanted to adjust the position of the X-rays in the screen by head movements, he lost the control of the system because he had problems with looking at both the HMD (to control the pointer) and the large screen (to see the X-rays) at the same time. The same problem happened when P2 wanted to adjust the MRI depth view.

5   Scenario 2: Tele-Presence

After adjusting the medical images on the screen (in the previous scenario) during the surgery, the surgeon encounters a complex situation and needs help from an expert colleague. The surgeon uses the WPA to start a tele-presence session with the remote colleague. The local surgeon takes a picture of the surgical site and calls the remote surgeon using the Glass. The remote surgeon answers the call. Then the local surgeon explains the situation and shares the taken picture with the remote surgeon. The remote surgeon provides some voice guidance while at the same time marking the shared photo on his tablet (Fig. 2c). The local surgeon sees the content provided by the remote surgeon on the Glass and also hears the voice of the remote surgeon in real-time (Fig. 2b) in real-time.

5.1   Apparatus

We developed a tele-presence app on the Google Glass for the local surgeon while for the remote surgeon, we developed an Android application on an Asus

Nexus 7 tablet. The audio communication is done over WIFI connection using UDP protocol. Due to the limitations in processing resources of the Google Glass and to avoid registration challenges in an augmented reality user interface, the Glass application shares a still picture (instead of video) of the local side, and the remote person is able to draw sketches on top of the shared image using the Android application on the tablet. The sketches are superimposed over the shared image in real-time on the Google Glass HMD of the local user.

5.2 Procedure

In the tele-presence simulation, we ran the scenario twice, and during each time one of the surgeons played the role of a remote expert and the other surgeon played the role a local surgeon. In the second run, the surgeons swapped their role and the surgery case was also changed from patient 1 to the patient 2. Before starting each run, we attached the printed image of the surgical site on the simulation doll. The remote surgeon sat on a chair in the hallway outside of the surgery room. After activating the Google Glass by head nudge gesture, the local surgeon opens the tele-presence application by voice command and takes a picture of the surgical site. Then the local surgeon calls the remote colleague by saying his/her name from a list on the HMD. The remote surgeon receives and accepts the call. As soon as the call is accepted the audio communication is possible and the taken picture is displayed on both sides. The local surgeon explains the situation and asks for the remote surgeon's opinion. The remote surgeon provides vocal and visual guidance by marking the shared image of the surgical site using different colors on his tablet device, markings that show up immediately in the Google Glass display carried by the local surgeon.

5.3 Results

Interview: We asked surgeons what other content they would like to share in a tele-presence session. P1 believes sharing still images of the surgical site (like our implementation) is very useful for orthopedic surgeries while live videos can be useful in emergency cases. Also sharing medical images such as X-rays or MRIs can be valuable in cases where a junior surgeon needs an approval from a senior surgeon. Currently the senior surgeon needs to come personally to the surgery room and have a look at the X-rays or the junior surgeon sends the X-ray using a smartphone. P2 thinks the quality of the image on the HMD is not good enough for complex surgeries with a lot of soft tissues. He suggested to add a zoom-in functionality to overcome the limited resolution of the HMD.

Observations: The communication between the two surgeons was smooth. There was about half a second delay in the audio communication due to the WIFI-based communication. But the surgeons got used to it after a while. Also during the tele-presence scenario, when the local surgeon was talking to the remote surgeon, Google Glass detected the "Ok Glass" command by mistake and the surgeon needed to deactivate the voice command and continue the session.

6   Scenario 3: Mobile Access to Electronic Patient Records

It is one day after the surgeries. Patients are lying down in the bed in the ward. The surgeons should visit two patients who got surgery. The surgeons use the WPA to review the new X-rays and the latest state of the patients while walking to the ward together with a nurse. The surgeon searches for the patient records on the Glass by saying the patients name. After finding the patient records, the surgeon reads the updated EPR and looks at the recent X-rays and MRIs on the Glass. The surgeon zooms in/out, rotate, and navigate through the medical images. The nurse reports the latest state of the patient (last blood test, etc.) to the surgeon. The nurse answers the questions that the surgeon might ask during the ward round. The surgeon visits the patients and asks some questions about their pain, etc. Also the surgeon might need to use the EPR system for answering patients' questions. After visiting the patients, the surgeon prescribes the next treatments and the nurse writes down the prescriptions.

6.1   Apparatus

For this scenario, we only needed an EPR app on the Google Glass. Since in the ward round, the clinicians' hands do not necessarily need to be sterilized, the EPR app supports also touch-based interaction on the Google Glass side touchpad. Table 1 shows the ways surgeons can interact with the EPR app. We used different touch-gestures for interaction with text pages and medical images: swipe front/back for browsing EPR and X-rays, short tap for zoom in, long tap for zoom out, swipe up for 90 ° rotation, and swipe up to exit from an active card to the previous menu. Since it was not possible to connect the Google Glass to the EPR in the hospital, the patients data was hard-coded into the EPR app.

6.2   Procedure

In the ward round simulation, each surgeon performed the ward round scenario once where both patients (human actors) lying in the patient bed (Fig. 1-a) were visited. A nurse accompanied the surgeon during the ward round and provided necessary information. The surgeons used the WPA to see the recent EPR and X-rays while talking to the patients (see Fig. 2-d). They tried both voice commands and touch gestures to interact with the WPA. The patients also asked some questions about the result of the surgery.

6.3   Results

Interview: The surgeons were asked about the pros and cons of the EPR module during ward rounds. P1 mentioned that the most obvious advantage of using the EPR on the Glass is to reduce unnecessary moving between a stationary computer and the ward to check the EPR. However, P2 thinks the small screen in Google Glass makes it hard for the surgeon to read the EPR texts, while a stationary computer is more convenient for such intensive readings. P1 also mentioned that getting an overview of the EPR is much faster using a desktop computer since in Glass the text is distributed over several pages.

The other question was about the content that surgeons might need to have access to during a ward round in addition to the EPR and medical images. P2 mentioned that the main information the doctors need during a ward round is lab results that can also be provided on the Glass. However, due to the small size of the HMD in Google Glass, the lab results should be visualized in a way that the interesting results (important abnormal values) are highlighted, and the surgeon can get what s/he wants at a glance. P2 indicated that aside from the medical data, patients usually ask a lot of practical questions about e.g. when they can leave the hospital, when they have their next appointment, etc. The WPA should also provide such practical information to the surgeon.

We also asked about the modality they prefer to use during ward rounds. P1 mentioned that he prefers touch gestures since the voice commands interfere with communication with the patient. P2 said *"I also prefer touch gestures because the head movements look bizarre!"*. All participants (two surgeons, a nurse, and two patients) were asked about the social acceptance of the Google Glass. P2 said: *"Some people might think wearing such a [smart] glasses is arrogant since you are not present with the patient"*. The nurse mentioned that sometimes the surgeon was looking at the HMD but she thought the surgeon is looking at her. Moreover, the patients mentioned that they did not feel good when the surgeon was trying to interact with the Google Glass instead of talking to them.

Observations: During the ward round, P1 spent more time for interaction with the WPA compared to P2 and sometimes there was a long silence until the surgeon read the EPR on the Google Glass. The reason was that P2 was familiar with the medical cases used in the simulation while both cases were new for P1.

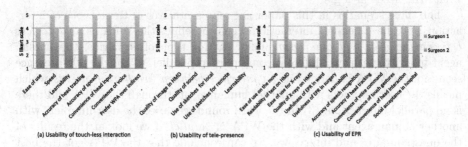

Fig. 3. (a) Usability of the touch-less interaction module of the WPA, (b) usability of the tele-presence module of the WPA, and (c) usability of the EPR module of the WPA.

7   Discussion and Conclusions

Our study indicates that using the WPA for touch-less interaction with medical images can save surgeons time and energy for the surgery. Moreover, by using the WPA for touch-less interaction, there is no need for a dedicated nurse to control the mouse for surgeons. However, there are some limitations in both voice commands and head movements for touch-less interaction. Using voice commands is a relatively reliable modality but due to the slow speed of the discrete voice commands, it is not an appropriate modality for providing a lot of commands within a short time. In contrast to the voice commands, the head movements can be useful for continuous interactions; however, due to the perceptual overlap between seeing the large screens and the pointer on the HMD, it is not easy to use the head movements as a mouse to control the pointer on the HMD. The lowest scores in Fig. 3-a are related to the accuracy of head tracking specially by P2. This reveals the challenge of using head movements for touch-less interaction.

Apart from the low quality of the image on the HMD indicated in both questionnaire (Fig. 3-b) and the complementary interview, the WPA was successfully used in the tele-presence scenario. As both surgeons mentioned, the tele-presence scenario was the best application for the WPA. However, in this scenario we observed the problem of overlapping between human to human conversation and voice commands to the system. This indicates a need for more touch-less input modalities (e.g. gaze) to avoid overlap between the input modality (voice commands) and surgeons' conversation. The most challenging scenario was the ward round which revealed the social problems of using Google Glass in parallel with human to human interactions. Apart from the social problems, the small HMD of the Glass turned out to be a limitation for intensive text readings which is in line with the concept of microinteractions [15] where interacting with the device should not exceed 4 s. To achieve such fast interactions, the WPA needs to prepare the information for the surgeons in a way that the surgeon can get what s/he needs at a glance.

The three scenarios in this paper are representatives of three types of interaction. (1) The touch-less interaction scenario defines the WPA as an *interface between the user and other computers*. In this type of scenarios, the human agent interacts with two different computers in parallel. (2) In the tele-presence scenario, the WPA is defined as an *interface between two human agents* which means the user interacts with another human agent through the WPA and there is no parallel interaction. (3) In the ward round scenario, the user interacts with another human agent and with the WPA *in parallel*. If we look at the results of the questionnaires and interviews, we can conclude that the WPA got the best scores in the tele-presence scenario where there was no parallel interaction, and the user interacts sequentially with the WPA and the other human agent. In the touch-less interaction scenario, the usability of the WPA is evaluated as average. In this scenario, the user interacts with two computers in parallel: the WPA and X-ray/MRI systems. The most challenging scenario is the ward round where the user needs to interact in parallel with the WPA and a human agent.

Acknowledgements. We thank Sanne Jensen at the ITX hospital simulation facility as well as MD Ulrik Kaehler Olesen, Dept. of Traumatology and Orthopedic Surgery, Rigshospitalet, Copenhagen. This work was supported by the EU Marie Curie Network iCareNet under grant number 264738.

References

1. Marshall, J., Tennent, P.: Mobile interaction does not exist. In: CHI EA 2013, pp. 2069–2078. ACM, New York (2013)
2. Jalaliniya, S., Pederson, T.: Designing wearable personal assistants for surgeons: an egocentric approach. IEEE Pervasive Comput. **14**(3), 22–31 (2015)
3. Windyga, P., Wink, D.: A wearable computing based system for the prevention of medical errors committed by registered nurses in the intensive care unit. In: 24th Annual Conference of Engineering in Medicine and Biology, vol. 3, pp. 1940–1941, October 2002
4. Adamer, K., Bannach, D., Klug, T., Lukowicz, P., Sbodio, M.L., Tresman, M., Zinnen, A., Ziegert, T.: Developing a wearable assistant for hospital ward rounds: an experience report. In: Floerkemeier, C., Langheinrich, M., Fleisch, E., Mattern, F., Sarma, S.E. (eds.) IOT 2008. LNCS, vol. 4952, pp. 289–307. Springer, Heidelberg (2008). doi:10.1007/978-3-540-78731-0_19
5. Liu, D., Jenkins, S., Sanderson, P.: Clinical implementation of a head-mounted display of patient vital signs. In: ISWC 2009, pp. 47–54, September 2009
6. Drugge, M., Hallberg, J., Parnes, P., Synnes, K.: Wearable systems in nursing home care: prototyping experience. IEEE Pervasive Comput. **5**(1), 86–91 (2006)
7. Thomas, B.H., Quirchmayr, G., Piekarski, W.: Through-walls communication for medical emergency services. Int. J. Hum. Comput. Interact. **16**(3), 477–496 (2003)
8. Cheng, J., Bannach, D., Adamer, K., Bernreiter, T., Lukowicz, P.: A wearable, conductive textile based user interface for hospital ward rounds document access. In: Roggen, D., Lombriser, C., Tröster, G., Kortuem, G., Havinga, P. (eds.) EuroSSC 2008. LNCS, vol. 5279, pp. 182–191. Springer, Heidelberg (2008). doi:10.1007/978-3-540-88793-5_14
9. Levin-Sagi, M., Pasher, E., Carlsson, V., Klug, T., Ziegert, T., Zinnen, A.: A comprehensive human factors analysis of wearable computers supporting a hospital ward round. In: IFAWC 2007, pp. 1–12, March 2007
10. Brent, A., Lasun, O., Phani, K., et al.: Emerging technology in surgical education: Combining real-time augmented reality and wearable computing devices. Orthopedics **37**(11), 751–757 (2014)
11. Widmer, A., Schaer, R., Markonis, D., Muller, H.: Facilitating medical information search using google glass connected to a content-based medical image retrieval system. In: Proceedings of EMBC 2014, pp. 4507–4510, August 2014
12. Muensterer, O.J., Lacher, M., Zoeller, C., Bronstein, M., Kbler, J.: Google glass in pediatric surgery: an exploratory study. Int. J. Surg. **12**(4), 281–289 (2014)
13. Vorraber, W., Voessner, S., Stark, G., Neubacher, D., DeMello, S., Bair, A.: Medical applications of near-eye display devices: an exploratory study. Int. J. Surg. **12**(12), 1266–1272 (2014)
14. Ahmed, K., Jawad, M., Abboudi, M., Gavazzi, A., Darzi, A., Athanasiou, T., Vale, J., Khan, M.S., Dasgupta, P.: Effectiveness of procedural simulation in urology: a systematic review. J. Urol. **186**(1), 26–34 (2011)
15. Ashbrook, D.L.: Enabling Mobile Microinteractions. Ph.D. thesis, Georgia Institute of Technology, Atlanta, GA, USA, AAI3414437 (2010)

A Multi-agent Approach to Assist with Dressing in a Smart Environment

Claire Orr[(✉)], Chris Nugent, Haiying Wang, and Huiru Zheng

Computer Science Research Institute and School of Computing
and Mathematics, University of Ulster, Newtownabbey
Co. Antrim BT37 0QB, Northern Ireland
orr-c2@email.ulster.ac.uk,
{cd.nugent,hy.wang,h.zheng}@ulster.ac.uk

Abstract. This paper proposes an approach to offer assistance with dressing for those persons with a form of cognitive impairment. The main underlying technical component in the solution is the use of a multi-agent system. A prototype was implemented, consisting of six agents, which received input in the form of simulated data. The system then has the ability to offer a recommendation as a person leaves their home environment in the form of a clothing suggestion. The decision for this is based partially on the external temperature and their current apparel. The long term aspiration of this work is to support persons with cognitive impairment to dress appropriately for environmental and social conditions.

Keywords: Activities of Daily Living · Cognitive impairment · Dressing · Multi-Agent System · Smart environment

1 Introduction

One of the biggest challenges in current research is to find ways to allow the growing population of elderly people to live more independently for longer within their own homes. Previous research has considered the use of technology as a popular solution to assist those with cognitive impairment [1]. Systems can be developed that aim to monitor and track Activities of Daily Living (ADLs) and subsequently remind or alert users or carers if required. This has the benefit of taking the burden off family members or carers who would otherwise have to personally assist the patient more frequently in addition to providing an increased level of independence for the person suffering from the impairment [2]. Through researching current systems and assistance already available to help in these cases, the ADL of dressing has to date received very little attention, from a technology solution perspective.

Systems developed make use of sensors and actuators to identify and monitor the environment to recognise the actions taking place and to adapt the environment accordingly. In order to do this they have assigned goals and decisions to fulfil; this also enables them to be known as software agents [3]. When agents are combined in order to work together to solve problems, they become a Multi-Agent System (MAS). As a result more complex, effective systems, providing improved scalability and

© ICST Institute for Computer Sciences, Social Informatics and Telecommunications Engineering 2017
K. Giokas et al. (Eds.): eHealth 2016, LNICST 181, pp. 220–223, 2017.
DOI: 10.1007/978-3-319-49655-9_29

cooperation, can be developed [4]. This paper proposes a solution to assisting with the ADL of dressing through the use of a MAS.

In Sect. 2 a review of related work and relevant studies is provided. Work carried out to date is presented in Sect. 3 followed by a discussion of limitations faced and Future Works in Sect. 4.

2 Related Work

A study by Benhaji *et al.* developed a MAS dedicated to manage and control the movement of patients in medical care facilities. Patients and hospital resources, such as physicians and nurses, were represented by agents with their focus on creating a patient-centred system. A heterarchical architecture was used to ensure communication was achieved through negotiation, cooperation and coordination and that agents could be added or removed without major impact on structure or performance. Within this there are only two levels, the top containing the patient agent as the central component of the system and the bottom containing all other agents. The system allows the hospital to see where patients are assigned to and where free places may be. Limitations with this approach lay amongst the negotiation mechanism as conflict issues were found to cause problems for the system [4].

Matic *et al.* devised a system to monitor the activity of dressing and to identify common failures using a combination of RFID and computer vision. The 'AID-ME' system, standing for 'Automatic Identification of Dressing failures through Monitoring of patients and activity Evaluation' aimed to non-intrusively recognise and evaluate the accuracy of dressing through using information gained from the RFID tags and vision combined. They found that there were limitations when these systems were used on their own, however, once fused they found it provided a 10% higher recognition rate for detecting the incorrect order of dressing. In conclusion they stated that the integration of the two systems was required for the improvement in efficiency [5].

This research proposes a MAS to assist dementia patients with dressing in a smart environment. Whilst MAS have been used for processing data within smart environments, most have concentrated on low abstraction levels or domain-specific tasks [6]. Nevertheless, it would offer additional advantages to be able to build the context at a higher level, via the processing of raw data. This allows the agents to understand the semantic information, in turn enabling them to make the relevant decisions required to meet their goals.

3 Methodology

To date, a software solution has been created to expedite the prototyping, consisting of six agents: Decision, GUI, Door, Coat, Temperature and Template (Fig. 1 shows the methods and attributes of each agent). The Decision agent receives information from the Door, Coat and Temperature agents, making decisions based on their current states. The GUI agent's focus relates to the layout of the user interface as it contains buttons representing the door and coat, in addition to an input for temperature. Through the

Door, Coat and Temperature agents' information, the Decision agent will decide upon an alert or action to be taken. Both the Door and Coat agents contain rules for their corresponding tasks. The state of these tasks is communicated to the Decision agent. If the state is 'true', this indicates that the door has been opened and 'false' if it is closed. The states of the Coat are represented as 'true' for taken and 'false' if it has not been taken. The Temperature agent contains the rules required to identify if the temperature input values exceed a predefined threshold value. It is set to represent 'true' if it is over 23° and 'false' if it is below, indicating that it is cold. Finally the template agent, which simply exists to assign the layout and size of the GUI. An example of the system in action is as follows: if the Decision agent is told that the Coat state is true whilst the Temperature is true and the Door state is also true, the GUI will be told by the Decision agent to alert the user that it is too warm for a coat. These agents will communicate in order to make a joint decision on the appropriate alert or action to take (Fig. 2 shows the communication flow between each agent). Looking at the scenario where patients may dress inappropriately for the weather; for example, if the patient prepares to leave their home on a cold day without their coat, they would be alerted to lift a coat before they leave. This infrastructure has been put in place and example tested upon, using simulated data input by a human expert, in order to validate that everything is working as expected.

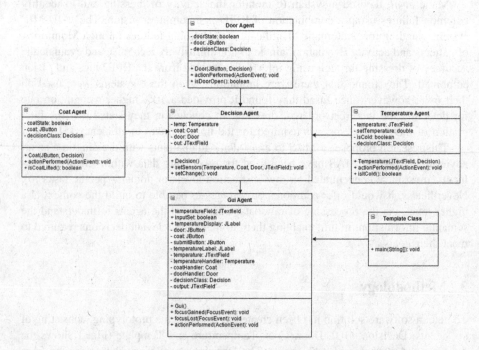

Fig. 1. Class diagram showing the methods and attributes within each agent.

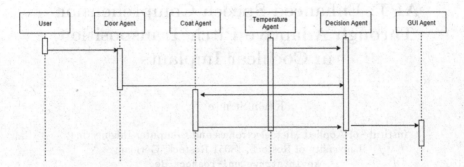

Fig. 2. Sequence diagram showing the communication between each agent and the user.

4 Discussion and Conclusion

This research aims to develop a MAS in a smart environment that will be able to assist with dressing for persons with cognitive impairment. It is hoped that it will advance not only help with dressing, however, also the implementation and use of MAS in smart environments on a large scale. Due to this work being at an early stage, limitations are present. This system is only partially created, before being able to implement this in a real life environment, sensors are the next step. The proposed solution will include a thermometer in place of the thermometer input; an RFID tag in a coat in place of the simulated coat event and a movement sensor on a door in place of the simulated door event. Once implemented, this system should address the issues previously highlighted in the Related Work section in that no conflicts should occur and the system will work efficiently with good coordination and communication among agents.

References

1. Rodríguez, S., De Paz, J.F., Villarrubia, G., Zato, C., Bajo, J., Corchado, J.M.: Multi-agent information fusion system to manage data from a WSN in a residential home. Inf. Fusion **23**, 43–57 (2014)
2. McNaull, J., Augusto, J.C., Mulvenna, M., McCullagh, P.: Multi-agent system feedback and support for ambient assisted living. In: Proceedings of 8th International Conference on Intelligent Environments. IE 2012, pp. 319–322 (2012)
3. Niazi, M., Hussain, A.: Agent-based computing from multi-agent systems to agent-based models: a visual survey. Scientometrics **89**, 479–499 (2011)
4. Benhajji, N., Roy, D., Anciaux, D.: Patient-centered multi agent system for health care. IFAC-PapersOnLine **48**, 710–714 (2015)
5. Matic, A., Mehta, P., Rehg, J.M., Osmani, V., Mayora, O.: AID-ME: automatic identification of dressing failures through monitoring of patients and activity Evaluation. In: 2010 4th International Conference on-NO PERMISSIONS Pervasive Computing Technologies for Healthcare (PervasiveHealth) (2010)
6. Alfonso-Cendón, J., Fernández-de-Alba, J.M., Fuentes-Fernández, R., Pavón, J.: Implementation of context-aware workflows with multi-agent systems. Neurocomputing **176**, 91–97 (2016)

APT: Enhanced Speech Comprehension Through Adaptive Pitch Transposition in Cochlear Implants

Kevin Struwe[✉]

Institute of Applied Microelectronics and Computer Engineering,
University of Rostock, 18051 Rostock, Germany
kevin.struwe@uni-rostock.de

Abstract. Cochlear Implants are a marvelous option for hearing-impaired patients to perceive sound again, yet some people still cannot benefit from their implant. The resulting problem is a suboptimal pitch discrimination, which in turn is a vital factor for vowel identification. As an approach to solve this problem, this paper proposes an adaptive pitch transposition, which transposes a given signal to a fixed pitch in which the implant patient has the best comprehension. This pitch is called comfort pitch and has to be determined in a patient test. As a result of these considerations, APT was prototypically implemented in Octave/Matlab and serves as an evaluation platform for the quality of the produced signals. Furthermore, the comfort pitch is a new measure to tune the performance of a cochlear implant patient. The entire concept can be used as a preprocessing stage for state-of-the art speech processing algorithms in cochlear implants.

Keywords: Cochlear Implants · Pitch transposition · Speech processing

1 Introduction

Cochlear implants (CI) are a marvelous way for patients with severe sensorineural hearing loss to gain or regain the ability to perceive sound from their surroundings. In a CI, the sound is captured by a microphone and processed by a speech processor, which transforms the analog sound wave into digital pulses. These pulses are then transmitted to an electrode array in the cochlea, where they invoke an electric field to stimulate the hearing nerve at the electrode's position. However, in spite the success of these implants, some patients still cannot comprehend speech. Low speech comprehension is caused by a variety of circumstances: among others, shallow insertion depth of the electrode array and a low brain plasticity are limiting factors [5]. That leads to a residual hearing range, which is shifted upwards and prohibits the perception of lower frequencies.

To tackle this problem, this paper proposes an adaptive pitch transposition, or APT for short, for transposing the input speech signal to the frequency range in which a particular patient has the best comprehension with his existing

© ICST Institute for Computer Sciences, Social Informatics and Telecommunications Engineering 2017
K. Giokas et al. (Eds.): eHealth 2016, LNICST 181, pp. 224–228, 2017.
DOI: 10.1007/978-3-319-49655-9_30

cochlear implant. The perceived speech frequency is called Pitch. The frequency range for best comprehension is thus called comfort pitch and is an empirically determined value that describes the Pitch in which a patient has the best comprehension.

APT uses the optimal range of frequencies for each individual patient, even with a drastically reduced number of active electrodes. Furthermore, by reducing pitch variance by fixing the pitch not to a range but a single value, APT provides the brain with always the same stimulus. This makes it easier for the patient to learn and adapt to the new sound experience.

The remainder of the paper is organized as follows. Section 2 covers the actual problem and how it fits into the context of current research. This leads to the concept of APT, which is explained in depth in Sect. 3. This section describes the individual parts of the concept in detail. The achieved results are presented and discussed in Sect. 4, which concludes the paper.

2   Problem Description

Even with todays sophisticated algorithms, not everyoné can understand speech with his CI. The standard insertion depth of a CI electrode array does not allow the patient to perceive frequencies lower than 1000 Hz [3]. With a reduced insertion depth, this limit raises even further. Because of this, and CIs coarse frequency representation, CI patients may have up to 24-times worse pitch perception than a hearing control group [6].

However, research aiming at enhancing pitch perception was recently done by Laneau et al. [2], which developed f0mod. f0mod modulates the electrode signal with the fundamental frequency, which has been shown to be beneficial for frequencies up to 1000 Hz. Francart et al. [1] have shown that pitch related tasks can benefit from the f0mod approach. Vandali et al. developed a training program for pitch and timbre discrimination improvement in [4]. Improvements were shown, but only in environments with little variations. But even with all available improvements, not all patients receive a comprehensible hearing sensation.

Another problem, this paper is addressing, is the impact of low brain plasticity from some of the patients. Brain plasticity means that the brain is able to adapt to new and different stimuli by changing its "wiring". While aging, the plasticity of the brain degrades. CI users of old age, who are severely hearing impaired, have thus problems when using their devices.

These problems led to the concept of adaptive pitch transposition (APT). The shallow insertion depth and therefore the reduced number of electrodes limit the accessible range of frequencies to a minimum. From there, it is obvious that a shift of the most interesting region of sound to the remaining frequencies should be a way to enhance speech perception. This also inherently reduces the influence of a low brain plasticity, since the main cues for comprehension are now always in focus.

3   Adaptive Pitch Transposition

The APT concept works as follows: It assumes that a particular patient has a certain voice pitch where he or she obtains the best recognition rates. This particular pitch is called comfort pitch. Then it transposes all incoming sound samples into that pitch frequency. This approach requires the following processing stages: (1) determine the current pitch, (2) determine the required shift amount, and (3) shift and transpose all incoming signals to the targeted best pitch frequency. The resulting transposed signal may then be relayed into an arbitrary CI simulation model.

The comfort pitch is the first necessity for each patient. This paper defines it as the one Pitch, with that a particular listener has the best speech recognition rates among a given set of pitches. The relationship of comfort pitch and voice pitch range are depicted in Fig. 1.

The comfort pitch can be determined by a patient test. This test could be comprised of voices of different pitch, uttering randomized phrases from a fixed set. Pitch-score pairs are then ranked for best speech recognition rates on the patients side. The voice pitch with the best score will be the new comfort pitch for optimal recognition when using the system. With this test, the comfort pitch adapts to the patient.

Since the goal is to transpose a given signal to a specific comfort pitch, the pitch of the current input signal has to be determined to calculate a transposition coefficient, which in turn defines how much shift has to be applied.

The Autocorrelation function (ACF) is an algorithm for this very purpose. Pitch is defined by the signals fundamental frequency and its harmonics, which are equally spaced in the frequency spectrum. The ACF slides a portion of data with a varying offset lag over itself to determine a similarity measure. This measure can then be interpreted as fundamental frequency under certain conditions.

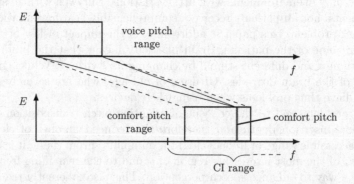

Fig. 1. Different pitch ranges in the frequency domain. The voice range of possible voice pitches is spacial disjunct from the range, a CI can address. Therefore the pitch has to be transposed into the CI range.

For input signals which actually have a pitch, the ACF gives a good estimate. These signals are called *voiced*. However, for signals that do not have a pitch (*unvoiced* signals), the ACF results appear pseudo-random. Therefore, it is necessary to verify these results. This process is called voice-activity-detection (VAD) for speech audio signals, and is used in speech recognition software or other speech related tasks.

Comfort pitch and determined pitch now allow for the calculation of the transposition coefficient.

Pitch transposition is usually seen as a combination of time stretching and re-sampling of an audio signal. First the signal is time-stretched while maintaining the original signal pitch. Then it is re-sampled to the original signal length. A signal stretched by the factor of two, re-sampled to the original length, will thus have a pitch at the double frequency. As an example one can imagine a glass of water, where the fill level of the water is the pitch and the diameter of the glass is the signal length. If we can make the diameter bigger while keeping the fill level, and afterwards make the diameter small again, we will have a raised fill level (thus: pitch).

4   Conclusion

This paper has presented a concept for preprocessing signals for cochlear implants. The complexity of an input sound signal in terms of pitch gets reduced to benefit the brains ability to adapt to stimuli.

This approach is only applicable, if an improvement in speech recognition can be observed for specific pitches. The extent to which the proposed system enhances the speech recognition rates in patients is subject of future research.

One major drawback of the current approach is the loss of speaker differentiation through the pitch fixing. Nevertheless, in prospect of regaining the ability to understand speech, this seems negligible.

The APT concept has been prototypically implemented in Octave/Matlab. The resulting system has yet some drawbacks regarding quality and computing time, but it acts as a foundation for a testbed to evaluate the effect on speech recognition compared to a simulation of a pure speech processing algorithm. Furthermore, the comfort pitch constitutes an additional parameter to tune the efficacy of speech processing algorithms.

Future research will be directed to the evaluation and testing with hearing people as well as CI users. Performance and quality increase are desired for real time usage.

Lastly APT is a powerful preprocessing stage, which is adaptable to any other speech processing strategy. It thus yields the potential to theoretically enhance the speech recognition rate for every CI user.

Acknowledgments. The author thanks the welisa graduate school for its support. Part of this research was funded by the German Research Foundation (DFG) grant number GRK 1505.

References

1. Francart, T., Osses, A., Wouters, J.: Speech perception with f0mod, a cochlear implant pitch coding strategy. Int. J. Audiol. **54**(6), 424–432 (2015)
2. Laneau, J., Wouters, J., Moonen, M.: Improved music perception with explicit pitch coding in cochlear implants. Audiol. Neurotol. **11**(1), 38–52 (2006)
3. Shannon, R.V., Fu, Q.J., Galvin, J., Friesen, L.: Speech perception with cochlear implants. In: Zeng, F.-G., Popper, A.N., Fay, R.R. (eds.) Cochlear Implants: Auditory Prostheses and Electric Hearing, pp. 334–376. Springer, New York (2004)
4. Vandali, A., Sly, D., Cowan, R., van Hoesel, R.: Training of cochlear implant users to improve pitch perception in the presence of competing place cues. Ear Hear. **36**(2), e1–e13 (2015)
5. Wilson, B.S., Dorman, M.F.: Cochlear implants: a remarkable past and a brilliant future. Hear. Res. **242**(12), 3–21 (2008). http://www.sciencedirect.com/science/article/pii/S0378595508001251, frontiers of auditory prosthesis research: Implications for clinical practice
6. Zeng, F.G., Tang, Q., Lu, T.: Abnormal pitch perception produced by cochlear implant stimulation. PloS One **9**(2), e88662 (2014)

A Wireless Sensor-Based System for Self-tracking Activity Levels Among Manual Wheelchair Users

Alexandre Grillon[1,4]($\boxtimes$), Andres Perez-Uribe[1,4], Hector Satizabal[1,4], Laurent Gantel[2,4], David Da Silva Andrade[2,4], Andres Upegui[2,4], and Francis Degache[3,4]

[1] Institute for Information and Communication Technologies IICT, HEIG-VD, Yverdon-les-Bains, Switzerland
{alexandre.grillon,andres.perez-uribe,
hector-fabio.satizabal-mejia}@heig-vd.ch
[2] Institute on Information Technologies InIT, Hepia, Geneva, Switzerland
{laurent.gantel,david.dasilva-andrade,andres.upegui}@hesge.ch
[3] University of Health Sciences, HESAV, Lausanne, Switzerland
francis.degache@hesav.ch
[4] University of Applied Sciences and Arts of Western Switzerland (HES-SO), Delémont, Switzerland

Abstract. ActiDote —activity as an antidote— is a system for manual wheelchair users that uses wireless sensors to recognize activities of various intensity levels in order to allow self-tracking while providing motivation. In this paper, we describe both the hardware setup and the software pipeline that enable our system to operate. Laboratory tests using multi-modal fusion and machine learning reveal promising results attaining a F1-score classification performance of 0.97 on five different wheelchair-based activities belonging to four intensity levels. Finally, we show that such a low cost system can be used for an easy self-monitoring of physical activity levels among manual wheelchair users.

Keywords: Self-tracking · Wheelchair · Handicap · Wireless sensors · Wearables · Machine learning

1 Introduction and Motivation

Physical inactivity has been identified as a major contributor to the exacerbation of physical illnesses [9]. The WHO identified it as the fourth leading risk factor of global mortality after high blood pressure, tobacco use and high blood glucose. Therefore, in recent years, many actions against inactivity have come to the fore [12]. For instance, diverse pedometer devices have been developed to help people reach various physical activity goals, like walking 30 min per day or completing 10'000 steps per day. Moreover, many smartphone applications attempt to help people self-track their physical activity and motivate them to

© ICST Institute for Computer Sciences, Social Informatics and Telecommunications Engineering 2017
K. Giokas et al. (Eds.): eHealth 2016, LNICST 181, pp. 229–240, 2017.
DOI: 10.1007/978-3-319-49655-9_31

continuously exercise. Unfortunately, an equivalent application for people using wheelchairs is missing and there is a clear absence of motivational devices that can support the self-tracking of physical activity among people with spinal cord injury. The few studies that have dealt with this issue concluded that current commercial physical activity measurement devices are not appropriate for wheelchair users [7], and to make things worse, those users very often adopt sedentary habits as a consequence of their disability. The result is that obesity rates for adults with disabilities are higher than for adults without disabilities [17].

In this paper we present ActiDote —activity as an antidote— a system based on wearable and wheelchair-attached sensors that wirelessly communicate with a smartphone to allow the tracking of the physical activity of people with motor disabilities using wheelchairs. Our system integrates machine learning algorithms that analyse the sensor data to identify the intensity of the physical activity being realized, and provides a daily (and weekly) summary of activities as a feedback to the user. This paper is organized as follows: in Sect. 2, we present the state-of-the-art in the domains of physical tracking and activity recognition among disabled people. In Sect. 3, we describe the Actidote system, namely the hardware setup, the activity recognition approach and the feedback visualization. Section 4 presents experimental tests and results and finally, Sect. 5 presents our conclusions and future work.

2   Related Work

The increasing availability of wearable sensors embedded in smartphones, watches and physical activity trackers has opened the door to a wide number of applications, mainly in health and wellness improvement. Many devices and services help with tracking physical activity, caloric intake, sleep quality, posture, and other factors involved in personal well-being (e.g., the so-called Quantified-Self movement[1]). One typically collects data by means of sensors like GPS, accelerometers, gyroscopes, barometers, heart rate meters, thermometers, microphones, etc. As far as the physical activity monitoring is concerned, recent research and development has allowed to leverage the power of accelerometers for building systems capable of estimating energy expenditure and to achieve mass market penetration (e.g., Jawbone, Fitbit, Nike+, Polar Loop, Garmin vivofit). Unfortunately, it has been found that these general public devices do not provide accurate estimates of the energy expenditure of people using wheelchairs, in particular, during wheelchair propulsion [3,7]. Even the SenseWear Armband (SWA), which has been validated as a means to estimate energy expenditure in overweight children, in patients with cancer, and healthy children, has provided inaccurate measures among the disabled population [15].

Researchers have thus attempted to estimate energy expenditure of manual wheelchair users using activity-dependent models [6], increasing the sampling frequency and computing features of the raw data [5], and by fusing multiple modalities (e.g., accelerometry and heart rate monitoring) [15]. In [5], Garcia-Masso

---

[1] http://quantifiedself.com.

et al., obtained accurate estimations of energy expenditure on paraplegic persons using a cumbersome system with four wearable sensors (Actigraph GT3X accelerometers), one on each wrist, one on the waist and one on the chest. Finally, there has been some work attempt to better estimate energy expenditure with the use of Machine Learning techniques to derive data-driven models that exploit data from accelerometers or multiple sensors [10,13,14,16], but without involving people with spinal cord injury.

3   A Data-Driven Approach to Physical Tracking

The amount of energy spent by a person during a given activity can be assessed using a mechanistic approach if the right physiological variables are measured. However, these measurements are not easy to perform due to different practical constraints (e.g., sensors are expensive and not portable). Data-driven approaches offer an alternative to the mechanistic analyses which have been traditionally used for modelling complex metabolic phenomena. Data-driven models try to discover the relationships between the variables involved in the analysis from the data, while in mechanistic approaches these relationships are based on prior theoretical knowledge about the phenomenon. Indeed, in a data-driven approach, the variables used do not necessarily have a physiological meaning, and in most of the cases they are mere surrogates to a quantity that is difficult to measure. One of the main strengths of a data-driven approach is its robustness. The fact of using the acquired data to build the model provides a better tolerance to sensor imprecision given its non-dependence on sensor calibration or precise sensor positioning and orientation. While mechanistic analysis relies on the understanding of a physical phenomena that requires well defined inputs for obtaining an accurate solution, data-driven approaches accept not to understand the phenomena, making it less dependent on the accuracy of the inputs. Our approach is thus to acquire as much pertinent sensor data as possible for further identification of the required inputs to build the model.

3.1   Hardware Setup

In order to acquire the pertinent data to build our data-driven model, we have designed a set of wireless sensors to be embedded on an ordinary wheelchair. Our main goal is to accurately estimate the energy expenditure of the user, specifically focusing on the expenditure due to physical activity. The type of physical activity can be estimated through different motion sensors placed on the wheelchair and on the user body. However, activity intensity is impossible to infer from inertial motion sensors only. For instance, displacing a wheelchair on a regular surface will require much less energy than on a sandy surface, even if motion sensors read similar data. Static effort is another example: it can be more physically intensive to stay static on an uphill than to move on a downslope. Force sensors on the wheels can help estimate such physical intensity.

We have thus equipped an ordinary wheelchair with a set of several Bluetooth Low Energy (BLE) sensors in order to build a complete physical activity

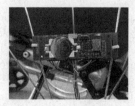

Fig. 1. Wireless sensor board

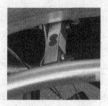

Fig. 2. Load cell coupled to the wheel

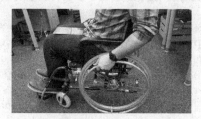

Fig. 3. Modified wheel

monitoring system (PAMS). The system is composed of five sensors allowing to collect data regarding the movements and the effort done by the wheelchair user.

We have designed a wireless sensing board to be fixed on the wheel. It contains a gyrometer and accelerometer device used to determine the wheel speed and an amplifying circuitry for connecting the strain gauges of three load cells (Fig. 1). The wheel has been modified in order to assess the forces applied to it through measuring with load cells the mechanical deformation between the hand rim and the wheel. We have thus replaced the hand rim separators by three load cells in order to measure the tangential force applied to the wheel. Figure 2 depicts how each load cell has been coupled to the wheel. The strain gauges on each load cell are connected to form a Wheatstone bridge topology. The two output signals from the bridges are then amplified, compared and filtered. Finally, the result is read by an embedded microcontroller through an analog-to-digital converter to get the strength value. Figure 3 and Table 1 the complete hardware setup.

Table 1. Summary of the sensors used

Location	Device	Sensors
Wrist	Smartwatch Moto360	Accelerometer & Heart Rate
Chair bottom	BLE113	Accelerometer & Gyroscope
Wheel	BLE113	Accelerometer & Gyroscope
Wheel push ring	Load Cells (3x)	Strain gauges

A second wireless sensing board is directly fixed to the chair. This one is also equipped with accelerometer and gyrometer but without strain gauge interfaces. Its goal is to measure wheelchair inclination for discriminating between upslope, downslope and flat surfaces as well as rotations of the wheelchair.

Both sensing boards are equipped with a Bluetooth Low Energy (BLE) module. The module is the BLE113 developed by Bluegiga. It integrates a calibrated antenna at 2.4 GHz and a low consumption microcontroller. The main interest in this all-in-one module is the reduction of the development time on the hardware design and the full implementation of the Bluetooth stack usable with a simple script language named BGScript. Finally, a commercial smartwatch (i.e., the Moto 360) is fixed on the user's wrist. It is also equipped with motion sensors and is used to detect arm motions in order to improve the model with the detection of other gestures, like auto-propulsing his chair, playing ping-pong or lifting weights. Moreover, this smartwatch is also equipped with a photoplethysmogram sensor used to monitor the users heart rate (HR). HR measurements should help to enhance the model by directly using physiological data for estimating specific users caloric expenditures needs and capacity. All the above described collected data from custom sensors and the commercial smartwatch are transferred through BLE to an Android handheld device carried by the wheelchair user in order to further perform data analysis.

3.2 Activity Recognition

In our project, activity recognition was first envisioned as an intermediate objective, given that we aim at estimating energy expenditure in the end. However, in this paper we present a system that allows for self-tracking of physical activity levels taking already advantage of the activities being recognized, as in [4]. Indeed, as we will show in Sect. 3.3, a graphical summary of the amount of time spent on activities of different levels of intensity can be exploited in a straightforward way to motivate more regular physical exercise. The processing chain of the sensor data [2] starts with the sensor-data acquisition: a stream of sensor samples is obtained and the sensor data stream is preprocessed. A detailed explanation of this activity recognition chain is described in Sect. 4.

3.3 Feedback Visualization

We found important for the end user to have some kind of feedback available. We developed a front-end web interface that shows both the current day summary and a history of the previous week. The interface in its current state is depicted in Fig. 4. All statistics are related to the following intensity levels: Sleeping (or None), Light, Moderate, and Vigorous. For now, this interface is in a beta test state. In a future version of this project, we envision that the users will be able to log on to this interface and see these statistics in near real time.

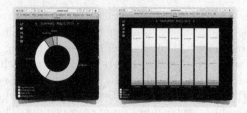

Fig. 4. The web interface for the end user feedback

4   Experiments and Results

4.1   Data Collection

In order to recognize different activities, we started by determining the activities that should be detected and learned. This list contained activities such as: resting, moving (e.g., at different speeds, on different ground types, given different slopes, self-pushed, pushed by a caretaker), desk-work-like (e.g., desk work, browsing on computer, eating, being on the phone) or even replacements (e.g., in the chair, from the wheelchair to the toilet). Moreover, these activities were grouped in several classes of intensity ranging from sleeping (or None) to vigorous. This was done to pave the way for the energy expenditure predicting model that we will develop in a future phase of this project. For the machine learning to take place, the first step was to collect data corresponding to the goal that needs to be achieved. In this case, it meant to use the sensors we described to collect the data of the activities we mentioned above. This operation was performed by an Android handheld device. The data captures followed a protocol that encompassed five activities: resting, desk work, self-pushing at medium speed on a standard flat indoor floor, self-pushing on an ascending slope, and external pushing by a caretaker. Therefore, each activity defined in the list had an intensity level of respectively: none, light, moderate, and vigorous. The protocol required no predefined order for doing the activities, but defined that each activity was to be performed for five minutes straight. This was a precaution to make sure that the model had enough examples for each activity and was therefore able to learn all of them correctly. This protocol was obviously only designed for laboratory purposes and was used to train a model to recognize such activities. The long term goal was to be able to classify captures free from any protocol, such as captures that any person with Spinal Cord Injury would do in a normal day. To ensure that our model performed well, we chose to train it on a specific data capture, and then to test it on another data capture and the other way around. This way, we could be sure that our predictive model generalized well on the activities themselves and not on a spurious setup depending on some day-dependent variables. Furthermore, we grouped the obtained data following an early fusion pattern. We downsampled the Moto 360 accelerometer data by decimation from 50 Hz to 15.63 Hz and upsampled the Moto 360 heart sensor from 1 Hz to 15.63 Hz by repetition. Therefore, at the end of the data collection step, we had two fully labelled datasets of roughly 25 min with 5 min by activity and a 15.63 Hz sampling rate (therefore with a sample for each sensor every 64 ms).

4.2 Feature Extraction

To perform the feature extraction, we chose to roll two windows of respectively 5000 and 1000 ms over the data, in order to have two order of magnitudes of what we can consider a context for every sample. We computed the median, standard deviation and energy of the signal of the windows leading to each sample (included). We extracted these values for the three axes-accelerometer on the wrist, the three axes-accelerometer on the chair, the three axes-gyroscope on the wheel and the three load cells on the pushing ring. Unfortunately, the heart rate sensor from the Moto 360 on the wrist proved to be too noisy and we had to drop it from our analysis. We were therefore left with two captures of respectively 22471 samples (24 min) and 23439 samples (25 min), with the 72 same features. As a lot of these features are probably redundant and correlated, the best choice for an off-the-shelf model is random forest. This is a model introduced by Breiman in 2001 [1] that bags (short for bootstrap aggregates) classification and regression trees (CART) and randomly samples a subset of the features at each split. In doing so, the model averages many noisy but approximately unbiased models, and hence reduces the variance. For classification, a committee of trees each cast a vote for the predicted class. As trees are invariant under linear modification of input, this also speeds up the activity recognition chain since no further preprocessing is required.

4.3 Analysis and Results

As stated before, we wanted to make sure that our model performed well by training it on a specific data capture and testing it on the other one. We also had to do it the other way around to make sure that the model performs equivalently, otherwise it would indicate an inherent problem with the training step. Regarding the temporal resolution, we decided that in order to assess the intensity, it made no sense to predict very short activities. We decided to refine the predictions by rolling a modal filter of 1 min length over them. Indeed, the end user will have no interest in knowing every activity he did at a very high resolution (64 ms); he will be more interested in a more global feedback about his day. In doing so, we make sure that a very short change of activity will be erased. This can both improve or worsen the predictions depending on the conjuncture, but it will always enhance the feedback we can give to the end user.

Experiment 1: All Features. The first experiment we tried was to feed into our model all of the features we extracted. For both ways of training and predicting (train on first capture and predict on second capture, and the other way around), we repeated the training step ten times and we computed both the

Table 2. F1-scores on training, raw predictions and refined predictions for both training orders

Training Set	Prediction Set	Train	Test (raw)	Test (refined)
Capture 1	Capture 2	0.9998 ± 0.00	0.7754 ± 0.01	0.7678 ± 0.03
Capture 2	Capture 1	0.9999 ± 0.00	0.9314 ± 0.00	0.9874 ± 0.00

normalized confusion matrices and the weighted F1-scores of the raw resulting classification and of the refined predictions as described in Sect. 4.3 with the modal filter. We used the ensemble package of scikit-learn [11] for building our random forest classifier. For the parameters, we used 1000 trees, the entropy criterion, and used the square root for selection of the maximum number of features at each split. These are standard parameters when using a Random Forest classifier.

The results of this first experiment are described in Table 2. Each row in the table represents a different order for training and predicting, each column contains results on the training set (by out-of-bag score), on the testing set with raw predictions and on the testing set with refined predictions.

As we see in Table 2, both ways of training and predicting are not equivalent. Indeed, the score on the test set when trained of the first capture drops dramatically compared to the same score when trained on the second one. This indicates a disparity between the two captures. This is a recurring problem in machine learning: when not enough data is available, the noise can sometimes be mistaken as signal. The more data we have, the more the noise gets averaged among captures and the easier the signal can be recognized.

In our case, we analyzed this problem as being caused by proxy features. Proxy features are features that seem to be discriminant in a given dataset but are not in reality. We included an example for illustration: In Fig. 5, we see that if we look at the first capture, this variable —the energy of the chair accelerometer signal in the x-axis over the last 5000 ms— seems excellent to separate activity classes *Still* and *Work*. On the other hand, we see in the second capture that this variable has actually no importance and does not separate these two activities at all. In this case, we can deduce that the proxy variables used did not accurately represent both activities. A classifier, even a human one, trained on the first capture will obviously make mistakes when predicting the second capture. Conversely, a classifier trained on the second capture will select another variable to separate these activities and will probably separate correctly these activities. This example explains the dispaired results shown in Table 2.

This problem is caused by lack of data and should disappear as we collect more data, but in the meantime, a good way of overcoming that issue is to manually select features that we know from expert knowledge and bio-medical modelling are relevant for characterizing the activities we defined.

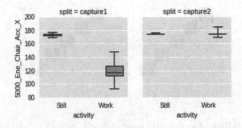

Fig. 5. A "proxy" feature in first (left) and second (right) capture, in activities Still and Work

Experiment 2: Manually Selected and Engineered Features. In this experiment, we crafted and hand-picked features that we know are important for the resolution of this problem. We therefore ensured that our model only got features that are relevant in every case. Indeed, every feature is certified by expert knowledge to be of influence in the activity we hope to recognize. These features were namely: the sum of the standard deviation of the three load cells over the last 5000 ms, the sum of the standard deviation of the wrist three-axis accelerometer values over the last 5000 ms, the median orientation of the chair in the longitudinal plane over the last 5000 ms, the standard deviation of the wheel angular speed in the z-axis (longitudinal ground speed) over the last 5000 ms, the median wrist acceleration in the x-axis (longitudinal acceleration) over the last 5000 ms, and the median wrist acceleration magnitude (norm of the three axis vector) over the last 1000 and 5000 ms. We built models and estimated their performance as explained in Sect. 4.3. These results are presented in Table 3. The model is now working as expected, with training orders being equivalent in terms of performance. To illustrate this, Fig. 6 depicts the confusion matrices of ground truth against raw (left) and refined (right) predictions with the first capture used as training and second capture used as testing, while Fig. 7 shows the same matrices but with the reverse training order.

We highlighted the effect, positive in this case, of the modal filter in Figs. 8 and 9. These figures present the raw (top) and refined (middle) predictions on the second capture (when the model was trained on the first one) in Fig. 8 and on the first capture (when the model was trained on the second one) in Fig. 9.

Table 3. F1-scores on training, raw predictions and refined predictions for both training orders with manually selected features

Training Set	Prediction Set	Train	Test (raw)	Test (refined)
Capture 1	Capture 2	0.9995 ± 0.00	0.8923 ± 0.00	0.9550 ± 0.00
Capture 2	Capture 1	0.9985 ± 0.00	0.8844 ± 0.00	0.9933 ± 0.00

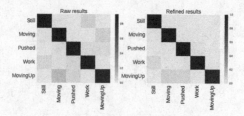

Fig. 6. Confusion matrices of raw (left) and refined (right) predictions using first capture as train test and second capture as test set

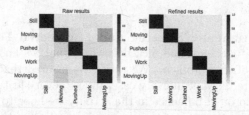

Fig. 7. Confusion matrices of raw (left) and refined (right) predictions using second capture as train test and first capture as test set

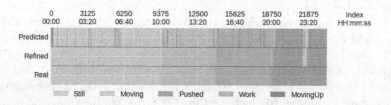

Fig. 8. Timeline of ground truth (bottom) against raw (top) and refined (middle) predictions using first capture as train test and second capture as test set

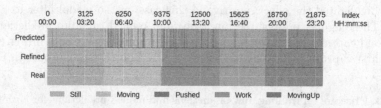

Fig. 9. Timeline of ground truth (bottom) against raw (top) and refined (middle) predictions using second capture as train test and first capture as test set

We also see that this filter has a lag effect causing the detection of a start of a new activity to be slightly delayed comparing to its real start. This lag is approximately equal to 30 s (half the filter size), which is a negligible error.

We can therefore conclude that the system in its basic version can recognize the defined activities with a F1-score of roughly 0.9, which is already an excellent score for an activity recognition task similar to what is currently achieved in [8]. In its refined version, with a 1 min modal filter applied to it, the results seem to climb around 0.97. Of course, this is an even better score, but its contribution does not only encompasses the score enhancement, but also —and more importantly— gives a much clearer feedback to the user. Knowing the system is able to correctly classify such activities, it is therefore also able to separate activities with different intensities, since the activities are grouped into intensity levels.

5   Conclusions and Future Work

In this paper, we presented our ActiDote —activity as an antidote— system which in its current state can accurately detect and recognize activities of different intensity levels. Indeed, a weighted F1-score of 0.97 has been attained on two different data captures. This means that with the training and the testing data belonging to different experiments, the model was still able to perform well. In order to have a robust model that can adapt to different wheelchairs and different users, it is mandatory to train it on more data. This is why one of the next step is to capture labelled data for a larger group of user with the current setup. This should also avoid having to select the features to feed into our model. Indeed, the noise contained in each individual capture should theoretically be averaged out.

The system as described is available at a lower cost compared to similar setups and gives the end user a very accurate feedback. Therefore, not only does it provide a means for self-tracking physical activity and self-motivation, but it can also be used for potential continuous monitoring of patients during rehabilitation. Last but not least, the development of self-tracking devices and continuous monitoring should indirectly contribute to reduce health costs.

We are currently working on improving the system accuracy by developing new hardware and software. On the hardware side, we are currently developing our own strength sensors based on strain gauges. The main improvement will consist in measuring the force applied on a radial axis in addition to the tangential axis already measured. Other sensing elements are also being evaluated like pressure sensors on the chair surface in order to track posture and activities like switching chairs (transfer on public bathrooms, etc.) or adjusting seat position (pressure relief, etc.). As for the software side, we do not only aim at making this system near real-time, but also capable of recognizing more activities. The next steps encompass extrapolating an energy expenditure measurement, in order for the user or caregivers to have a quantitative estimation as feedback.

Acknowledgements. This project has been supported by the HES-SO grant IA-INTERDISC14-01. We would like to thank all the members of the ACTIDOTE consortium for fruitful discussions and collaboration and Eric Henchoz for developing the web-based visualization interface. We thank Julien Rebetez and Aitana Lebrand for comments and suggestions on the manuscript.

References

1. Breiman, L.: Random forests. Mach. Learn. **45**(1), 5–32 (2001)
2. Bulling, A., Blanke, U., Schiele, B.: A tutorial on human activity recognition using body-worn inertial sensors. ACM Comput. Surv. (CSUR) **46**(3), 33 (2014)
3. Conger, S.A.: Physical activity assessment in wheelchair users (2011)
4. Ding, D., Hiremath, S., Chung, Y., Cooper, R.: Detection of wheelchair user activities using wearable sensors. In: Stephanidis, C. (ed.) UAHCI 2011. LNCS, vol. 6767, pp. 145–152. Springer, Heidelberg (2011). doi:10.1007/978-3-642-21666-4_17
5. Garcia-Masso, X., Serra-Ano, P., Garcia-Raffi, L., Sánchez-Pérez, E.A., López-Pascual, J., Gonzalez, L.: Validation of the use of actigraph gt3x accelerometers to estimate energy expenditure in full time manual wheelchair users with spinal cord injury. Spinal Cord **51**(12), 898–903 (2013)
6. Gendle, S.C., Richardson, M., Leeper, J., Hardin, L.B., Green, J.M., Bishop, P.A.: Wheelchair-mounted accelerometers for measurement of physical activity. Disabil. Rehabil. Assist. Technol. **7**(2), 139–148 (2012)
7. Hiremath, S.V., Ding, D.: Evaluation of activity monitors in manual wheelchair users with paraplegia. J. Spinal Cord Med. **34**(1), 110–117 (2011)
8. Hiremath, S.V., Intille, S.S., Kelleher, A., Cooper, R.A., Ding, D.: Detection of physical activities using a physical activity monitor system for wheelchair users. Med. Eng. Phys. **37**(1), 68–76 (2015)
9. Kokkinos, P., Sheriff, H., Kheirbek, R.: Physical inactivity and mortality risk. Cardiol. Res. Pract. **2011**, 924–945 (2011)
10. Pande, A., Zeng, Y., Das, A., Mohapatra, P., Miyamoto, S., Seto, E., Henricson, E.K., Han, J.J.: Accurate energy expenditure estimation using smartphone sensors. In: Proceedings of the 4th Conference on Wireless Health, p. 19. ACM (2013)
11. Pedregosa, F., Varoquaux, G., Gramfort, A., Michel, V., Thirion, B., Grisel, O., Blondel, M., Prettenhofer, P., Weiss, R., Dubourg, V., et al.: Scikit-learn: machine learning in python. J. Mach. Learn. Res. **12**, 2825–2830 (2011)
12. Rooksby, J., Rost, M., Morrison, A., Chalmers, M.C.: Personal tracking as lived informatics. In: Proceedings of the 32nd Annual ACM Conference on Human Factors in Computing Systems, pp. 1163–1172. ACM (2014)
13. Ruch, N., Joss, F., Jimmy, G., Melzer, K., Hänggi, J., Mäder, U.: Neural network versus activity-specific prediction equations for energy expenditure estimation in children. J. Appl. Physiol. **115**(9), 1229–1236 (2013)
14. Staudenmayer, J., Pober, D., Crouter, S., Bassett, D., Freedson, P.: An artificial neural network to estimate physical activity energy expenditure and identify physical activity type from an accelerometer. J. Appl. Physiol. **107**(4), 1300–1307 (2009)
15. Tanhoffer, R.A., Tanhoffer, A.I., Raymond, J., Hills, A.P., Davis, G.M.: Comparison of methods to assess energy expenditure and physical activity in people with spinal cord injury. J. Spinal Cord Med. **35**(1), 35–45 (2012)
16. Vyas, N., Farringdon, J., Andre, D., Stivoric, J.I.: Machine learning and sensor fusion for estimating continuous energy expenditure. AI Mag. **33**(2), 55 (2012)
17. Weil, E., Wachterman, M., McCarthy, E.P., Davis, R.B., O'Day, B., Iezzoni, L.I., Wee, C.C.: Obesity among adults with disabling conditions. Jama **288**(10), 1265–1268 (2002)

Non Invasive Detection of Coronary Artery Disease Using PCG and PPG

Rohan Banerjee[1]([✉]), Anirban Dutta Choudhury[1], Shreyasi Datta[1],
Arpan Pal[1], and Kayapanda M. Mandana[2]

[1] Innovation Labs, Tata Consultancy Services Ltd., Kolkata, India
{rohan.banerjee,anirban.duttachoudhury,shreyasi.datta,arpan.pal}@tcs.com
[2] Fortis Hospital, Kolkata, India
kmmandana@gmail.com

Abstract. Coronary Artery Disease (CAD) kills more than a million of
people every year. However, there is no significant marker for identifying
CAD patients unobtrusively. In this paper, we propose a methodology
for non invasive screening of CAD patients from heart sound analysis.
Instead of segregating the diastolic heart sound as mentioned in prior
arts, the proposed methodology extracts spectral features from the entire
phonocardiogram (PCG) signal, broken into small overlapping windows.
Support vector machine (SVM) is used for classification. Our methodology produces 80% classification accuracy on a dataset of 25 subjects,
containing PCG data of both cardiac an non cardiac patients as well as
healthy subjects. Results also reveal that a simple transfer function can
be formed to identify the CAD patients if photoplethysmogram (PPG)
signal is available simultaneously along with PCG.

Keywords: Coronary Artery Disease · Phonocardiogram · Classification · Photoplethysmogram · Transfer function

1 Introduction

Simple, low cost and non-invasive solutions for health monitoring are increasingly gaining attention in both developed and developing nations. Such solutions
deploy a set of low cost sensors to extract meaningful information regarding physical condition of a person. Although the performance of those solutions is not
comparable to the costly medical devices and investigations, they can be useful
for day to day monitoring, preventive health care and alert generation. Off the
shelf solutions to estimate physiological vitals like heart rate, blood pressure,
ECG are already available in the market. Some of them use dedicated wearable
sensors (Fitbit[1]), whereas some utilize the inbuilt sensors of smart phones along
with some extra attachments (Alivecor[2]) to increase their affordability.

---

[1] https://www.fitbit.com/.
[2] http://www.alivecor.com/home.

© ICST Institute for Computer Sciences, Social Informatics and Telecommunications Engineering 2017
K. Giokas et al. (Eds.): eHealth 2016, LNICST 181, pp. 241–252, 2017.
DOI: 10.1007/978-3-319-49655-9_32

Coronary Artery Disease (CAD) is a leading cause of death, killing more than a million of people across the world every year [8]. The reason of CAD is building up of fatty deposits (plaque) on the walls of coronary arteries [8]. This makes the cavity inside arteries narrower, restricting the blood flow, causing heart attack and death. As the natural elasticity of arteries deteriorates with ageing, the elderly population is more prone to the disease. However, proliferation of sedentary life style and unhealthy diet are exposing the young generation also towards CAD.

The most common symptom to identify CAD is angina or chest pain [8]. However, there is no definite marker for CAD. Typically the doctors advise various investigations after considering self and family history and life style of the patients, complaining of angina. Which is followed by echo cardiogram, angiography or exercise stress test to diagnose early or sense CAD. However, these are all costly and invasive medical tests. Thus the importance of non-invasive CAD markers comes into the scenario.

A coarse detection of CAD is possible from different physiological signals. The most commonly used non-invasive marker is the heart rate variability (HRV) [3,6,9]. Gold standard for HRV is to measure the R-R interval distance from the ECG waveform. Research shows that CAD patients typically have a reduced HRV, compared to a normal person [6]. However, this requires the analysis of ECG signal for a prolonged time interval. The other popular marker is to analyse the heart sound [12,13]. The heart sound signal, also known as phonocardiogram (PCG), is generally recorded using a digital stethoscope. The sounds generated from a healthy heart during opening and closing of heart valves is different than that of an abnormal heart. The power spectrum of the diastolic part of PCG signal was analysed in [4] and found that the spectral energy is more at a frequency region higher than 130 Hz for the CAD patients. However PCG is extremely vulnerable to ambient noise and thus a clear segregation of diastolic heart sound is a tricky task. Moreover patients having cardiac murmur, generally have a noisy heart sound, making the segregation task further difficult. Certain prior arts [2] claimed to identify heart disease from photoplethysmogram (PPG) signal. However the dataset used by [2] is too small to take any conclusive decision. PPG is a simple non-invasive technique that measures the volumetric blood flow in capillaries [1]. PPG signal is periodic in nature whose fundamental frequency indicates the heart rate.

In this paper, we propose a methodology to identify CAD patients from spectral features of PCG signal. Instead of segregating the diastolic heart sounds, the proposed methodology splits the entire signal into small overlapping windows, each having at least one complete heart cycle. We used our in-house low cost digital stethoscope [14] to collect the PCG data in order to cut down the overall cost of the system. Also we explore the feasibility of classifying CAD patients by forming a transfer function from simultaneously recorded PPG and PCG signals. It is important to mention that, our objective is not to replace the established clinical techniques for identifying CAD, but to propose a screening system, to be used by the physicians before subjecting a patient for an invasive medical diagnosis.

The rest of the paper is organized as follows. The transfer function based approach is explained in Sect. 2. Our proposed PCG based methodology is detailed in Sect. 3. Experimental dataset is explained in Sect. 4. Followed by results and conclusion in Sects. 5 and 6 respectively.

2   Transfer Function from Simultaneously Recorded PCG and PPG Signals

Human cardiovascular system can be considered as a closed loop system, where the heart acts as a source to pump blood to the end capillaries. In this approach, we consider PCG as the input to the cardiovascular system, representing the function of opening and closing of heart valves (source) and PPG as the output signal, representing the blood flow at end capillaries (sink). Thus a simple transfer function of the system can be formed from them. As both PCG and PPG signals of a CAD patient is different from a non CAD person, the same is expected to reflect in the transfer function. In this paper we use an adaptive filter to get the same.

An adaptive filter is a kind of digital filter, whose transfer function is adjusted over time to adapt the properties of the output signal. Adaptive filters are commonly used for noise cancellation, identification of response of an unknown system, inverse system identification etc. The block diagram of an adaptive filter is shown in Fig. 1. Here u denotes the filter input, which is the PCG signal in our case. The desired signal d is the PPG signal. Our job is to adjust the tap weights of the adaptive filter in such a way, that the filter output y matches the desired signal d, minimizing the error e, where $e = d - y$. Normalized Least Mean Square (NLMS) algorithm [5] is popularly used for calculating the filter coefficients of an adaptive filter. In this iterative process, the output (y) of the FIR filter is calculated by convolving the input signal (u) and filter taps $(\hat{w})$. The overall error, estimated from the difference between the filter output (y) and the desired output (d) is used to adjust the tap weights based on the principle of steepest descent. NLMS guarantees the stability of LMS algorithm by normalizing the learning rate with respect to the input signal.

Simultaneously recorded PPG and PCG signals are required for the validation of the above-mentioned approach. We used a freely available dataset [11], that contains both the signals sampled at 1000 Hz. The dataset contains, 2 normal adult subjects and 2 CAD patients. The CAD patients include an 11 year old female subject having cardiac murmur with aortic stenosis and a 14 months old female subject having pulmonary stenosis, ventricular septal defect and pulmonary hypertension. Tap size of the filter is chosen as 1024. Frequency response of the transfer function for all 4 subjects present in the dataset is shown in Fig. 2(a). It can be visualized that, the overall spectrum is much noisier for the CAD patients due to the presence of high frequency components in their PCG signals due to cardiac murmur. For a detailed inspection, we divide the entire

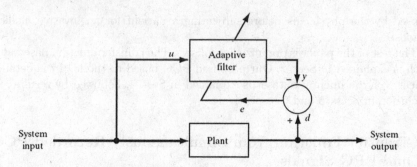

Fig. 1. Block diagram of adaptive filter

spectrum shown in Fig. 2(a) into 16 bins and the variance of spectral amplitude at each bin is shown in the bar chart of Fig. 2(b) for all the subjects. This clearly shows that above bin 5, the amplitude variance of the CAD patients is significantly higher compared to the normal subjects.

3   Proposed Methodology

In spite of its simplicity and robustness, The method discussed in Sect. 2 has the following limitations,

- PPG and PCG signals, need to be completely synchronized
- Both signals should have equal sampling rate

However, in practical scenario, the task of synchronizing multiple biomedical signals recorded at different sampling rates has severe deployment issues. Sampling rate of a commercial pulse oximeter, that captures PPG signal is around 100 Hz. On the other hand, raw audio signals are sampled at several KHz of sampling rate in a digital stethoscope. Up-sampling of PPG signal and/or downscaling of PCG signal introduce noise in both the signals, making the transfer function unreliable. Thus we propose an alternative approach, to identify CAD patients using PCG as the only source of input. Block digram of the proposed methodology is shown in Fig. 3. Different components are further illustrated in the following subsections.

3.1   Preprocessing

Being a wide band signal, PCG is highly susceptible to noise. Ambient signals present in the audible range is the major source of such noise. Noise, generated due to friction at the contact region of the diaphragm of stethoscope and the subject body also heavily corrupts the signal. Important information regarding heart sound is typically confined within 150 Hz. Thus, we remove all frequency components above 500 Hz using a low pass filter. Subsequently the signal is down sampled at 1000 Hz before further processing.

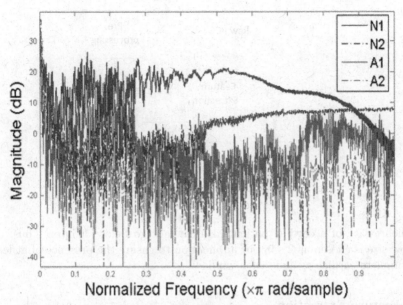

(a) Frequency Response of Transfer Function N1, N2:Normal, A1, A2: CAD

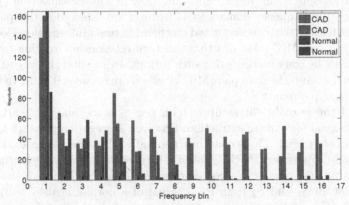

(b) Variation of Spectral Amplitude at Different Frequency Bins

Fig. 2. Results of transfer function based approach on dataset [11]

3.2 Windowing

A PCG signal is non-stationary in nature due to heart rate variability. Thus the raw signal is broken into rectangular windows with 50% overlapping to restore the temporal information. Selecting of the optimum window length is a tricky task. A prolonged window size may end up in mixing up multiple cardiac cycles in a single window. Thus the window size should be short enough to preserve the temporal information corresponding to individual cycle. We can safely assume

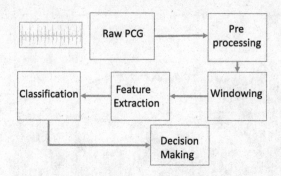

Fig. 3. Block diagram of proposed methodology

that heart rate of a cardiac patient also can not go below 30 bpm. Thus, the window size is chosen as 2 s in our application to ensure the presence of at least one complete cardiac cycle in each window.

3.3   Feature Extraction

Feature extraction is the most important task in any classification problem. Several time and frequency domain PCG features are explored in this paper and the relevant feature set is chosen based on their Maximal Information Coefficient (MIC) [10] scored. MIC measures the statistical relationship existing between a pair of dataset by constructing grids with various sizes to find the largest mutual information between the data pair. MIC gives a score between 0 and 1 to indicate that relationship strength.

Most of the available literatures [4,13] segregate S_1 and S_2 heart sounds from PCG signal for feature extraction. However, segregation of heart sounds is not always very trivial. The second heart sound (S_2) is often suppressed due to ambient noise. Moreover, PCG signal of a cardiac patient having murmur may contain extra heart sounds (S_3, S_4) corrupting S_1 and S_2. Figures 5 and 6 show the detection of S_1 and S_2 from PCG signal of a normal healthy subject and a subject having cardiac murmur using the state of the art approach presented in [7]. Results show that detection of S_2 is often missed especially in case of cardiac murmur. Thus instead of segregating the S_1 and S_2 regions, we attempt to process the entire signal, by splitting into small overlapping windows.

For extracting frequency domain features, we compute short-time Fourier transform (STFT) of every window to get the spectrum. For k^{th} time window $W_k(t)$, if $S_k(\omega)$ be the corresponding amplitude of spectral power in frequency domain and N be the length of the window, then the optimum feature set based on top 5 MIC scores includes

(1) Ratio of spectral power between 0–100 Hz and 100–150 Hz
(2) spectral centroid ($cen = \sum_{\omega=1}^{N} \omega * S_k(\omega) / \sum_{\omega=1}^{N} \omega$)
(3) spectral roll-off ($SR = 0.85 * \sum_{\omega=1}^{N} S_k(\omega)$)

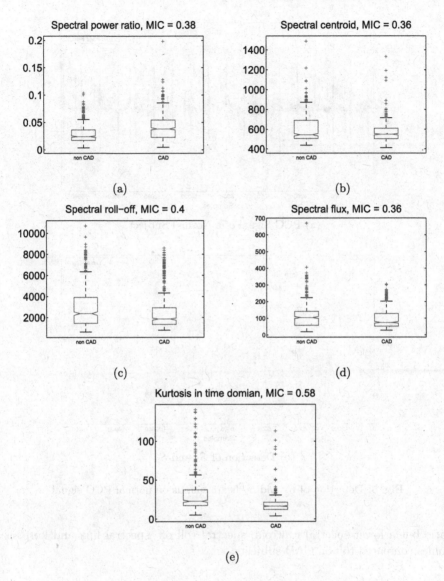

Fig. 4. Box plots of PCG features for CAD and non CAD subjects

(4) spectral flux ($\|S_k(\omega) - S_{k-1}(\omega)\|$)
(5) kurtosis of the signal window in time domain

In descriptive statistics, box plot is a standardized graphical way of display-ing the distribution of data, based on five metrics e.g. minimum, first quartile, median, third quartile, and maximum. Figure 4, shows the box plots as well as MIC scores of different PCG features applied on our dataset detailed in Sect. 4. It can be observed that CAD patients typically have a higher spectral power

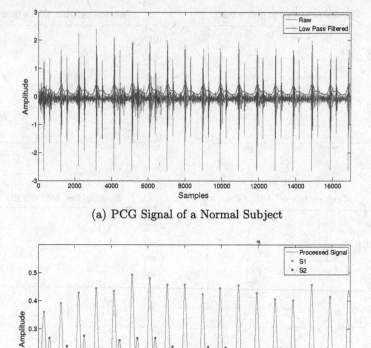

(a) PCG Signal of a Normal Subject

(b) Detection of S_1 and S_2

Fig. 5. Detection of S_1 and S_2 heart sounds on normal PCG signal

ratio but a lower spectral centroid, spectral roll off, spectral flux and kurtosis values compared to non CAD subjects.

3.4 Classification

Support Vector Machine (SVM) is used for classification. Both linear and non linear SVM were explored and it is found that non-linear SVM with Radial Basis Function (RBF) kernel produces the optimum classification performance. Like feature extraction, classification is also performed on individual window. The final decision making (CAD or non CAD) is done based on majority voting across all the windows present in a particular test signal.

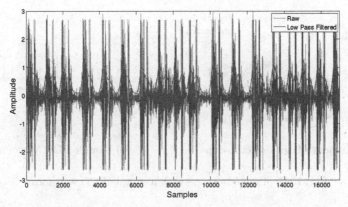

(a) PCG Signal of a Subject having Cardiac Murmur

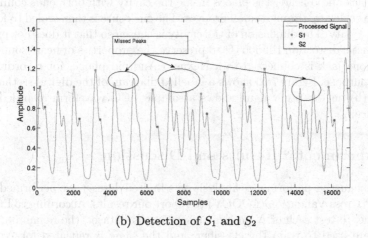

(b) Detection of S_1 and S_2

Fig. 6. Detection of S_1 and S_2 heart sounds on murmur PCG signal

4   Experimental Dataset

We created a corpus of CAD and non CAD subjects to conduct our experiments. A total of 11 healthy individuals, aged between 24 ± 2 years, having no known cardiovascular disease and 4 patients (aged 56 ± 11 years) being treated for non cardiovascular diseases in a large urban hospital in Kolkata, India participated as non CAD subjects. Another 10 angiography-proven patients (aged 61 ± 12 years), were selected from the same hospital as CAD subjects. According to their consultant physicians, out of 10 CAD subjects, 2 subjects had a marginal 30% blockage and the rest having a blockage of 70% or higher.

. Heart sound was collected using our in-house digital stethoscope [14], which is a low cost replacement of a commercial digital stethoscope. The metal earpiece of a clinical stethoscope is removed and its tube ends are inserted into a 3-D printed rectangular cavity. In order to hear the heart sound, the microphone of a

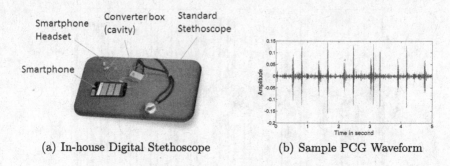

(a) In-house Digital Stethoscope   (b) Sample PCG Waveform

Fig. 7. Digital stethoscope with a sample PCG waveform

3.5 mm jack audio headset is placed inside the cavity with both ends coming out from the enclosure through small grooves. The enclosure is then sealed to form an air-tight cavity. The dimension of the cavity is chosen so that it does not produce any acoustic distortion till 500 Hz to preserve the properties of heart sound. The microphone jack is connected to a Nexus 5 Android phone, for recording and storage purpose. Figure 7(a) shows a labelled diagram of the digital stethoscope. Figure 7(b) on the other hand shows a sample PCG waveform recorded using the device.

5   Experimental Results and Discussion

For an exhaustive performance analysis on a limited dataset, we performed Leave One Out Cross Validation (LOOCV) to report our results. According to LOOCV technique, to test each of N entries present in the dataset, the remaining $N - 1$ entries are used to train the classifier, and the same is repeated for N times, making N different training-testing scenarios.

First we tested the performance of our proposed methodology on the freely available dataset in [11]. Being a very clean dataset, We got the confusion matrix shown in Table 1 with 100% detection accuracy. However as we move on to the dataset captured using our in-house digital stethoscope, containing some noisy PCG signal, the performance of the proposed methodology drops. The confusion matrix is shown in Table 2. Results show that, the proposed methodology can detect the non CAD subjects more accurately compared to CAD patients. A detailed observation further reveals that, out of 4 false negative cases (actually CAD but predicted as non CAD), the proposed classifier failed to detect 2 borderline CAD patients, having 30% blockage (mentioned in Sect. 4). Inclusion of more such patients might be required in the training set in order to correctly detect such cases. The only false positive (actually non CAD but detected as CAD) occurrence, was a male subject who was being treated in the hospital for asthma related disease. It is remained to be seen, whether the PCG signal of a asthmatic patient contains any signature similar to a CAD patient.

Table 1. Confusion matrix on dataset [11]

Predicted	Actual	
	CAD	Non-CAD
CAD	2	0
Non-CAD	0	2

Table 2. Confusion matrix on our dataset

Predicted	Actual	
	CAD	Non-CAD
CAD	6	1
Non-CAD	4	14

Sensitivity and specificity are popularly used for measuring the performance of a binary classifier. In our application, sensitivity or true positive rate measures the fraction of CAD patients being correctly identified whereas specificity or true negative rate measures the fraction of non CAD subjects being correctly identified by the classifier. For an ideal system both sensitivity and specificity should be closer to 1. In our case the overall sensitivity and specificity of detecting CAD patients are found to be 0.6 and 0.93 respectively, with an overall 80% classification accuracy. A high specificity of the classifier indicates that, there is a very little chance of declaring a non CAD patients as CAD, which helps the doctor to prescribe lesser number of invasive medical tests to angina patients. However, due to low sensitivity, there is a high chance that a CAD patient might be classified as non CAD. This needs a significant improvement in order to realize the screening system.

6   Conclusion and Future Work

In this paper we propose a non invasive methodology to classify CAD patients. The proposed methodology extracts time and frequency domain features from PCG signal to perform the task. Results show that, in spite of performing well on a clean dataset, the sensitivity of the proposed algorithm still needs improvement before actual system deployment. Results also show that if PPG and PCG signals are available simultaneously at an equal sampling rate, a transfer function can be formed to detect CAD patients. Our future work will focus on cleaning of the noisy PCG data, as well as fusion of PCG signal with other non-invasive biomedical signals (PPG, ECG etc.) to boost up the overall confidence score of the system. Also we are experimenting the feasibility of estimating the percentage blockage in coronary artery of a cardiac patient in a non invasive manner, enhancing the proposed methodology.

References

1. Allen, J.: Photoplethysmography and its application in clinical physiological measurement. Physiol. Meas. **28**(3), R1 (2007)
2. Angius, G., Barcellona, D., Cauli, E., Meloni, L., Raffo, L.: Myocardial infarction and antiphospholipid syndrome: a first study on finger ppg waveforms effects. In: Computing in Cardiology (CinC), 2012, pp. 517–520. IEEE (2012)

3. Dua, S., Du, X., Sree, S.V., Vi, T.A.: Novel classification of coronary artery disease using heart rate variability analysis. J. Mech. Med. Biol. **12**(04), 1240017 (2012)
4. Gauthier, D., Akay, Y.M., Paden, R.G., Pavlicek, W., Fortuin, F.D., Sweeney, J.K., Lee, R.W., Akay, M.: Spectral analysis of heart sounds associated with coronary occlusions. In: 6th International Special Topic Conference on Information Technology Applications in Biomedicine, ITAB 2007, pp. 49–52. IEEE (2007)
5. Hayes, M.H.: Statistical digital signal processing and modeling. Wiley, New York (2009)
6. Krittayaphong, R., Cascio, W.E., Light, K.C., Sheffield, D., Golden, R.N., Finkel, J.B., Glekas, G., Koch, G.G., Sheps, D.S.: Heart rate variability in patients with coronary artery disease: differences in patients with higher and lower depression scores. Psychosom. Med. **59**(3), 231–235 (1997)
7. Kuan, K.L.: A framework for automated heart and lung sound analysis using a mobile telemedicine platform. Ph.D. thesis, Massachusetts Institute of Technology (2010)
8. MedlinePlus: Coronary artery disease (2016). https://www.nlm.nih.gov/medlineplus/coronaryarterydisease.html. Accessed 5 Feb 2016
9. Mironova, T., Mironov, V., Antufiev, V., Safronova, E., Mironov, M., Davydova, E.: Heart rate variability analysis at coronary artery disease and angina pectoris. Recent Pat. Cardiovasc. Drug Discov. **4**(1), 45–54 (2009)
10. Reshef, D.N., Reshef, Y.A., Finucane, H.K., Grossman, S.R., McVean, G., Turnbaugh, P.J., Lander, E.S., Mitzenmacher, M., Sabeti, P.C.: Detecting novel associations in large data sets. Science **334**(6062), 1518–1524 (2011)
11. Ridha, S.A.: Simulation Recording of an ECG, PCG, and PPG for Feature Extractions (2014). https://doaj.org/article/81af935cef6841ad99361ff1dbc53049
12. Schmidt, S.E., Hansen, J., Zimmermann, H., Hammershøi, D., Toft, E., Struijk, J.J.: Coronary artery disease and low frequency heart sound signatures. In: Computing in Cardiology, 2011, pp. 481–484. IEEE (2011)
13. Schmidt, S., Holst-Hansen, C., Graff, C., Toft, E., Struijk, J.: Detection of coronary artery disease with an electronic stethoscope. In: Computers in Cardiology, 2007, pp. 757–760. IEEE (2007)
14. Sinharay, A., Ghosh, D., Deshpande, P., Alam, S., Banerjee, R., Pal, A.: Smartphone based digital stethoscope for connected health - a direct acoustic coupling technique. In: 2016 the IEEE 1st International Conference on Connected Health: Applications, Systems and Engineering Technologies (IEEE CHASE 2016), June 2016

Detection and Assessment of Behaviours Associated with the Risk of Obesity in Adolescents

Filip Velickovski[1](✉), Silvia Orte[1], Marc Sola[1], Sarah A. Tabozzi[2], and Claudio L. Lafortuna[2]

[1] Eurecat, Barcelona, Spain
{filip.velickovski,silvia.orte,marc.sola}@eurecat.org
[2] IBFM-CNR, Segrate, Milano, Italy
{sarah.tabozzi,claudio.lafortuna}@ibfm.cnr.it

Abstract. Obesity in younger age groups has been recognized as an alarming key predictor for obesity in adulthood. PEGASO aims to develop a solution involving wearable devices and an mHealth based application running on a smartphone and cloud computing infrastructure, with the capability of gradually changing harmful behaviours and encouraging healthy habits in adolescents. We present an assessment strategy in the short and long term to evaluate behaviours associated with the risk of adolescent obesity from scientifically informed indicators.

Keywords: Obesity · Physical activity · Adolescents · mHealth · Wearable · Behaviour recognition

1 Introduction

Obesity in younger age groups has been recognized as an alarming key predictor for obesity in adulthood [13], beside having a serious negative impact on health and social and psychological well-being also during juvenile age. Appropriate levels of physical activity, and adequate nutrition are recognised as having a key role for obesity prevention, furthermore the adoption of healthy habits in eating, and an active lifestyle determine in children and adolescents a reduction of the risk for developing obesity [9,12,14]. Therefore, the leveraging of behaviour change towards positive lifestyles is a primary component of a preventive approach.

The rapidly growing availability of wearable devices, and mobile phones connected to the internet has allowed for research into newer innovative and scalable solutions for personalised interventions for the prevention of obesity [5], which may overcome the limitations deriving from face-to-face interventions (small effects and limited reach) or disseminated through mass media approaches (generic content and poor personal relevance of feed-backs) [11]. However, a prerequisite for widespread efficacy of health behaviour change interventions is the

© ICST Institute for Computer Sciences, Social Informatics and Telecommunications Engineering 2017
K. Giokas et al. (Eds.): eHealth 2016, LNICST 181, pp. 253–258, 2017.
DOI: 10.1007/978-3-319-49655-9_33

exploitation of a behaviour detection and assessment approach based on objectively measured parameters and scientifically evidenced criteria for evaluation [2].

The *Personalised Guidance Services for Optimising lifestyle management in teenagers through awareness, motivation and engagement* system (PEGASO) [3] is built upon mobile health (mHealth) and cloud computing technologies, which are articulated to analyse adolescents' behaviours and trigger personalized actuations that foster behaviour change. For physical activity and resting attitudes (sleep included) which are the focus of the present paper, the analysis of user's behaviour detected through objectively measured variables (with smartphone sensors and wearable devices) relies upon evidence-based criteria and takes advantage of cloud solutions to perform a two-stage processing of the user-generated data at distinct interval durations: into daily aggregated summaries (24 h timespan), and uploaded into a cloud based data repository for further processing. This analysis will provide the user with different levels of feedback and interaction. Data collected in the smartphone is continuously analysed to provide almost real-time response to detected events such as behavioural abnormalities. In the cloud, the data is analysed over a longer timespan (1 month) so that the system can identify the user's behavioural trends and evaluate her progress on the long term goals set in the platform.

2   Method

A number of behaviours whose correlation to obesity is representative and measurable have been identified by recent biomedical research [7,14]. In PEGASO, the behaviours of interest are referred as targets, so the term **target behaviour** defines an absence of a healthy habit that is susceptible to be changed, and represents a threat to the health of the adolescents in a short and long-term period. On the basis of their coherence and relevance with PEGASO requirements (i.e. strength of correlation with obesity onset and measurability through wearables) ten target behaviours were selected. Common to all selected behaviours is the characteristic that they are amenable to positive change. Among the behaviours, six that refer to physical activity, sedentariness and sleep attributes are the focus of this work. Different sources of information throughout PEGASO produce the necessary data to model and quantify the behaviour of the user. The Sensing System, designed and implemented within PEGASO, is composed of a smart bracelet, a smart garment and smartphone embedded sensors. They collect information about human kinetics and cardiovascular activity which, after a post-processing phase, provide data about the time spent doing activities of different intensity (walking, running, biking, swimming, etc.), the number of steps done throughout the day, the distance, the energy expended and other parameters related to sleep. The design of each wearable was completed within the project, and took into account quality control assessments to ensure the reliability of the measured parameter. Furthermore a data fusion algorithm (beyond the scope of this paper) to enhance reliability was implemented when the same parameter (e.g. steps walked) was measured by more than one wearable sensor.

Assessment of Target Behaviours in the Short-Term. Short-term behaviour is defined as the sum of the actions that PEGASO is able to detect during the shortest period of assessment (generally one day), evaluated and converted into a score. Experts in the project used the indications contained in the international guidelines and evidence-based literature to set referenced cut-offs permitting a classification of each behaviour and building a scoring system for the behaviour assessment in the short-term. Table 1 summarises the translation into scores the objectively detected behaviours, which are measured according to the degree to which the user adheres to the recommendations. In the system, 0 indicates the compliance with recommendations (and hence also the lowest risk for obesity) and 2 indicates the worst adherence to recommendations (and hence the highest risk).

Assessment of Target Behaviours in the Long-Term. Long-term behaviour is the sum of short-term behaviour assessments that captures the general trend over a longer period (initially defined as 4 weeks). This allows the system to assess if behaviour change has indeed occurred in the user, and is not just a temporary fluctuation of their habit. The long-term score for target behaviours is calculated from the daily (short-term) scores calculated over the long-term period. As in the short-term scores, a score of 0 indicates the lowest risk level and the presence of the healthy habit, conversely a score of 2 indicates the highest risk level and the absence of the healthy habit. Figure 1 shows the relationship

Table 1. Short-term behaviour scoring system

Target behaviour	Cut-offs	Risk score
Exercising [15]	$\geq$ 60 min/day of moderate-vigorous activity	0
	$\geq$ 30 and < 60 min/day	1
	< 30 min/day	2
Walking [6]	$\geq$ 12000 steps/day	0
	$\geq$ 6000 and < 12000 steps/day	1
	< 6000	2
Active transportation [8] to school	Walking, cycling, skateboarding both journeys	0
	Motorised means on one journey	1
	Motorised means both journeys	2
Non-sedentary lifestyle [1]	$\leq$ 45% of total daily activity < 1.5 METS	0
	> 45% and $\leq$ 55%	1
	> 55%	2
Sleeping enough [10]	$\geq$ 8 hrs of sleep per night	0
	$\geq$ 7 hrs and < 8 hrs of sleep per night	1
	< 7 hrs of sleep per night	2
Sleeping well [10]	sleep time is $\geq$ 95% of overall time in bed	0
	sleep time is, $\geq$ 90% and < 95% of overall time in bed	1
	sleep time is < 90% of overall time in bed	2

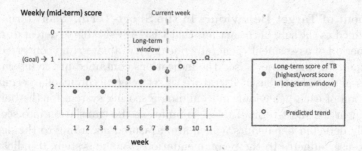

Fig. 1. Long-term (monthly) and mid-term (weekly) assessment of a target behaviour

between long-term and intermediate mid-term weekly score (mean of a week of daily scores). The long-term score is defined as the maximum (or worst) of the weekly scores, thus to increase in this score, the user must sustain the good behaviour over the full period of the long-term window, rather than have variable behaviour (e.g. time spent in sedentary activity some weeks of high performance, and some weeks of low performance).

Use of Behaviour Assessment. The user interacts with PEGASO through a centralised app called the *Companion* [4], which is an advanced interface that assist, and entertains the user providing her with education on healthy habits, and motivating to comply with personalised goals. After an initial assessment period, the Companion uses the long-term scores to help a user select a target behaviour to improve, offering her a choice of the poorer performing ones. The goal of the user would be then to improve in the long-term score by one level before having the choice to select a different behavioural goal. The system module implementing short-term assessment provides instantaneous detection of positive or negative performance prompting the Companion to trigger an appropriate action, for example, giving virtual points and congratulating the user for reaching the step count goal 5 days in a row.

3   Conclusion

This paper has presented a method for assessing behaviours (physical activity and resting attitudes) in the short (daily), medium (weekly) and long term (monthly) based on indicators derived from wearable sensors. We have developed a scientifically informed system of scoring that is associated to the degree of obesity risk each individual target-behaviour conduces. These scores are to be used by components of PEGASO further down the pipeline in order to instigate change in the most relevant behaviours affecting obesity risk. A pilot is scheduled to start in September 2016 involving 400 adolescents. Although nutritional behaviours are also pertinent, and are included in the system, the scope of this paper is limited to behaviours that were inferable from the wearable sensors.

We plan a full study including all aspects of the obesity risk behaviour recognition strategies employed in PEGASO to be published in the near future.

Acknowledgement. The research described in this paper is partly supported by the PEGASO European project (FP7-ICT-2013-10), whose members we would like to thank. The opinions expressed in this paper are those of the authors and are not necessarily those of the project partners or the European Commission.

References

1. Arundell, L., Salmon, J., Veitch, J., OConnell, E., Hinkley, T., Hume, C.: Standardising the after-schoolperiod for childrens physical activity and sedentary behaviour. Health Promot. J. Aust. **24**(1), 65–67 (2013)
2. Bastawrous, A., Armstrong, M.J.: Mobile health use in low-and high-income countries: an overview of the peer-reviewed literature. J. Roy. Soc. Med. **106**(4), 130–142 (2013)
3. Caon, M., Carrino, S., Guarnieri, R., Andreoni, G., Lafortuna, C.L., Khaled, O.A., Mugellini, E.: A persuasive system for obesity prevention in teenagers: a concept. In: Proceedings of the Second International Workshop on Behavior Change Support Systems (BCSS 2014), Padova, Italy (2014)
4. Carrino, S., Caon, M., Abou Khaled, O., Andreoni, G., Mugellini, E.: PEGASO: towards a life companion. In: Duffy, V.G. (ed.) DHM 2014. LNCS, vol. 8529, pp. 325–331. Springer, Heidelberg (2014). doi:10.1007/978-3-319-07725-3_32
5. Chen, J.L., Wilkosz, M.E.: Efficacy of technology-based interventions for obesity prevention in adolescents: a systematic review. Adolesc. Health, Med. Ther. **5**, 159–170 (2014)
6. Colley, R.C., Janssen, I., Tremblay, M.S.: Daily step target to measure adherence to physical activity guidelines in children. Med. Sci. Sports Exerc. **44**(5), 977–982 (2012)
7. Committee, P.A.G.A., et al.: Physical activity guidelines for Americans. Washington, DC: US Department of Health and Human Services, pp. 15–34 (2008)
8. Dentro, K.N., Beals, K., Crouter, S.E., Eisenmann, J.C., McKenzie, T.L., Pate, R.R., Saelens, B.E., Sisson, S., Spruijt-Metz, D., Sothern, M.S., et al.: Results from the united states' 2014 report card on physical activity for children and youth. J. Phys. Act. Health **11**, S105–S112 (2014)
9. Flynn, M., McNeil, D., Maloff, B., Mutasingwa, D., Wu, M., Ford, C., Tough, S.: Reducing obesity and related chronic disease risk in children and youth: a synthesis of evidence with best practice recommendations. Obes. Rev. **7**(s1), 7–66 (2006)
10. Hirshkowitz, M., Whiton, K., Albert, S.M., Alessi, C., Bruni, O., DonCarlos, L., Hazen, N., Herman, J., Hillard, P.J.A., Katz, E.S., et al.: National sleep foundations updated sleep duration recommendations: final report. Sleep Health **1**(4), 233–243 (2015)
11. Lau, P.W., Lau, E.Y., Wong, D.P., Ransdell, L.: A systematic review of information and communication technology-based interventions for promoting physical activity behavior change in children and adolescents. J. Med. Internet Res. **13**(3), e48 (2011)
12. Martinez-Gomez, D., Ruiz, J.R., Ortega, F.B., Veiga, O.L., Moliner-Urdiales, D., Mauro, B., Galfo, M., Manios, Y., Widhalm, K., Béghin, L., et al.: Recommended levels of physical activity to avoid an excess of body fat in european adolescents: the helena study. Am. J. Prev. Med. **39**(3), 203–211 (2010)

258   F. Velickovski et al.

13. Simmonds, M., Llewellyn, A., Owen, C.G., Woolacott, N.: Predicting adult obesity from childhood obesity: a systematic review and meta-analysis. Obesity Rev. **17**, 95–107 (2016)
14. World Health Organization: Global strategy on diet, physical activity and health: a framework to monitor and evaluate implementation (2006)
15. World Health Organization: Global recommendations on physical activity for health (2010)

Towards Stress Detection in Real-Life Scenarios Using Wearable Sensors: Normalization Factor to Reduce Variability in Stress Physiology

Bishal Lamichhane[1(✉)], Ulf Großekathöfer[1], Giuseppina Schiavone[1], and Pierluigi Casale[2]

[1] Holst Center/imec, Eindhoven, The Netherlands
lamichhane.bishal@gmail.com
[2] Philips Lighting Research, Eindhoven, The Netherlands

Abstract. Wearable physiological sensors offer possibilities for the development of continuous stress detection models. Such models need to address the inter-individual and intra-individual differences in stress physiology. In this paper we propose and evaluate a normalization factor, *Stress Response Factor* (*SRF*), to address such differences. *SRF* is computed using physiological features and the corresponding stress level at a reference point. The proposed normalization factor is evaluated in a dataset obtained from a free-living study with 10 participants, where each participant was monitored for 5 days during their working hours using different physiological sensors. We obtain an average reduction of mean squared error by up to 32% in models with *SRF* compared to the models without *SRF*.

Keywords: Stress detection · Wearable sensors · Physiology normalization · Machine learning

1 Introduction

Stress, in particular stress in the workplace, is a growing issue of concern worldwide. Recent studies provide evidence for this. In a survey conducted by the American Psychology Association [3], up to 60% of the Americans reported workplace as a significant source of their stress. Also in Europe, up to 25% of the workers have been found to be at the risk of health problems due to stress generated in the workplace [10]. It is important to develop an objective measure to reliably monitor stress in order to enable workplace stress management solutions. Wearable sensors are able to provide a sensing paradigm for continuous monitoring of stress-related physiological variables. Machine learning techniques can then be used to develop stress detection models which relate the physiological state to a stress level. However, it is challenging to build such models due to the variability in stress physiology. The changes in physiology, i.e., the physiological reaction, and the corresponding perception of stress, i.e., the psychological reaction, in response to a stressor, will depend upon various personal,

© ICST Institute for Computer Sciences, Social Informatics and Telecommunications Engineering 2017
K. Giokas et al. (Eds.): eHealth 2016, LNICST 181, pp. 259–270, 2017.
DOI: 10.1007/978-3-319-49655-9_34

contextual and psychological factors. These factors lead to differences in stress physiology across the individuals (inter-individual differences) and even within the same individual over time (intra-individual differences).

Most of the stress-related research studies are conducted in controlled laboratory conditions. As the duration of monitoring is short, only inter-individual differences have to be accounted for when developing the stress detection model. This, if addressed by the study, is generally done by normalizing the data from each individual by their baseline physiological response measured in the rest condition, at the start of the monitoring. However, controlled studies do not adequately represent the challenges of free-living conditions [25]. Further studies and validation of stress detection models in free-living conditions are required. In such free-living studies, the individuals need to be monitored for multiple days so as to capture various instances of responses to natural stressors which generally occur at a low frequency. Therefore, stress detection models for free-living conditions have to address the intra-individual differences also, in addition to the inter-individual differences in stress physiology.

The aim of our study is to investigate the development of machine learning models for stress detection in real-life conditions using wearable sensors. In this paper we show that machine learning models perform no better than a trivial model (a model with no learning capability) when differences in stress physiology are not accounted for. To address this, we propose normalization using *Stress Response Factor* (*SRF*) which is computed with physiological features at a reference point scaled by the stress level for the corresponding period. Different reference points for the calculation of *SRF* are comparatively evaluated in this work. The proposed *SRF* leads to an improvement of up to 32% in the model performance, on an average across different machine learning models.

The paper is organized as follows. In Sect. 2, we outline previous works on stress detection using physiological sensors. This is followed by the discussion of stress physiology and the proposed *Stress Response Factor* (*SRF*) for normalization in Sect. 3. In Sect. 4, we describe the dataset and the analysis method used for the evaluation. We present the experimental results in Sect. 5, followed by the discussion and conclusion in Sect. 6.

2   Previous Work

Stress detection based upon physiology has mostly been investigated in controlled studies [1,8,11,13,19,20,24,28]. Only few stress-related works have been conducted in free-living conditions. In [12], the authors studied stress detection in drivers. However, the study protocol was designed to create stressful conditions based upon the route driven, instead of having natural stressors. The authors of [18,26] investigated stress detection in free-living but do not address the model development and evaluation in subject-independent or day-independent settings. Therefore, the issue of intra-individual or inter-individual differences in stress physiology has not been investigated in either of those studies.

Some studies conducted in controlled conditions have acknowledged the presence of differences in stress physiology. In [8], the authors reported 20% reduction in classification accuracy, for a binary classification problem of detecting stress from non-stress state, with a between-subject model (affected by inter-individual differences) compared to a within-subject model (not affected by inter-individual differences). The authors in [17] noted that, within an individual, physiological data from the same day were clustered more cohesively in comparison to the data across the days, for a given affective state. They proposed various approaches to address the observed differences across the days, such as: include information about the day in the model, subtract the day-dependent baseline, or use features that are less influenced by the daily variability. In [21], the authors developed a stress detection model using heart rate variability features. They proposed to normalize the feature values with standardization and include the data from the baseline physiology for each subject, in order to account for the inter-individual differences. Authors in [19] addressed the inter-individual differences by developing a personalized model based upon the modification in the machine learning algorithm used to train the model. This is done by using the physiological data of the individual from the neutral state when no stressors are applied. Authors in [27] proposed to cluster the individuals based upon their baseline physiological features and develop cluster-specific stress detection model as the stress physiology is non-homogeneous across the individuals. In [11], the authors used subject's baseline physiological recordings to normalize the measured physiological data and suppress the inter-individual variability. This lead to an increment of up to 9% in the classification accuracy, for a binary classification problem of detecting stress from non-stress state. However, all these proposed methods for the correction of the differences in stress physiology cannot be translated directly to free-living studies. Majority of the solutions depend on the use of physiological baseline from the individual. The controlled studies, spanning few tens of minutes with an explicit baseline measurement phase in the protocol, facilitate the establishment of baseline physiology. Identification of such baseline is non-trivial in free-living studies where monitoring spans multiple days.

3   Stress Physiology and Normalization

Every individual has a different body physiology and varying responses to similar stressors. As an example, in Fig. 1a, stress profile (distribution of reported stress levels on a day) of two individuals is shown on the left-hand side. The stress profile of these individuals is similar, but their respective heart rate profile (distribution of the mean heart rate in the corresponding period) deviate significantly from each other (shown on the right-hand side). We have used mean heart rate as an example, it being one of the most commonly used features in stress detection models [12,20,21,25]. Individuals generally have differences in stress physiology. Physiological and psychological response to a stressor differ between the individuals due to a multitude of factors. Moreover, even within an individual, different physiological responses can be elicited for similar stressors (Fig. 1b). A stress detection model that works in real-life conditions should be able to account for these differences.

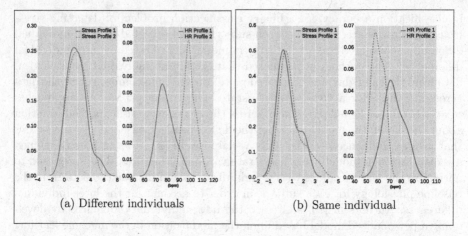

(a) Different individuals   (b) Same individual

Fig. 1. In the figure, distribution of stress level and heart rate (referred to as stress profile and HR profile respectively) measured over a day is shown. In (a), the profile for two individuals is shown. Even though they report similar stress profile on these days, their heart rate profile differs. In (b), profile of an individual on two different days is shown. As it can be seen from the figure, there can be physiological differences across the days for an individual, even though the reported stress is similar.

The variability in stress physiology can be corrected by normalization. Let PV be the physiological feature vector representing the physiological state and l represent the stress level. An optimal normalization factor could be the value of PV, when l is at some fixed reference value. The variability of this factor encompasses the inconsistency in stress physiology. However, it is not possible to obtain such common reference point across the days and for different individuals in real-life conditions. The possible values for l on a given day for an individual are completely uncontrolled. Therefore, there is not one fixed value of l which is guaranteed to occur on each day for different individuals. We propose to obtain the reference point based upon some characteristic features in the stress physiology profile of the day and include scaling with the value of l in the normalization factor. This allows to compute a factor that accounts for the variability in the stress physiology, while l can have different values at the selected reference point. In this work, we empirically evaluate and compare different reference points that can be used to compute the normalization factor, using linear scaling by l. If PV^{ref} is the physiological feature vector and l^{ref} is the corresponding stress level at a given reference point, the factor for normalization, defined as *Stress Response Factor (SRF)*, is computed as:

$$SRF = PV^{ref}/(1 + l^{ref}) \qquad (1)$$

where ref represents the selected reference point. Normalization with SRF computed for a particular day is able to factor the day's stress physiology profile in the model. This makes the stress physiology comparable over days and across individuals. We evaluate different reference points for computing SRF which are: (i). Ref_{minstr}: Minimum stressful period of the day (ii). Ref_{maxstr}: Maximum stressful period of the day (iii). Ref_{minhr}: The period of the day for which the heart rate is minimum (iv). Ref_{arbit}: An arbitrary period from the day.

These reference points have been chosen on the basis of insights from the research in stress and other application domains. Ref_{minstr} is the closest point of the day to a baseline rest phase, based upon the reported stress level as an evidence. As discussed earlier, baseline rest phase has been used to compute the normalization factor for stress detection model in many controlled studies. Ref_{maxstr} is the closest point of the day to a hypothetical maximum point in stress physiology. Normalization based upon maxima is commonly used in other applications like energy expenditure estimation [15]. Ref_{minhr} is the closest point of the day to a baseline rest phase based upon the physiological evidence, as lower heart rate is one of the indicator of a calm and resting state. Finally, Ref_{arbit} provides a comparison to establish the merit of using other reference points for computing SRF. A period from a given day is selected randomly as the reference point, from among the period for which the user reported their stress level.

4   Materials and Methods

4.1   Data Collection

Study Population: We evaluate our stress detection model using a dataset collected in free-living conditions [25]. A total of 10 healthy participants, 7 females and 3 males took part in the study. Mean age of the participants was 31.1 ± 11.9 years. All participants were researchers, typically sedentary during the work day. They were monitored continuously during their working hours for 5 days. The entire study protocol was communicated to each participant and they were asked to sign an informed consent form, before the start of the study. The participants were allowed to discontinue their participation in the study at any time, should they decide to do so for any reason.

Sensor Modalities: Wireless body area network developed within the Human++ program [7] was used for synchronous physiological signal acquisition from each participant. The system consisted a necklace-based device measuring ECG and 3D acceleration, a chest band for respiration monitoring, an EMG device measuring muscle activity at the upper trapezius muscle, and a wrist-band device measuring GSR, 3D acceleration, skin temperature, relative humidity, ambient temperature and ambient humidity. This system has been used before for physiological monitoring in various applications like energy expenditure estimation [2], emotion monitoring [7] etc. We refer to [25] for the details on the sensor setup used in the study. On the first day of the study, sensors were handed over to the participants and they were given instructions about its usage. On each day of the study, participants wore the sensors at the start of the day and took them off at the end of the working day. For the analysis in this paper, ECG, GSR, respiration and accelerometer signals (measured from the necklace-based device) are used. These signals were acquired at a sampling frequency of 256 Hz, 128 Hz, 256 Hz and 32 Hz respectively by the corresponding sensors.

Reference Stress Level: Various reference measures for the stress level were obtained from the participants. A smartphone, with an application to collect annotations every 30 min, was provided to each participant. The participants annotated their perceived stress level (for the past 30 min period and at the current moment) on a Visual Analog Scale (VAS), from 0 (not at all stressed) to 10 (totally stressed). Participants also provided annotations for their activities, postures, and food consumptions. Cortisol level, a bio-chemical marker of stress level, was also measured from the participants four times per day using saliva sampling equipment Salivettes (Sarstedt, Germany). Participants also filled in the Daily Stress Inventory [5] each day. For the analysis in this paper, only the self-reported perceived stress level has been used as the reference, it being the less intrusive probe into the stress level for free-living conditions.

4.2 Features Computation from Sensor Modalities

We use features that have been commonly used in other studies for stress detection [25]. The features are extracted from the 30 min window corresponding to the period for which the participant reported their stress levels. All the signals are processed without any sampling rate conversion.

ECG: We compute different features from the ECG signal based upon the R-peaks detected using the Pan-Tompkins algorithm [14]. The features extracted are: i. mean heart rate (mhr) ii. standard deviation of R-R peak intervals (sdnn) iii. root mean of sum of squared difference of consecutive R-R peak intervals (rmssd) iv. low frequency component of the spectrum of R-R peak intervals (lf): power in the 0.04 Hz–0.15 Hz band v. high frequency component of the spectrum of R-R peak intervals (hf): power in the 0.15 Hz–0.4 Hz band vi. ratio of LF to HF (lfhf) vii. percentage of R-R peak intervals that are greater than 50 ms (pnn50) viii. approximate entropy of R-R peak intervals (apen) ix. poincare plot based features. As suggested in [23], we extract the following features from the poincare plot: sd1 (length of the major axis), sd2 (length of the minor axis), sd1/sd2 (ratio of the axes).

GSR: The features extracted from the measured GSR signal are: i. skin conductance level (scl) ii. signal power of the skin conductance (scp) iii. skin conductance response rate (scrr) iv. signal power in the second order difference of the skin conductance (scdiff2).

Respiration: We extract respiration rate (resprate), the number of respiration cycles per minute, as a feature from the respiration signal.

Accelerometer: We extract the magnitude of motion (mom) feature from the measured 3-D accelerometer signal. This is computed as the mean of the magnitude of the 3-D motion vector, $mom = \frac{1}{N}\sum_{i=1}^{N}\sqrt{accx_i^2 + accy_i^2 + accz_i^2}$.

4.3   Data Analysis

We use regression models for the prediction of the stress level using physiological features, as the reported stress levels are in a continuous scale. *Random Forest (Rforest)* [6] for regression, *Lasso* [22], *Support Vector Regression (SVR)* [9] with epsilon-insensitive loss function, and *k-Nearest Neighbours (k-NN)* have been used in our analysis.

4.4   Evaluation Method and Metrics

We use leave-one-participant-out cross-validation to evaluate the performance of the models, using mean squared error (mse) as the performance metric. A trivial regression model is evaluated to obtain a baseline against which the performance of other regression models is compared. A trivial regression model is defined as a model which provides the mean of the labels for the data in the training set, as the constant prediction output. Unlike classification problems, where baseline performance can be established with the class prior (e.g. 50% accuracy on a balanced binary classification problem), no such prior-based baseline can be established for regression problems. The performance of a trivial model helps to establish an alternate baseline. Using mse or rmse (root mean squared error) as a model evaluation metric to compare with the baseline from a trivial or other regression models has been used in other studies [4,16].

SRF is used for normalization in a model by scaling all sample points from the day with the factor. The reference point used to compute SRF is excluded from the analysis for all the models. Thus each model, regardless of its usage of SRF, is evaluated with the same training and test set for comparison. We also compare other standard normalization methods, namely a min-max scaler (scales the data between 0 and 1) and a standard-scaler (removes the mean and scales the data to have a unit variance) applied to the data from each day.

The effect of SRF on model performance is summarized with the within-model and over-baseline gain. If mse_{model} is the mse obtained from a model when no normalization is used, $mse_{modelSRF}$ is the mse obtained from the model when SRF is used for normalization, and $mse_{trivial}$ is the mse obtained from a trivial regression model, then the within-model gain is defined as: $\frac{mse_{model} - mse_{modelSRF}}{mse_{model}} * 100$ and over-baseline gain is defined as: $\frac{mse_{trivial} - mse_{modelSRF}}{mse_{trivial}} * 100$.

We tune the parameters of regression models with cross-validation within the training set. For *Rforest*, the number of estimators ($\{101, 201, 301\}$) and the maximum number of features ($\{sqrt(total\ number\ of\ features), log2(total\ number\ of\ features)\}$) to be used for the split of decision trees are tuned. In *Lasso*, α (the regularization parameter) is tuned automatically with iterative fitting. For SVR, we use a RBF kernel and tune ϵ ($\{i/10\}_{i=1}^{10}$), γ ($\{2^i\}_{i=-8}^{8}$) and C($\{2^i\}_{i=-8}^{8}$). In the k-NN model, the number of neighbors k ($\{3, 5, 7, 9, 11\}$), weights ($\{uniform, distance\}$) and distance-metric ($\{'euclidean', 'manhattan', 'chebyshev'\}$) are tuned.

In all evaluations, data in the training set is scaled with a min-max scaler to restrict the feature space between 0 and 1 and these scaling parameters are also propagated for scaling data in the test set. All tests for significance are evaluated with a paired t-test at a significance level of 0.05.

5   Experimental Results

In our evaluation setting, the training and test set, on an average, consist of 630 samples and 70 samples respectively. In Fig. 2, the evaluation results for different regression models with and without normalization are shown. Significant reduction in mse is obtained with our proposed normalization method. The model performances for SRF computed with different reference points are shown in Fig. 3.

We proposed to compute SRF based upon the reference point from each day. This is compared with the model performance when a single SRF is computed per participant with an assumption that there is no variability in stress physiology within an individual. Two different methods for computing a single SRF per participant are evaluated. The first method pools all the data of a participant from across the multiple days together, establishes a single reference point in the pooled data and computes SRF based upon this reference point. The second method computes SRF from the reference point in the first day.

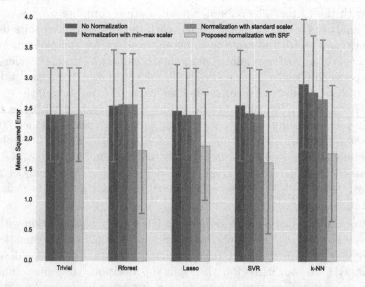

Fig. 2. mse obtained for different regression models evaluated in leave-one-participant-out setting. The performance of models without normalization and with different normalization methods is compared. The model performance for the normalization with SRF is reported with the reference point considered at the minimum stressful period of the day (Ref_{minstr}).

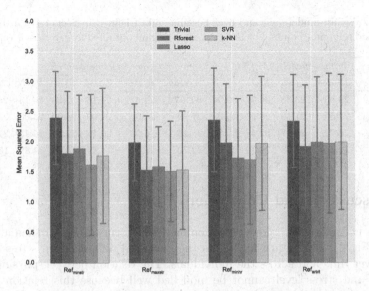

Fig. 3. Performance of the models with normalization factor computed from different reference points. For Ref$_{arbit}$, the average performance from 8 runs is reported.

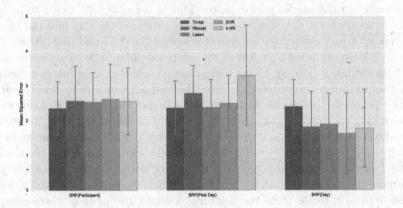

Fig. 4. Performance of the models with a single SRF per participant by pooling data of the participant from all the days: RF(participant), a single SRF per participant based upon the reference point obtained from the first day: RF(first day) and a SRF for each day of the monitoring: RF(day). The results are reported with Ref$_{minstr}$ as the considered reference point.

The comparison result is shown in Fig. 4. An improvement in the model performance is obtained only when SRF is computed for each day per participant. In Table 1, we report the obtained improvement in the model performance due to SRF, using within-model and over-baseline gain metrics.

Table 1. Within-model gain and over-baseline gain (defined in Sect. 4.4) for different models and reference points. For Ref_{arbit}, average gain obtained from 8 runs is reported.

	Within-model gain (%)					Over-baseline gain (%)				
	Rforest	Lasso	SVR	k-NN	Average	Rforest	Lasso	SVR	k-NN	Average
Ref_{minstr}	28.90	23.38	36.57	39.04	**31.97**	24.4	21.16	32.36	26.14	**26.01**
Ref_{maxstr}	24.50	21.10	28.97	35.02	27.39	23.00	20.00	24.00	23.00	22.50
Ref_{minhr}	20.71	28.97	32.41	30.76	28.21	16.03	26.58	27.84	16.45	21.73
Ref_{arbit}	22.40	18.03	22.35	28.05	22.70	17.87	14.89	15.74	14.89	15.85

6   Discussion and Conclusion

Without normalization, stress detection model performs no better than a trivial model (Fig. 2). This result highlights the discussed differences in stress physiology, over time and across the individuals. The relation between physiological features and stress level cannot be modelled well because this relation is not comparable across the days and individuals. With min-max scaler and standard scaler to normalize the data from each day, still no improvement in the model performance is obtained. The use of SRF for normalization leads to a significant improvement in the model performance. This is because SRF helps to include some characterization of the stress-physiology profile of the day into the model, thus making stress physiology comparable across the days and individuals. The characterization obtained from any of the reference point in the day improves the model performance (Fig. 3). Using within-model and over-baseline gain metrics as the comparison criteria, Ref_{minstr} gives the best performance in our evaluation setting (Table 1). The results shown in Fig. 4 depict that the SRF needs to be computed for each day, highlighting the presence of intra-individual differences across days. Stress detection in free-living requires periodic identification of the normalization factor to account for the temporal variations in stress physiology.

One limitation of the proposed SRF is that the normalization factor is dependent upon the availability of labeled data points. Normalization factor which can be derived directly from the features, without the need of corresponding label, would be desirable for deployment scenarios. For future work, it would be interesting to investigate the temporal characteristics of the features at different label-independent reference points or ranges (e.g. during morning period) for such normalization factor. Nonetheless, the analysis presented here makes first step towards robust stress detection models in free-living conditions identifying the differences in stress physiology as one of the key challenges for such models.

To conclude, stress physiology shows variability due to the effects of different personal and temporal factors. A stress detection model needs to account for the differences stemming from these factors. The *Stress Response Factor (SRF)* proposed in this paper helps in addressing these differences by characterizing the stress physiology profile of the day into the model. We were able to validate its contribution to the stress detection model, using a dataset collected in free-living conditions. It is desirable to further investigate and validate stress detection models with a study involving long-term monitoring of a larger number of individuals.

References

1. Alamudun, F., Choi, J., Gutierrez-Osuna, R., Khan, H., Ahmed, B.: Removal of subject-dependent and activity-dependent variation in physiological measures of stress. In: Proceedings of the 6th International Conference on Pervasive Computing Technologies for Healthcare (2012)
2. Altini, M., Penders, J., Amft, O.: Energy expenditure estimation using wearable sensors: a new methodology for activity-specific models. In: Proceedings of the conference on Wireless Health (2012)
3. Association, A.P.: Stress in America: paying with our health. Technical report, American Psychological Association (2014). http://www.apa.org/news/press/releases/stress/2014/stress-report.pdf
4. Bennet, J., Lanning, S.: The Netflix prize. In: KDD Cup and Workshop (2007)
5. Brantley, P.J., Waggoner, C.D., Jones, G.N., Rappaport, N.B.: A daily stress inventory: development, reliability, and validity. J. Behav. Med. **10**, 61–73 (1987)
6. Breiman, L.: Random forests. Mach. Learn. **45**, 5–32 (2001)
7. Brown, L., Grundlehner, B., van de Molengraft, J., Penders, J., Gyselinckx, B.: Body area network for monitoring autonomic nervous system responses. In: Pervasive Computing Technologies for Healthcare (2009)
8. Choi, J., Ricardo, G.O.: Using heart rate monitors to detect mental stress. In: Sixth International Workshop on Wearable and Implantable Body Sensor Networks (2009)
9. Drucker, H., Bruges, C.J.C., Kaufman, L., Smola, A.J., Vapnik, V.N.: Support vector regression machines. In: Advances in Neural Information Processing Systems (1996)
10. Eurofound, E.-O.: Psychological risks in Europe: prevalance and strategies for prevention. Technical report, Publications Office of the European Union, Luxemborg (2014)
11. Giakoumis, D., Tzovaras, D., Hassapis, G.: Subject-dependent biosignal features for increased accuracy in psychological stress detection. Int. J. Hum Comput Stud. **71**, 425–439 (2013)
12. Healey, J., Picard, R.W.: Detecting stress during real-world driving tasks using physiological sensors. IEEE Trans. Intell. Transp. Syst. **6**, 156–166 (2005)
13. Hjortskov, N., Rissen, D., Blangsted, A.K., Fallentin, N., Lundberg, U., Søgaard, K.: The effect of mental stress on heart rate variability and blood pressure during computer work. Eur. J. Appl. Physiol. **92**, 84–89 (2004)
14. Jiapu, P., Tompkins, J.W.: A real-time QRS detection algorithm. IEEE Trans. Biomed. Eng. **32**, 230–236 (1985)
15. Keytel, L., Goedecke, J., Noakes, T., Hiloskorpi, H., Laukkanen, R., van der Merwe, L., Lambert, E.: Prediction of energy expenditure from heart rate monitoring during submaximal exercise. J. Sports Sci. **23**, 289–297 (2005)
16. Nadeau, D., Sabourin, C., Koninck, J.D., Matwin, S., Turney, P.D.: Automatic dream sentiment analysis. In: Proceedings of the Workshop on Computational Aesthetics at the 21st National Conference on Artificial Intelligence (AAAI) (2006)
17. Picard, R.W., Vyzas, E., Healey, J.: Toward machine emotional intelligence: analysis of affective physiological state. IEEE Trans. Pattern Anal. Mach. Intell. **23**, 1175–1191 (2001)
18. Sano, A., Picard, R.W.: Stress recognition using wearable sensors and mobile phones. In: Humaine Association Conference on Affective Computing and Intelligent Interaction (2013)

19. Shi, Y., Ngyuen, M., Blitz, P., French, B., Frisk, S., Torre, F., Smailagic, A., Siewiorek, D., al'Absi, M., Kamarck, T., Kumar, S.: Personalized stress detection from physiological measurements. In: Proceedings of the 2nd International Symposium on Quality of Life Technology (2010)
20. Sun, F.-T., Kuo, C., Cheng, H.-T., Buthpitiya, S., Collins, P., Griss, M.: Activity-aware mental stress detection using physiological sensors. In: Gris, M., Yang, G. (eds.) MobiCASE 2010. LNICST, vol. 76, pp. 211–230. Springer, Heidelberg (2012). doi:10.1007/978-3-642-29336-8_12
21. Tanev, G., Saadi, D., Hoppe, K., Sorensen, H.: Classification of acute stress using linear and non-linear heart rate variability analysis derived from sternal ECG. In: 36th Annual International Conference of the Engineering in Medicine and Biology Society (EMBC) (2014)
22. Tibshirani, R.: Regression shrinkage and selection via the Lasso. J. Roy. Stat. Soc. B **58**(1), 267–288 (1996)
23. Tulppo, M., Makikallio, T., Takala, T., Seppanen, T., Huikuri, H.V.: Quantitative beat-to-beat analysis of heart rate dynamics during exercise. Am. J. Physiol. Cell Physiol. **271**, H244–H252 (1996)
24. Wijsman, J., Grundlehner, B., Penders, J., Hermens, H.: Trapezius muscle EMG as predictor of mental stress. ACM Trans. Embed. Comput. Syst. **12**, 99:1–99:20 (2013)
25. Wijsman, J.: Sensing stress: stress detection from physiological variables in controlled and uncontrolled conditions. Ph.D. thesis, University of Twente (2014)
26. Wu, M., Cao, H., Nguyen, H.L., Surmacz, K., Hargrove, C.: Modeling perceived stress via HRV and accelerometer sensor streams. In: 37th Annual International Conference of the IEEE Engineering in Medicine and Biology Society (2015)
27. Xu, Q., Nwe, T.L., Guan, C.: Cluster-based analysis for personalized stress evaluation using physiological signals. IEEE J. Biomed. Health Inform. **19**, 275–281 (2014)
28. Zhai, J., Barreto, A.: Stress detection in computer users through non-invasive monitoring of physiological signals. Biomed. Sci. Instrum. **42**, 495–500 (2006)

Personalized Characterization of Sustained Attention/Vigilance in Healthy Children

Paruthi Pradhapan[1]([✉]), Richard Griffioen[2], Marcel Clerx[2],
and Vojkan Mihajlović[1]

[1] Holst Centre/imec, 5656 AE Eindhoven, The Netherlands
{paruthi.pradhapan,vojkan.mihajlovic}@imec-nl.nl
[2] SAM Foundation, 1181 DB Amstelveen, The Netherlands
sam@euronet.nl, marcel.clerx@stichtingsam.nl

Abstract. Baseline shifts in electroencephalography (EEG) spectral response, in combination with phasic activity, can result in poor performance in sustaining attention. To explore the contribution of tonic response changes, we studied the 10 s segments preceding cues of correct and incorrect responses during target stimuli of an attention paradigm. The goal was to determine metrics that indicate tonic differences in spectral response between error and no error trials while performing a Sustained Attention to Response Task (SART) in a non-clinical setting. Data was recorded on 9 healthy children using IMEC's 8-channel wearable EEG headset with conductive polymer electrodes. In addition to fixed frequency bands, personalized bands based on individual alpha peak frequencies, were computed to account for inter-subject variability. The results indicate that relative theta and alpha power, along with their ratios, is a reliable metric indicating periods of attention or its lapses. The current results are a promising step towards understanding the cognitive responses of a healthy brain and potentially using them to assess the mental health of subjects undergoing training or treatment. Obtaining these results would not be possible without the use of a wireless dry electrode EEG headset, which demonstrates the essential role wearable devices have in monitoring cognition outside the clinical environment.

Keywords: Electroencephalography · SART · Sustained attention · Vigilance · Personalization · Children · Cognition

1 Introduction

Sustained attention/vigilance is defined as the ability to sustain conscious processing of random, repetitive stimuli without succumbing to habituation or distraction by other trivial stimuli. The ability to measure sustained attention/vigilance in response to events or tasks is essential in determining cognitive state and memory processes associated with the brain. Such objective means of measuring vigilance level is a vital step in the diagnosis and treatment of cognitive disorders that usually affect attention, learning or perception abilities in

© ICST Institute for Computer Sciences, Social Informatics and Telecommunications Engineering 2017
K. Giokas et al. (Eds.): eHealth 2016, LNICST 181, pp. 271–281, 2017.
DOI: 10.1007/978-3-319-49655-9_35

an individual. Several studies have investigated physiological correlates of attention, often comparing normal and population with cognitive disabilities [1–4], to determine whether these indices vary in different cognitive disease states. However, in order to understand the attention/inattention processes in a diseased population, it is essential to first understand a normal brain's response to sustained attention tasks in a daily life setting.

Researchers have explored a range of electroencephalography (EEG) features derived from data collected during experimental paradigms that involve cued responses to trials while anticipating a target stimulus. Orienting responses (phasic neurophysiological processes), which is described as the immediate, short-term response elucidated in the brain as a result of target stimulus, are often investigated to understand the cognitive processes related to attention. However, it has been reported that EEG changes cycle at lengths in the order of 15 s to minutes (i.e. tonic response) [5], which leads to the hypothesis that poor tonic activity, in combination to phasic processes, might result in poor task performance. Oken and colleagues [6] observed an increased slow frequency activity during decreasing attention and attenuation of alpha frequencies during maximal attention. In a series of investigations by Makeig and coworkers [7,8], poor performance was marked by relative increase in theta band power approximately 10 s prior to stimulus onset. The often encountered limitations in assessing these changes is the inter-subject variability of spectral responses, especially in children, since the alpha peak frequency matures progressively with age [9]. Moreover, these evaluations are performed in a clinical setting, which does not truly reflect the cognitive state in an uncontrolled environment where other external stimuli could dissolve the attention process. The fact the traditional EEG devices use wired systems limits the possibilities of conducting experiments that elucidate natural brain processes.

To determine whether sustained attention or its deficits can be distinguished in an uncontrolled environment, we designed a pilot study to assess the tonic spectral response while performing a sustained attention task. A random Sustained Attention to Response Task (SART) was chosen as the basis for the evaluation, due to its simple and straight-forward protocol in measuring attention. The original protocol, which involves displaying random digits between (1–9), was marginally modified. In order to keep the subjects engaged to the experiment, the numbers were replaced by pictures of cartoon characters as cues during the measurement. EEG data was collected from healthy children between 6–18 years age group while performing the modified SART. A wireless wearable EEG system, designed by IMEC, was used in the study as it allows unrestricted mobility to the subjects. Personalized frequency bands based on the individual alpha peak frequency (IAF), were evaluated in addition to traditional fixed frequency band definition of the EEG spectrum to investigate whether such means of normalization leads to comparable results among different subjects. The aim of the current evaluation was to determine whether metrics based on tonic responses during attention tasks can provide meaningful information about the cognitive state of an individual. The results might facilitate improvement in learning or treatment methods, either directly (interventions or neurofeedback training) or indirectly (treatment design), in treating cognitive impairments.

This report is organized as follows: Sect. 2 describes the study cohort, data acquisition, measurement protocol and data analysis methods used. The results of the experiment are presented in Sect. 3, following which Sect. 4 discusses the outcomes and inferences. Finally, the motivation and derived conclusions of the study are summarized in Sect. 5.

2 Materials and Methods

2.1 Subjects

9 children (Age range: 6–18 years; Mean $\pm$ s.d $= 12.44 \pm 3.50$ years; 3 male), without any history of neurological disorders participated in the study. Since the subjects were below 18 years of age, measurements were performed only after written informed consent was obtained from their parent/guardian. Two subjects (female) could not complete the data acquisition due to improper fitting of the headset and were, therefore, excluded from analyses. Two subjects (1 male and 1 female; 10 years) completed two measurements during different sessions, further described in the *Measurement Protocol* section.

2.2 Acquisition Setup

The measurements were performed using IMEC's 8-channel wearable wireless EEG headset, designed to be used in cognition and emotion research. The headset (shown in Fig. 1) is a highly integrated EEG acquisition device, with electrodes

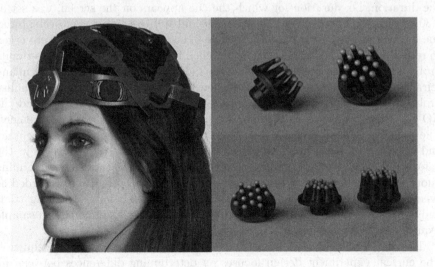

Fig. 1. EEG headset designed by IMEC for cognition monitoring studies. Figures on the right show the polymer electrodes with silver/silver-chloride coating used for data acquisition.

positioned at Fz, F3, F7, F4, F8, P3, P4 and A1 of the International 10–20 electrode positioning system. Patient ground is placed at Pz and the reference electrode at A2 (right mastoid). This configuration allows re-referencing each of the channels to a specific reference (if required). The headset can be mounted easily, without the need of expert intervention, and is fitted with conductive polymer electrodes [10] coated with silver/silver-chloride layer on the tips, as shown in the figure. Each polymer electrode consisted of 15 pins of either 5 mm or 8 mm length. The small and large pin electrodes were attached to different electrode sites based on the morphology of subjects' scalp. The use of dry electrodes overcome the need for any skin preparation prior to use. Overall, the use of a wireless, dry electrode EEG system minimized setup time and made it possible for measurements to be performed in an uncontrolled setting. In addition, such wearable EEG devices allows for futuristic applications such as self-tracking or brain activity monitoring in daily life scenarios.

2.3   Measurement Protocol

SART, a GO/NO-GO paradigm, was chosen as the voluntary attention task to determine metrics for sustained attention. SART protocol is a computer-based user response task designed to measure a person's ability to withhold responses to infrequent and unpredictable target stimuli while responding as quickly and accurately as possible. Traditionally, the SART protocol involves flashing numbers between 1–9 on a screen for a short and fixed duration for which the user responds, depending on the type of cue (target or non-target stimulus). In order to motivate the young subjects of the current study, traditional SART was modified to include 8 pictures of cartoon characters instead of numbers. The cue duration, i.e. duration for which the cue appears on the screen, was set at 0.30 s for subjects between 6–12 years of age and at 0.15 s for older subjects. Inter-cue interval was between 1–1.5 s, inclusive of cue duration. Subjects were asked to respond to the cues by mouse button click for GO trials (non-target stimuli; probability of occurrence 87.5%) using the index finger of the dominant arm and refrain from producing any response when the NO-GO trials (target stimulus; probability of occurrence 12.5%) appeared. The picture that represented the NO-GO trial was shown to the subjects prior to the start of the measurement. The subjects were specifically instructed to give equal importance to accuracy and speed while performing the tasks. The protocol was implemented in the data acquisition software used to record EEG data from the headset. Timing information of cues and user responses (mouse button clicks) were recorded as events on the software. This information was later used for segmenting trials and determining correct and incorrect responses. Figure 2 summarizes a sample sequence of events during SART.

Each measurement session involved 300 cues appearing in random sequence. The current experiment design focuses on determining differences between *no error*, i.e. when subjects successfully inhibited response to NO-GO trials, and *error*, i.e. when subjects failed to inhibit a response to NO-GO trials. Since the

Measurement 1			Dolphin game/dog training session	Measurement 2		
Baseline	SART	Baseline		Baseline	SART	Baseline

|← 10-12 minutes →|← 5-15 minutes →|← 10-12 minutes →|

Fig. 2. Sequence of events during a measurement session.

NO-GO trials appeared only 12.5% of 300 trials, each subject performed two sets of measurements with a short break in between. Baseline recording, each comprising 90 s of eyes closed and eyes open recording, were performed prior to and after each SART measurement and were used to determine the IAF of each subject for personalization of frequency bands. During the break, the participants were divided into two groups, each of which participated either in a dolphin game or dog training session which lasted about 10 min. This activity was part of another evaluation and is not in the scope of the current study. The sequence of activities during the measurement sessions is described in Fig. 3. Participants were instructed not to remove the headset until the entire measurement phase was completed. Two subjects (1 male and 1 female) participated in both sessions and therefore recorded two sets of SART measurements. The measurements, including the inter-session activities, were performed under normal room conditions and is illustrated in Fig. 3. The protocol was approved by SAM foundation.

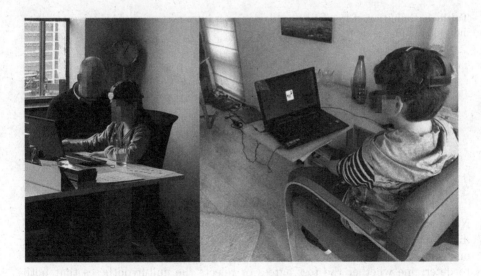

Fig. 3. Example acquisition setup during each measurement session

2.4 Data Analysis

Pre-processing: The pre-processing step involved band-pass filtering (3rd order Butterworth) in the 1–45 Hz frequency band and the use of 49–51 Hz notch filter (5th order Butterworth). Epochs of NO-GO trials starting 10 s prior to the cue and until the cue onset, were segmented based on cue timing information. An automatic artifact rejection method based on standard deviation and min-max of the signals within an epoch was used. By applying statistics based artifact rejection in the data analyses, epochs corrupted by noise and motion artifacts were rejected. After segmentation and artifact data exclusion, the epochs were classified as *no error* or *error* trials.

Feature Extraction: Power spectral densities were calculated using Welch method based on (i) fixed frequency bands and (ii) personalized frequency bands. The personalized frequency bands were computed based on methods described by Doppelymayr et al. [11], distributed around the IAF in order to account for the inter-subject variability. For personalization, the IAF was identified by analyzing 10 s epochs data from eyes closed baseline measurements. The spectral features were represented as both absolute and relative (ratio of power in specific frequency band to total power in the 1–30 Hz range) powers. The frequency bands for both feature extraction methods are described in Table 1. After spectral analyses, ratios between theta/alpha and theta/beta bands were computed for each channel.

Table 1. Definition of frequency bands during feature extraction. IAF corresponds to individual alpha peak frequency

Bands	Frequencies (Hz)	
	Fixed	Personalized
Theta	4–7.99	(0.4–0.6)*IAF
Alpha	8–12.99	(0.6–1.2)*IAF
Beta	13–29.99	1.2*IAF-29.99

3 Results

Non-parametric statistical tests were performed to establish differences since the distribution of each category and channel tested to be non-Gaussian (tested using one-sample Kolmogorov-Smirnov test). A significance level of 5% was chosen to determine whether the test agrees or rejects the null-hypotheses that both datasets come from the same population. The 1-tailed Mann-Whitney Wilcoxon (MWW) sign rank-sum tests revealed significant differences in relative theta power (U = 20768.0, p = .009) and alpha power (p = .001) in the frontal mid-line for fixed frequency bands. This contributed to the theta/alpha ratio (p = 0.027)

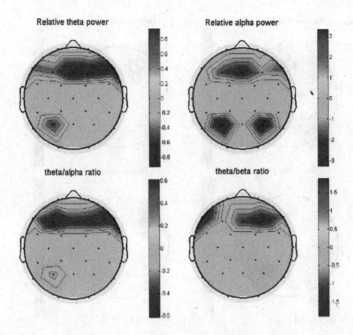

Fig. 4. Differences in fixed frequency bands' power distribution between *no error* and *error* trials.

and theta/beta ratio (p = 0.028) being significant indicators at the Fz channel. The personalized frequency bands revealed a significant difference in relative alpha power across the frontal positions of Fz (U = 20768.0, p = 0.024), F3 (U = 5742.0, p = 0.01) and F4 (U = 11040.0, p = 0.021) between the two test groups. Similarly, theta/alpha ratios were significant indicators of differences across the frontal electrodes (Fz: p = 0.001; F3: p = 0.007; F4: p = 0.009). Theta/beta ratio was significant for F3 (U = 5742.0, p = 0.005). Figures 4 and 5 represent the topographical power distribution for fixed and personalized frequency bands bands across different electrode positions.

4 Discussion

Several studies have focused on determining EEG spectrum correlates of attention deficit in cognitively challenged populations of different age groups [2,3,12]. Increased theta band power has been observed across ADHD subjects of all age categories during resting state [13–16]. This combined with the association of beta band activity to attentional arousal, implicates a high theta/beta ratio in frontal and central scalp regions in subjects with ADHD [12]. Reports by Ogrim et al. [17] suggests that an increase in theta band power and in turn, theta/beta ratio in ADHD population might be the result of inattention and executive problems rather than a direct manifestation of ADHD symptoms. However, the dynamics of band powers changes in ADHD is reported in the

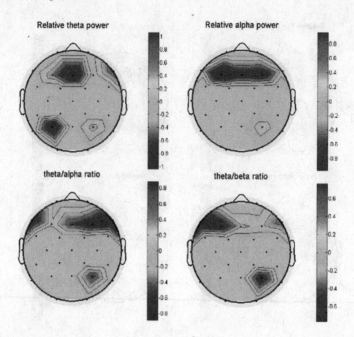

Fig. 5. Differences in personalized frequency bands' power distribution between *no error* and *error* trials.

resting state, unlike in normal subjects where differences were observed during lapses in attention while performing sustained attention tasks.

In order to understand the attention/inattention process in cognitively challenged population, it is essential to comprehend a normal brain's response to attention deficits. Several studies have focused on identifying event-related potentials (ERP) or response times correlates to attention tasks, but fail to address the contribution of baseline EEG in sustaining attention. The current study indicates that personalization of frequency bands, based on IAF, shifts the dominant frequency from beta to high alpha spectrum, thereby manifesting theta/alpha ratio as a marker for attention or its lapses. This is in line with reports by Dockree et al. [18], who performed dipole source analysis of alpha activity during fixed SART test on two subjects (Age range: 18–32 years), and reported that high tonic alpha power may be indicative of increased alertness towards task. In addition, under arousal or increased theta band power was observed in one or more of the frontal channels. Although this coincides with findings from subjects with ADHD, there is evidence to suggest that a similar increment in theta band power in frontal channels can be perceived during increased attentional loading [19]. The reason, both in the case of episodes of inattention in healthy subjects and pathophysiologies in ADHD, could be the result of under arousal marked by increased theta and decreased alpha activity in fronto-central regions of the scalp [12]. This is an interesting observation and calls for further exploration of personalized frequency bands.

Although the current study involved measurements during a static condition (i.e. attending to SART tasks in a seated position as shown in Fig. 3), other assessment or treatment modalities might require light to moderate movements, such as during animal interaction training which is commonly used in treating cognitive disabilities. The wireless headset design allows for data collection outside a clinical setting and use of polymer electrodes reduces the setup time and complexity. This is extremely beneficial, especially in studies involving children or cognitively impaired subjects, for whom adherence to stringent measurement protocols could prove challenging. By using sufficient signal cleansing mechanisms to exclude periods corrupted by motion artifacts, data from variety of protocols can be evaluated to determine attention lapses and in turn, learning/treatment efficacy. Moreover, the data visualization software can be run from a portable device making it easy to monitor personal cognitive state in real-time. This wearable solution opens new avenues in using EEG, such as monitoring attention lapses in children in a classroom, cognitive overload of air traffic controllers, etc.

5   Conclusion

This work demonstrates that a wearable and wireless EEG system can be used to monitor the brain activities while performing cognitive tasks in a regular classroom or home environment, providing a viable and convenient alternative to traditional gel-based systems. Moreover, the easy to *mount and monitor* headset provides a robust solution for performing brain signal analysis during different data acquisition protocols without any constraints on mobility or usability. To assess the attention level changes in healthy children, differences in spectral features computed for 10 s epochs preceding correct and incorrect SART trials were compared. The inter-individual differences in spectral response was accounted for by normalizing the frequency bands based on the IAF. The results have demonstrated that consistent differences in spectral power distribution can be observed between periods of sustained attention and its lapses. Although our evaluation has mainly focused on understanding the tonic responses as a result of attention lapses, it might be worthwhile to investigate phasic activity immediately prior to user response to identify similar metrics. Overall, the use of a wearable measurement system along with observations from the current study provide new avenues in assessing mental health or the effectiveness of therapy for subjects with cognitive disabilities.

The current study is unique in the aspect that cognitive functions evaluation was performed in a regular setting using a game-like protocol on healthy children. This combined with suitable intervention or neurofeedback training can be potentially used in a supervised environment for normal or cognitively impaired children alike, such that treatment is not bound to a clinical environment.

Acknowledgments. This study was supported by the EIT Digital Program (Activity N$^{\circ}$A15257) of the Playful Supervised Smart Spaces (P3S) project.

References

1. Johnson, K.A., Robertson, I.H., Kelly, S.P., Silk, T.J., Barry, E., Daibhis, A., Watchorn, A., Keavey, M., Fitzgerald, M., Gallagher, L., Gill, M., Bellgrove, M.A.: Dissociation in performance of children with ADHD and high-functioning autism on a task of sustained attention. Neuropsycholgia **45**, 2234–2245 (2007)
2. Lansbergen, M., Arns, M., van Dongen-Boomsma, M., Spronk, D., Buitelaar, J.K.: The increase in theta/beta ratio on resting-state EEG in boys with attention-deficit/hyperactivity disorder is mediated by slow alpha peak frequency. Prog. Neuropsychopharmacol. Biol. Psychiatry **35**, 47–52 (2011)
3. Bink, M., van Boxtel, G., Popma, A., Bongers, I., Denissen, A., van Nieuwenhuizen, C.: EEG theta and beta power spectra in adolescents with ADHD versus adolescents with ASD + ADHD. Eur. Child Adolesc. Psychiatry **24**, 873–886 (2015)
4. Mathewson, K.J., Jetha, M.K., Drmic, I.E., Bryson, S.E., Goldberg, J.O., Schmidt, L.A.: Regional EEG alpha power, coherence, and behavioral symptomatology in austism spectrum disorder. Clin. Neurophysiol. **123**, 1798–1809 (2012)
5. Makeig, S., Inlow, M.: Lapses is alertness: coherence of fluctuations in performance and EEG spectrum. Electroencephalogr. Clin. Neurophysiol. **86**, 23–35 (1993)
6. Oken, B., Salinsky, M., Elsas, S.: Vigilance, alertness, or sustained attention: physiological basis and measurement. Clin. Neurophysiol. **117**, 1885–1901 (2006)
7. Makeig, S., Jung, T.P.: Tonic, phasic, and transient EEG correlates of auditory awareness in drowsiness. Cogn. Brain Res. **4**, 15–25 (1996)
8. Makeig, S., Jung, T.P., Sejnowski, T.J.: Awareness during drowsiness: dynamics and electrophysiological correlates. Can. J. Exp. Psychol. **54**, 266–273 (2000)
9. Nidermeyer, E., da Silva, F.: Electroencephalography: Basic Principles, Clinical Applications, and Related Fields. Lippincott Williams and Wilkins, New York (2005)
10. Chen, Y.H., de Beeck, M.O., Vanderheyden, L., Carrette, E., Mihajlović, V., Vanstreels, K., Grundlehner, B., Gadeyne, S., Boon, P., Van Hoof, C.: Soft, comfortable polymer dry electrodes for high quality ECG and EEG recording. Sensors **14**, 23758–23780 (2014)
11. Doppelymayr, M., Klimesch, W., Pachinger, T., Ripper, B.: Individual differences in brain dynamics: important implications for the calculation of event-related band power. Biol. Cybern. **79**, 49–57 (1998)
12. Loo, S.K., Makeig, S.: Clinical utility of EEG in attention deficit/hyperactivity disorder: a research update. Neurotherapeutics **9**, 569–587 (2012)
13. Snyder, S.M., Quintana, H., Sexson, S.B., Knott, P., Hague, A.F., Reynolds, D.A.: Blinded, multi-center validation of EEG and rating scales in identifying ADHD within a clinical sample. Psychiatry. Res. **159**, 246–358 (2008)
14. Ogrim, G., Kropotov, J.D., Hestad, K.: The QEEG theta/beta ration in ADHD and normal controls: sensitivity, specificity, and behavioral correlates. Psychiatry. Res. **198**, 482–488 (2012)
15. Loo, S.K., Hale, T.S., Hanada, G., Macion, J., Shrestha, A., McGough, J.J., McCracken, J.T., Nelson, S., Smalley, S.L.: Familial clustering and DRD4 effects on electroencephalogram measures in multiplex families with ADHD. J. Am. Acad. Child Adolesc. Psychiatry **49**, 368–377 (2010)
16. Bresnahan, S.M., Barry, R.J.: Specificity of quantitative EEG analysis in adults with attention deficit hyperactivity disorder. Psychiatry. Res. **112**, 133–144 (2002)
17. Ogrim, G., Kropotov, J., Hestad, K.: The quantitative theta/beta ratio in attention deficit/hyperactivity disorder and normal controls: sensitivity, specificity, and behavioral correlates. Psychiatry Res. **198**, 482–488 (2012)

18. Dockree, P.M., Kelly, S.P., Foxe, J.J., Reilly, R.B., Robertson, I.H.: Optimal sustained attention is linked to the spectral content of background EEG activity: greater ongoing alpha (10 Hz) power supports successful phasic goal activation. Eur. J. Neurosci. **25**, 900–907 (2007)
19. Onton, J., Delorme, A., Makeig, S.: Frontal midline EEG dynamics during working memory. Neuroimage **27**, 341–356 (2005)

Increasing Quality of Life Awareness with Life-Logging

Floriano Zini[1(✉)], Martin Reinstadler[2], and Francesco Ricci[2]

[1] University of Bologna, Bologna, Italy
floriano.zini@unibo.it
[2] Free University of Bozen-Bolzano, Bolzano, Italy
martinreinstadler@gmail.com, fricci@unibz.it

Abstract. Life Meter is a health mobile application that helps users raise awareness of their quality of life by showing indicators derived from life-logs collected by commercial wearable trackers, smartphone sensors, and manual input. We describe the general infrastructure we developed for the collection and fusion of life-logs, how the quality of life indicators are calculated, and the GUI of Life Meter. The results of a live-user study show that our application has high functionality and subjective quality, and, according to the users, it increases their awareness of the importance of monitoring quality of life.

Keywords: Quality of life · Life-logging · Mobile app · User study

1 Introduction

Mobile applications have a great potential of becoming useful routine instruments for monitoring our health and quality of life (QoL). According to a recent survey conducted in the US and involving 500 healthcare professionals and 1,000 health mobile app users [7], healthcare professionals think health apps will improve healthcare, in particular for patients with chronic diseases. The survey also revealed that most people use the apps as a lifestyle choice to track their physical activity or to get help lose weight, and that the use of apps to support healthcare is growing. In general, more and more people are willing to use mobile devices and wearable trackers to acquire personal health data. They see mobile "personal agents", which are able to summarize the collected data into meaningful knowledge and present it when needed, as useful tools for achieving better self-management of their health conditions, in particular adherence to long-term therapies [12].

Despite this very promising scenario, also the most passionate members of the *Quantified Self*, a movement of people who use self-tracking technologies to collect and explore personal (numeric) data about their daily lives [4], encounter

---

The research presented in this paper was conducted while Floriano Zini was affiliated to Free University of Bozen-Bolzano.

barriers as lack of time and motivation as well as difficulty in data integration and interpretation [22]. Moreover, self-tracking is subject to several common pitfalls such as tracking too many things, not tracking triggers and context, and lack of scientific rigor [11].

Increased automation in tracking, fusion, analysis, summarization, storage, and context-dependent presentation of valuable personal data would certainly reduce barriers and risk of common pitfalls, and it would also contribute to the further diffusion of health apps. This can also be the basis for the development of innovative mobile healthcare *Proactive Advisory Systems (PASs)* [23], able to provide people with personalized information and advice, in order to promote healthier behaviors, well being, and adherence to medical treatments. This paper gives a contribution in both these directions. We describe a general infrastructure (a preliminary version is presented in [30]) able to acquire, fuse, and store life-log data from multiple channels (*Fitbit* [2] wearable trackers, *Android* smartphone sensors, and manual input); this infrastructure includes web services that third-party applications can invoke to retrieve various types of row data and inferred higher-level summaries. We also present *Life Meter*, a health mobile application that helps users better assess their QoL. *Life Meter* exploits the services of our generic infrastructure and presents personalized QoL indicators to users on a mobile GUI that shows the current values of the indicators, as well as their summaries over the last weeks. We focus on four QoL indicators that are useful for implementing PASs for healthcare: *activities* performed; *sleep* quality; level of *fatigue*; and *mood*. For example, a PAS for assisting allergic patients in the management of their disease treatment [23] could cross reference these QoL indicators with the treatment data in order to highlight the treatment efficacy or the negative effects of interrupting the treatment.

We present here the results of a live-user evaluation aimed at benchmarking *Life Meter* against the *Mobile App Rating Scale (MARS)* [28]. Our application proved to have higher functionality and subjective quality than the average of a benchmark of 50 health mobile applications. Moreover, the users indicated that *Life Meter* is likely to increase the awareness of the importance of monitoring QoL and the understanding of QoL indicators.

In the next section, we position our research with respect to the existing literature. Section 3 describes the generic infrastructure for multi-modal life-logging we have designed and implemented. Section 4 presents how the QoL indicators provided by *Life Meter* are calculated from users' life-logs, and how they are presented on the GUI. In Sect. 5, the evaluation of *Life Meter* is presented. Finally, Sect. 6 summarizes the lesson learned from this research and sketches future work.

2 Related Work

The research community has demonstrated a growing interest in the application of life-logging and mobile devices for the realization of healthcare services [21]. The provision of effective services should be based on the availability of robust and generic life-logging infrastructures, able to gather data from multiple devices and sensors, leverage it to infer higher-level knowledge of patient's health status, and present this knowledge to patients via usable user interfaces. Examples of infrastructures for life-logs acquisition that are not specifically dedicated to healthcare are *MyExperience* and *UbiqLog*. *MyExperience* [16] is a mobile system that uses both automatic logging from mobile phone sensors and applications, and context-triggered sampling of experiences by directly asking users. *UbiqLog* [25] is a lightweight, configurable, and extendable framework that uses the mobile phone for life-logging. Compared to these frameworks, our approach has the advantage of integrating data streams from smartphone sensors, wearable trackers, and manual input. This allow to have more comprehensive life-logs, able to better cover the users' activities during the day, also when the users do not carry the smartphone, for example when exercising.

Recently, projects have also focused on life-logging infrastructures dedicated to healthcare, with an approach similar to ours. For example, the research presented in [14] investigates the possibility of collecting and aggregating life-logging data with the use of wearable devices, mobile apps, and social media. Upon this infrastructure, *MyHealthAvatar* [27] is a web site built to empower citizens and patients through a number of health related services. A life-log collaboration framework on Android platform for the healthcare service infrastructure is proposed in [20]. The framework provides a collaboration mechanism between life-logging devices by different vendors and consists of three layers: the data logging layer, the data mining layer, and the data service layer. The framework was applied to develop health screening forms. *SenseSeer* [8] is a generic mobile-cloud-based life-logging framework that supports customizable services, such as personal health monitoring, location tracking, lifestyle analysis, and tourism focused applications. In particular, the *My Health* service is a personal healthcare-oriented web application that allows the user to track and visualize her physical activities. All these infrastructures were evaluated only performing some robustness test or by asking informal feedback to colleagues and not via a well structured user-study as we did for *Life Meter*. Performing rigorous user-study is fundamental for correctly adapting health mobile applications to users' needs [29], since it is increasingly difficult to readily identify and assess high quality apps [13].

Finally, it is worth mentioning that many commercial aggregators (e.g., *Zenobase* [6], *AddApp* [1], *TicTrac* [5], and *HealthVault* [3]) have been recently introduced, and this gives evidence of the popularity that self-monitoring is acquiring. These tools can usually aggregate and then show data from a wide range of sources. However, there is still need for extensive and rigorous user studies in order to evaluate their usability, efficacy and efficiency.

3   Life-Logging Infrastructure

The infrastructure we have developed for building users' life-logs integrates data continuously collected from wearable trackers, smartphone sensors, and manual

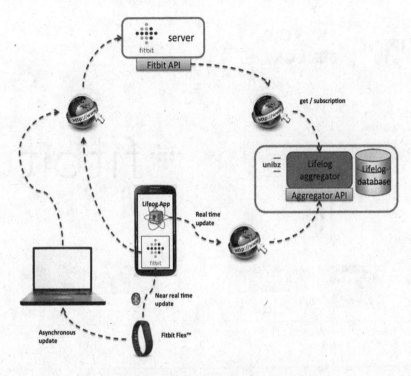

Fig. 1. Life-logging infrastructure.

input. For life-log, we intend the personal data generated by one's physical and digital activity (recorded by trackers and sensors) or manually entered by the user. The implemented system (see Fig. 1) automatically acquires information about what users do during the day. Data streams are collected from *Fitbit* [2] wearable trackers (we have experimented the infrastructure with *Fitbit Flex* and *Fitbit Charge HR*) and *Android* smartphones. While the tracker provides steps, burned calories, covered distance, heart rate, and sleep quality information, the smartphone collects information as performed calls, sent SMSs, position, and temperature. In addition, the user can manually input her mood in the system. All the collected data is exploited for the detection of QoL indicators. For example, phone calls to/from colleagues/work partners are signs that the user is probably working, or a variation of the resting heart rate from day to day can be used as a proxy of physical fatigue.

The life-logs are aggregated and stored on a dedicated server by two software components: a *Lifelog Service* and a server side *Lifelog Aggregator*. The *Lifelog Service* is developed for Android SDK 4.0+ and runs on the users' Android smart devices. It runs in the background, gathers life-log data from the device sensors, and periodically uploads it to the server. This is done by two always-active components (see Fig. 2(a)):

1. The *Sensordata Collector* monitors the sensors and stores their values in an internal database. In order to avoid draining the smartphone battery, the

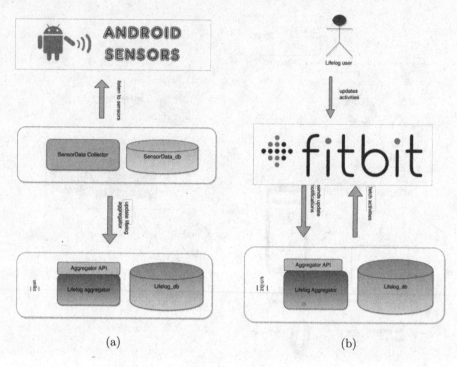

Fig. 2. Life-logs acquisition from smartphone sensors (a) and Fitbit server (b).

Sensordata Collector does not poll sensors for their status, but only reads new data when it is notified of a change in the sensor status.

2. The *Lifelog Uploader* starts at regular intervals (e.g., every hour) and uploads all data from the internal database to the *Lifelog Aggregator*.

The *Lifelog Aggregator* is made of two services:

1. The *Fittracker* is responsible for accessing the *Fitbit* server and fetching data from there (see Fig. 2(b)). It is based on a Java client library that facilitates the *Fitbit* authorization and resource access. As soon as new user's data is uploaded to the *Fitbit* server, a notification is sent to the *Lifelog Aggregator*, which starts the *Fittracker* service. Then, the *Fittracker* downloads the new data using the *Fitbit* API, invoked by the Java client library.

2. The second component of the *Lifelog Aggregator* provides REST web services with JSON responses. The services enable data storage and data retrieval to/from the *Lifelog Database*. The web services accept client requests, fetch or store data from the *Lifelog Database* and returns JSON responses. There are two types of web services: base data services are used to query/update low-level life-log data from the *Lifelog Database*; high-level data services are used to query the system for the values of QoL indicators.

4   Quality of Life Indicators

We now illustrate *Life Meter*, an *Android* mobile application developed on top of the infrastructure illustrated above. *Life Meter* helps users raise awareness of their QoL by showing them four specific indicators: *activities* performed; *sleep* quality; level of *fatigue*; and *mood*. In healthcare, the assessment of the QoL is extremely important to measure how a disease, disability, or disorder affects an individual's well-being over time [18]. The home screen of *Life Meter* (Fig. 3(a)) shows the values of the four indicators for today.

4.1   Mood

When their mood changes, the users can use the mood input tool, accessible by clicking on the smile icon in the home screen. The mood input tool is shown in Fig. 3(b). Users can express their mood using *Pick-A-Mood (PAM)* [15], a mood reporting and visualization tool, based on the circumplex model of affect [24]. The evaluation of *PAM* demonstrated that the use of cartoon characters enables people to unambiguously and visually report their mood in a rich and easy-to-use way. *PAM* consists of three characters (a man, a woman, and a robot) that are used to personalize the pictorial representations of the mood according to the gender of the user. The robot figure is used when the user prefers not to input the gender. Users can touch the point of the screen that corresponds to how they feel in that moment. The pictures help the users report typical moods of four main categories: energized-pleasant (*excited* and *cheerful*), energized-unpleasant (*irritated* and *tense*), calm-pleasant (*relaxed* and *calm*), and calm-unpleasant (*bored* and *sad*). In addition, there is a picture for *neutral* mood.

When users click below the mood picture in the *Life Meter* home screen, the view in Fig. 3(c) is opened. The interface shows, using again *PAM*, the mood

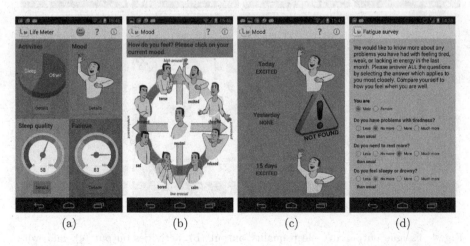

      (a)   (b)   (c)   (d)

Fig. 3. Home (a), mood input (b), mood output (c), and Chalder Fatigue Scale (d).

average value for today, yesterday, and over the last 15 days (or less if there is not enough data). In the calculation of the average, every mood is weighed by the time the user persisted in that mood. When the calculation of the average mood is not possible, because of lack of user input, a special exclamation mark icon is shown. For example, in Fig. 3(c), yesterday's average is not available.

4.2   Fatigue

Fatigue is a feeling of tiredness that can have physical or mental causes. Studies report a relation between fatigue and heart rate [26]. We experimented three fatigue indicators based on heart rate variability and two derived from simple heart rate. Heart rate variability is generally considered to be better correlated with fatigue over time, but *Fitbit* trackers are not precise enough to permit an accurate calculation of it. Therefore, we decided to use the resting heart rate directly measured by the *Fitbit* tracker as input value for calculating the fatigue indicator, measured as a number in the range $[0, 100]$.

In order to set up the initial value for the indicator when users start using *Life Meter*, the *Chalder Fatigue Scale* [10] is used to acquire their initial fatigue (see Fig. 3(d)). This survey has been selected because it allows the measurement of both dimensions (physical and mental) of fatigue, it is easy to administer (there are only 11 questions) and it has been validated for the general population. The survey is administered only once, when the users access *Life Meter* for the first time, and returns their fatigue values, in a range from 0 to 11. The values are rescaled in the $[0, 100]$ interval. Since the system also knows the value of the resting heart rate at the time when the *Chalder Fatigue Scale* is administered, this resting heart rate is associated to the measured fatigue. Assuming that the fatigue indicator varies linearly with the resting heart rate, we also need to define

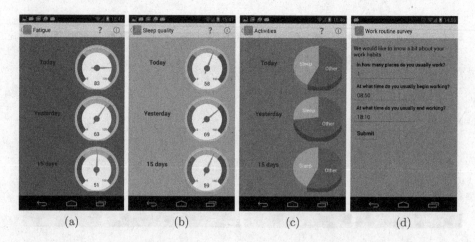

Fig. 4. Fatigue output (a), sleep quality output (b), activities output (c), and work habits survey (d).

the range for this variation and therefore to set up the heart rate corresponding to the minimum (0) and maximum (100) values for the fatigue indicator. In this set up, we assume that the resting heart rate has a variation range of 12 bpm, value that is derived from literature and from empirical measurement on some subjects.

When a user clicks below the fatigue chart in the *Life Meter* home screen, the view in Fig. 4(a) is opened. The interface shows the value of fatigue for today, yesterday, and over the last 15 days (or less if there is not enough data). Today's and yesterday's values are directly derived from today's and yesterday's resting heart rates and are proportional (on a scale from 0 to 100) to the differences between the user's resting heart rates and the heart rate corresponding to the minimum fatigue.

4.3 Sleep Quality

When users click below the sleep quality chart in the *Life Meter* home screen, the view in Fig. 4(b) is opened. The interface shows the average quality of sleep for today, yesterday, and over the last 15 days (or less if there is not enough data). We use the sleep quality indicator provided by *Fitbit* to estimate the sleep quality. This indicator, in the range $[0, 100]$, is the proportion of user's "deep" sleep (sleep without movements) over the total time the user spent in bed. We calculate the average sleep quality over a reference period by averaging the quality of the sleeps in that period. Each sleep quality is weighted by the duration of the sleep.

4.4 Activities

When a user clicks below the activities pie chart in the *Life Meter* home screen, the view in Fig. 4(c) is opened. From top to bottom, the three pie charts show the amount of time the user spent today, yesterday, and on average in the last 15 days (or less if there is not enough data) doing various types of activities. Three types of activity are shown: *Work*, *Sleep*, and *Other*. The time spent for work is calculated as follows:

1. The time stamped positions of the user during the day are clustered using *Expectation Maximization Clustering* [19], which performs optimization of the number of clusters; each cluster corresponds to a specific area the user visited during the day.
2. If the number of clusters in the time window indicated by the user as "usual" work period is the same as the number of "usual" work places indicated by the user, the working time is calculated as the difference between the max and min timestamps of positions belonging to the working clusters; otherwise, no working time is detected for the day.

The sleeping time is calculated by the *Fitbit* tracker. The time for other activities is calculated by subtracting the work time and the sleeping time from the total observed time. The average time spent every day working, sleeping, or doing other activities in the last 15 days is calculated by averaging the corresponding daily times. A simple survey (Fig. 4(d)) is used to acquire the users' work habits the first time they use *Life Meter*. The data acquired in this survey is used by the activity inference algorithm described above.

5   Life Meter Evaluation

We evaluated *Life Meter* using the *Mobile App Rating Scale (MARS)* [28], a new tool specifically designed for assessing the quality of health mobile applications. The quality dimensions included in *MARS* have been selected by a panel of experts after examining and clustering criteria proposed for assessing mobile healthcare applications by several authors. Among the dimensions, we decided to evaluate *functionality, aesthetic*, and *subjective quality* of *Life Meter*. Functionality and aesthetic refer to two fundamental aspects of mobile applications: being suited to serve their purpose well; and having an attractive GUI design. Subjective quality summarizes items as if the users would recommend the app to others, how frequently they would use the app in the future, or the overall star rating. We compared *Life Meter* with a benchmark obtained by evaluating 50 health mobile applications with the MARS tool.

We involved in the experiment 10 subjects (5 female, 5 male) recruited using convenience sampling [9] among researchers and students of our university and among our acquaintances. We adopted convenience sampling to be able to quickly run the experiment and draw conclusions on the *Life Meter* prototype. In order to mitigate the well known drawbacks of the sampling method, we payed attention that the sample was gender-balanced and included people with heterogeneous experience with mobile devices and wearable trackers. Two subjects had problems installing the system on their smartphones and drop the experiment[1], while 8 subjects completed it. The subjects registered on the *Fitbit* website and used the tracker for some days, in order to get familiar with it. In this period the tracker collected the data that was then used to initialize the QoL indicators. After some days, the subjects were informed how to download *Life Meter* from the Android marker, and how to install it on their smartphones. Then, they used *Life Meter* for about 15 days, in conjunction with the *Fitbit* tracker. At the end of the two weeks, the subjects were asked to fill in an online *MARS* survey.

The average rate given by the group of users to *Life Meter* functionality was 4.57 (max is 5), while the average functionality of the benchmark is 4.01. The functionality of *Life Meter* resulted to be significantly better than the benchmark (t-test, $p < 0.01$). The average rate of *Life Meter* aesthetic was 3.29, while the average aesthetic of the benchmark is 3.49. In this case, *Life Meter* underperformed the benchmark. The average rate of *Life Meter* subjective quality was 3.07, and resulted to be significantly better than the benchmark, which scores

---

[1] One had a too old version of Android and the other was not able to successfully follow the app installation instructions.

2.19 (t-test, $p < 0.01$). In summary, *Life Meter* demonstrated to outperform a benchmark composed by mobile health applications available on the market on two dimensions out of three. The reason for the inferior performance on aesthetic can be due to the fact that *Life Meter* is still a prototype and, at that point, the optimization of the look and feel was not a major priority.

In addition to rating the above quality dimensions, we measured the perceived impact of *Life Meter* on users' awareness of their QoL, their knowledge/understanding of it, and their inclination to improve it. We asked the users to judge if "Life Meter is likely to increase awareness of the importance of monitoring QoL indicators" and we obtained a score of 4.13 on a scale from 1 to 5. We obtained the same evaluation for the statement "Life Meter is likely to increase knowledge/understanding of QoL indicators", while the users agreed less (3.25) with the statement "Life Meter is likely to change attitudes toward improving QoL". These results indicate that *Life Meter* can be useful for rising the awareness of the users about the necessity of monitoring their QoL and can help them better understand the meaning of QoL indicators. As expected, users are less convinced that *Life Meter* can successfully support a life change that improves the users' QoL, probably because the current version of the system does not have any advisory functionality.

6   Conclusions

In this paper, we have presented a comprehensive system able to monitor the users' daily activity, build life-logs integrating data from multiple sources (wearable trackers, smartphone sensors, and manual input), calculate high-level QoL indicators from the life-logs, and show the indicators to the users via a dedicated mobile application. The system focuses on deriving high-level summaries from heterogeneous data, while other important aspects needed by a comprehensive life-logging framework, namely, long-term data preservation and privacy, are left as future work. The evaluation we performed demonstrated that our system is a solid starting point for the implementation of proactive advisory systems (able to take the initiative and propose information and advice) dedicated to various aspects of health care and well-being. In the future, we intend to integrate the system with *Smart Allergy Taming* [23] (a system supporting allergic patients to better manage their immunotherapy) in order to automatically provide indicators that help patients assess the efficacy of their therapy. Moreover, we also plan to exploit the developed infrastructure with *ChefPad* [17], a food recommender system that not only offers recipe recommendations that suit users' taste, but it also takes the users' health into account.

References

1. Addapp. website. https://addapp.io
2. Fitbit website. http://www.fitbit.com
3. Healthvault website. https://www.healthvault.com

4. Quantified self: self knowledge through numbers. http://quantifiedself.com/
5. Tictrac website. https://www.tictrac.com
6. Zenobase website. https://zenobase.com
7. Are mobile medical apps good for our health? A new study by research now reveals that doctors and patients say 'yes' (2015). https://goo.gl/AcKfX6
8. Albatal, R., Gurrin, C., Zhou, J., Yang, Y., Carthy, D., Li, N.: Senseseer mobile-cloud-based lifelogging framework. In: 2013 IEEE International Symposium on Technology and Society (ISTAS), pp. 144–146 (2013)
9. Battaglia, M.: Convenience sampling. In: Lavrakas, P.J. (ed.) Encyclopedia of Survey Research Methods, pp. 806–808. Sage Publications Inc., Thousand Oaks (2008)
10. Cella, M., Chalder, T.: Measuring fatigue in clinical and community settings. J. Psychosom. Res. **69**(1), 17–22 (2010)
11. Choe, E.K., Lee, N.B., Lee, B., Pratt, W., Kientz, J.A.: Understanding quantified-selfers' practices in collecting and exploring personal data. In: Proceedings of the SIGCHI Conference on Human Factors in Computing Systems, CHI 2014, pp. 1143–1152. ACM, New York (2014)
12. Choi, A., Lovett, A.W., Kang, J., Lee, K., Choi, L.: Mobile applications to improve medication adherence: existing apps, quality of life and future directions. Adv. Pharmacol. Pharm. **3**(3), 64–74 (2015)
13. Cummings, E.A., Borycki, E.M., Roehrer, E.: Issues and considerations for healthcare consumers using mobile applications. Stud. Health Technol. Inform. **183**, 227–231 (2013)
14. Deng, Z., Yang, P., Zhao, Y., Zhao, X., Dong, F.: Life-logging data aggregation solution for interdisciplinary healthcare research and collaboration. In: 2015 IEEE International Conference on Computer and Information Technology; Ubiquitous Computing and Communications; Dependable, Autonomic and Secure Computing; Pervasive Intelligence and Computing (CIT/IUCC/DASC/PICOM), pp. 2315–2320 (2015)
15. Desmet, P., Vastenburg, M., Bel, D.V., Herrera, N.R.: Pick-a-mood; development and application of a pictorial mood-reporting instrument. In: Out of Control: Proceedings of the 8th International Conference on Design and Emotion, London, UK, 11–14 September 2012 (2012)
16. Froehlich, J., Chen, M.Y., Consolvo, S., Harrison, B., Landay, J.A.: Myexperience: a system for in situ tracing and capturing of user feedback on mobile phones. In: Proceedings of the 5th International Conference on Mobile Systems, Applications and Services, pp. 57–70. ACM (2007)
17. Ge, M., Massimo, D., Ricci, F., Zini, F.: Integrating wearable devices into a mobile food recommender system. In: Mobile Computing, Applications, and Services: 7th International Conference, MobiCASE 2015, Berlin, Germany, November 12–13, 2015, Revised Selected Papers, vol. 162, pp. 335–337. Springer, New York (2015)
18. The WHOQOL Group: The world health organization quality of life assessment (whoqol): position paper from the world health organization. Soc. Sci. Med. **41**(10), 1403–1409 (1995)
19. Jin, X., Han, J.: Expectation maximization clustering. In: Sammut, C., Webb, G.I. (eds.) Encyclopedia of Machine Learning, pp. 382–383. Springer, New York (2010)
20. Kang, K., Kwon, Y., Kim, Y., Lee, J., Bae, C.: Lifelog collaboration framework for healthcare service on android platform. In: 2013 International Conference on ICT for Smart Society (ICISS), pp. 1–4 (2013)
21. Klasnja, P., Pratt, W.: Healthcare in the pocket: mapping the space of mobile-phone health interventions. J. Biomed. Inform. **45**(1), 184–198 (2012)

22. Li, I., Dey, A., Forlizzi, J.: A stage-based model of personal informatics systems. In: Proceedings of the SIGCHI Conference on Human Factors in Computing Systems, CHI 2010, pp. 557–566. ACM, New York (2010)
23. Nguyen, T.S., Ricci, F., Zini, F., Granconato, M.: Life-logging for healthcare proactive advisory systems. In: Cantador, I., Chi, M., Farzan, R., Jäschke, R. (eds.) Proceedings of UMAP 2014 Posters, Demonstrations and Late-Breaking Results. CEUR Workshop Proceedings, vol. 1181. CEUR-WS.org (2014)
24. Posner, J., Russell, J.A., Peterson, B.S.: The circumplex model of affect: an integrative approach to affective neuroscience, cognitive development, and psychopathology. Dev. Psychopathol. 17(3), 715–734 (2005)
25. Rawassizadeh, R., Tomitsch, M., Wac, K., Tjoa, A.M.: Ubiqlog: a generic mobile phone-based life-log framework. Pers. Ubiquitous Comput. 17(4), 621–637 (2013)
26. Schmitt, L., Regnard, J., Desmarets, M., Mauny, F., Mourot, L., Fouillot, J.P., Coulmy, N., Millet, G.: Fatigue shifts and scatters heart rate variability in elite endurance athletes. PloS One 8(8), e71588 (2013)
27. Spanakis, E.G., Kafetzopoulos, D., Yang, P., Marias, K., Deng, Z., Tsiknakis, M., Sakkalis, V., Dong, F.: Myhealthavatar: personalized and empowerment health services through internet of things technologies. In: 2014 EAI 4th International Conference on Wireless Mobile Communication and Healthcare (Mobihealth), pp. 331–334 (2014)
28. Stoyanov, S.R., Hides, L., Kavanagh, D.J., Zelenko, O., Tjondronegoro, D., Mani, M.: Mobile app rating scale: a new tool for assessing the quality of health mobile apps. JMIR mHealth and uHealth 3(1), e27 (2015)
29. Zapata, B.C., Fernández-Alemán, J.L., Idri, A., Toval, A.: Empirical studies on usability of mhealth apps: a systematic literature review. J. Med. Syst. 39(2), 1–19 (2015)
30. Zini, F., Reinstadler, M., Ricci, F.: Life-logs aggregation for quality of life monitoring. In: Proceedings of the 5th International Conference on Digital Health 2015, DH 2015, pp. 131–132. ACM, New York (2015)

SPW-1: A Low-Maintenance Wearable Activity Tracker for Residential Monitoring and Healthcare Applications

Xenofon Fafoutis[1]([✉]), Balazs Janko[2], Evangelos Mellios[1], Geoffrey Hilton[1], R. Simon Sherratt[2], Robert Piechocki[1], and Ian Craddock[1]

[1] Department of Electrical and Electronic Engineering,
University of Bristol, Bristol, UK
{xenofon.fafoutis,evangelos.mellios,geoff.hilton,r.j.piechocki,
ian.craddock}@bristol.ac.uk
[2] Department of Biomedical Engineering, University of Reading, Reading, UK
{b.janko,r.s.sherratt}@reading.ac.uk

Abstract. In this paper, we present SPW-1; a low-profile versatile wearable activity tracker that employs two ultra-low-power accelerometers and relies on Bluetooth Low Energy (BLE) for wireless communication. Aiming for a low maintenance system, SPW-1 is able to offer a battery lifetime of multiple months. Measurements on its wireless performance in a real residential environment with thick brick walls, demonstrate that SPW-1 can fully cover a room and - in most cases - the adjacent room, as well. SPW-1 is a research platform that is aimed to be used both as a data collecting tool for health-oriented studies outside the laboratory, but also for research on wearable technologies and body-centric communications. As a result, SPW-1 incorporates versatile features, such as external sensor support, various powering options, and accelerometer configuration options that can support a wide range applications from kinematics to long-term activity recognition.

Keywords: Wearable technologies · Bluetooth Low Energy · Internet of Things · eHealth · Healthcare technologies

1 Introduction

The increasing trends in elderly populations [8] and the continuous rise of chronic medical conditions, such as depression and diabetes, push the limits of national health systems [7]. Wearable technologies [5] and Ambient Assisted Living (AAL) infrastructures are widely considered promising directions that could encourage people to monitor their own well-being and facilitate timely interventions.

In addition to health-oriented applications, long-term activity monitoring with wearable technologies is a tool that facilitates health-oriented research. Avon Longitudinal Study of Parents and Children (ALSPAC) is a cohort study of children born in the county of Avon in England. During the first stage of

K. Giokas et al. (Eds.): eHealth 2016, LNICST 181, pp. 294–305, 2017.
DOI: 10.1007/978-3-319-49655-9_37

the study in the early 90s, thousands of pregnant women were monitored. More recently, the study continues; monitoring the grandchildren of the originally monitored subjects [19] and the researchers adopt wearable technologies to replace diaries. SPHERE (a Sensor Platform for Healthcare in a Residential Environment) is an interdisciplinary research collaboration that aims to monitor volunteers in their own home environment [25]. Wearable sensors are used, among other sensing modalities, to monitor the everyday behaviour of the users [10].

Long-term activity monitoring outside the laboratory, such as monitoring the activities of daily life in a residential environment, introduces important challenges that typically do not rise in controlled laboratory environments. The employed wearable devices need to be small, lightweight, comfortable and with low maintenance requirements. Contrary to fashionable wearable gadgets, health-oriented technologies cannot depend on the user for regular maintenance, such as recharging or replacing the battery. For instance, patients suffering from mental conditions are not in a position to maintain the technologies that support them. In addition, in health-oriented research studies outside the laboratory, long battery lifetime increases the reliability of data collection, as the problem of data loss, due to improper maintenance of the technologies used, is mitigated.

With the aforementioned requirements as the primary goal, this paper focuses on the design and evaluation SPW-1 (First SPHERE Wearable), a versatile wearable monitoring system shown in Fig. 1. The design is based on two triaxial accelerometers and uses Bluetooth Low Energy (BLE) [4] for wireless communication. Differential measurements from the two accelerometers enable the approximation of angular acceleration and hence an estimation of the angular velocity without the need of employing a power-hungry gyroscope.

SPW-1 is a research platform that is intended to be used both as a data collector for health-oriented studies and healthcare applications, but also for research on wearable computing and body-centric communications. To support long-term monitoring applications outside the laboratory, SPW-1 is small, lightweight, and ultra low power. At the same time, SPW-1 is a versatile research platform. It is fully programmable, compatible with various power sources - including energy harvesters - and supports external sensors and antennas. Moreover, different accelerometer configurations allow the user to trade battery lifetime for data quality, enabling a wide variety of applications ranging from kinematics to longterm activity recognition. The contribution of this work is twofold. Beyond offering a tool to the research community, we provide insight to researchers and engineers who are developing similar systems. In particular, we provide a thorough energy consumption study that is the basis of meaningful battery lifetime estimations for different sensor configurations. Moreover, we study SPW-1's wireless performance in the context of body-centric communications. The study includes measurements both in a controlled (i.e. anechoic chamber) and in a residential environment.

The remainder of the paper is organised as follows. Section 2 summarises the related work; Sect. 3 presents the system design of SPW-1; Sect. 4 evaluates its performance; and Sect. 5 concludes the paper.

2 Related Work

In recent years fashionable gadgets, such as Fitbit, Jawbone UP and Nike+ Fuelband SE, have appeared in the consumer electronics market [14]. Such fitness devices demonstrate the rise of a trend towards self-monitoring, as well as the willingness of users to wear them. However, commercial gadgets are of limited use for research or medical applications due to limited access to the raw data, their lack of interoperability with other healthcare systems and their limited expandability to new sensor technologies. Furthermore, their need for regular recharging (typical battery lifetime of less than a week) hinders their suitability for target groups that are uncomfortable with or physically unable of managing modern technologies.

The research community has also used several wearable devices for activity monitoring, a few of which are briefly reviewed in this paper. We refer the reader to [5] for an exhaustive survey on smart wearable technologies. Verity [24] is an AAL platform that is using a wearable device equipped with an accelerometer and a piezo-resistive sensor for fall detection and heart rate monitoring. In [11], the authors propose an AAL platform based on a waist-worn accelerometer that is able to identify basic activities, such as sitting, walking, running and jumping. Similarly, [6,26] perform identification of basic activities using multiple on-body accelerometers and gyroscopes. These platforms use off-the-shelf hardware and do not focus on their power consumption, resulting to wearable devices that require regular recharging. Other works present low power hardware that target various body sensing applications by incorporating different types of sensors, such as bio-impedance sensors [15], microphones [18] and inertial sensors [12].

On a different perspective, related work on Wireless Body Area Networks (WBANs) typically focuses on the networking aspects of body sensor networks [23].

3 System Design

SPW-1 is a research platform that is designed on two key principles. The primary design goal is ultra low power consumption and user acceptance. Indeed, a long battery lifetime may be considered fundamental for long-term monitoring. Furthermore, it is not desirable for the platform to depend on the user for maintenance. The secondary design goal is versatility. As a research platform, SPW-1 should be able to support different types of research that range from health-oriented studies to body-centric communications.

SPW-1 is designed with the wrist as the target body position. We consider a wrist-mounted device as the most socially-acceptable and least invasive choice to the subject's everyday routine, due to the fact that people of both sexes commonly wear wrist-worn gadgets, such as watches and bracelets. Alternative positions, such as the chest or the waist, can be realised via an appropriate enclosure, but hold the risk of being removed by the subject and compromising the effectiveness of the system. Social studies [3,27] have shown the importance

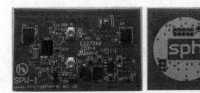

Fig. 1. SPW-1: Top view (left) and bottom view (right) of the circuit board.

of wearable devices being comfortable and not intrusive to the daily life activities. In [16], the authors assess various body positions and present comparison results in which the wrist ranks high in all the considered activities in terms of classification accuracy.

Figure 1 shows the printed circuit board (PCB), with dimensions of $24 \times 39 \times 3.8$ mm. The core component is a nRF51822 system-on-chip (SoC) which incorporates a ARM Cortex M0 microcontroller unit (MCU), 32 KB of RAM, 256 KB of non-volatile flash memory, and a BLE radio (a comparison study of BLE and ZigBee can be found in [20]). Two ADXL362 accelerometers are interfaced, over SPI (Serial Peripheral Interface), to the nRF51822 core. The ADXL362 is a micro-power triaxial digital accelerometer that has 12-bit resolution, a maximum sampling frequency of 400 Hz, and supports measurement ranges of ± 2 g, ± 4 g, ± 8 g. It also employs a 512-sample FIFO buffer (First In First Out). We refer the reader to [2] for figures on the measurement noise levels and their variation with temperature. The incorporation of two accelerometers, at a distance of 30 mm, provides a low power alternative to a gyroscope. Indeed, differential measurements from multiple accelerometers can be used to derive the angular acceleration [21]. The accelerometers are powered by the MCU through its GPIO (General Purpose Input Output) pins and hence is able to power them on and off individually. Therefore, the use of the second accelerometer is optional. The ADXL362 also provides two interrupt pins (INT1 and INT2) that can be used either to generate interrupts on events, or to generate events based on external triggers. The two INT1 pins of the accelerometers are connected to GPIO pins of nRF51822 with the purpose of generating interrupts that wake up the MCU. The two INT2 pins are connected, over the same bus, to a GPIO of the MCU as an input. Using INT2, the MCU generates a square wave signal that synchronises the accelerometers by triggering the measurements. The use of the interrupts is also optional.

Regarding powering options, SPW-1 is compatible with various sources. Ultra low power consumption is partially achieved by using the MCU in low power mode, *i.e.* at 1.8 V. The system employs the LTC3388 DCDC (Direct Current to Direct Current) converter that efficiently converts any voltage source from 2.7 V to 6 V, to the required 1.8V. Thus, converter supports multiple options, including 3 V coin cell batteries (such as CR2032), 3.7 V rechargeable Lithium-Polymer (Li-Po) batteries, and super capacitors. Moreover, SPW-1 is energy harvesting ready, in the sense that any harvester that works at the appropriate voltage

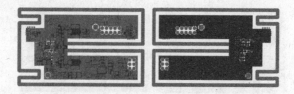

Fig. 2. SPW-1: Top copper layer (left) and bottom copper layer (right) of the circuit board. The differentially-fed loop antenna is printed around the other components.

level, is compatible. The converter can be also bypassed, as the board provides direct access to the 1.8 V trail. SPW-1 also employs an MCP73831, a 500 mA linear charge management controller with 4.2 V output that is compatible with single cell 3.7 V Li-Po batteries. The battery charger is, by default, isolated from the remaining of the circuit and can be optionally connected.

With regard to input and output interfaces, SPW-1 employs one button and two LEDs (Light Emitting Diodes). The button and one of the LEDs are controlled by the MCU and, thus, are available to the application. The other LED is connected to the battery charger indicating when the battery is charging. Moreover, external sensors can be connected to SPW-1, using 7 available GPIOs (all support digital inputs; 2 of them also support analogue inputs). The INT2 line of the accelerometers is also externally available, so that external sensors can be synchronised to the embedded accelerometers. Lastly, the board also employs a Serial Wire Debug (SWD) interface for programming and debugging.

Energy awareness is also considered in the design. With a potential divider, the high voltage of the source is appropriately conditioned to the requirements of the MCU's analogue-to-digital converter (ADC). When a battery (*e.g.* CR2025) is used, this feature can be used to issue low-battery warnings. In case of energy harvesting, energy-awareness allows the system to adapt to the available ambient energy.

As far as wireless is concerned, SPW-1 employs a meandered loop antenna printed on the FR4 substrate, matched to the differential RF output of the nRF51822 (shown in Fig. 2). The loop antenna was measured to have an efficiency of about 60% (relative to a high-efficient reference antenna) and a maximum directivity of 7 dBi (computed from the measured 3D radiation pattern). The antenna was measured in isolation in an anechoic chamber. A comparison of the wireless performance of SPW-1 to the reference design that employs a printed monopole antenna (and hence not using the differential RF output of the chip) is discussed in Sect. 4.2. Furthermore, SPW-1 supports external antennas by incorporating u.FL connectors. Using solder-bridges, the user can select either the embedded loop antenna or external antennas. The radio of the nRF51822 supports 7 transmission power levels ranging from −20 dBm to 4 dBm. The experiments, presented in Sect. 4, quantify the effect of this setting with respect to trade-off between energy consumption and wireless coverage.

4   System Evaluation

In this section, we evaluate the performance of SPW-1. First, we focus on measuring the energy consumption of fundamental system events, and on providing realistic battery lifetime estimations. Then, we measure the wireless performance in both an anechoic chamber and a house. The latter identifies the wireless coverage capabilities of SPW-1 in residential environments with thick brick walls.

4.1   Energy Consumption and Battery Lifetime Estimations

In this section, we benchmark SPW-1 against the reference design of the nRF51822 radio, *i.e.* the nRF51822-DK [17]. By incorporating the LTC3388 DCDC converter, SPW-1 yields lower power consumption than the reference design. The nRF51822-DK uses, instead, the nRF51822's internal linear regulator.

For the nRF51822-DK, the continuous idle power consumption is measured with a multimeter, configured as an ammeter and positioned in series with the positive side of the power supply. For this test, the nRF51822 is programmed to be in sleep mode and both accelerometers are disabled through the GPIOs. We measured a constant current of $5\,\mu A$. Because of its linear voltage regulation, the power consumption scales linearly with the supply voltage. Considering the typical battery voltage levels $3\,V$ and $3.7\,V$, the idle power consumption is $15\,\mu W$ and $18\,\mu W$, respectively. For SPW-1, the idle power consumption is not continuous. Instead, the DCDC converter consumes energy periodically keeping its output voltage above the target threshold. Hence, we measured the idle power consumption by measuring and multiplying the energy consumed during one duty cycle by their frequency. The energy of a duty cycle of the converter was measured with a series $10\,\Omega$ resistor and an oscilloscope, as in [9]. At both voltage levels, we measure a constant idle power consumption of $8.4\,\mu W$, 46% less than the reference kit, when using a $3\,V$ coin cell battery.

To measure the processing power consumption, both platforms were programmed to perform some dummy processing cycles (integer multiplication and addition). In a similar fashion, the current was measured with a series $10\,\Omega$ resistor on the positive side of the power supply. The results demonstrate again the benefits of the DCDC converter. Considering a $3\,V$ and a $3.7\,V$ battery, the reference kit consumes $18\,mW$ and $22.2\,mW$ for processing respectively. SPW-1, on the other hand, consumes $9.5\,mW$ at both voltage levels.

Next, we measure the energy required by the radio for transmitting data. In particular, we measure the energy consumption of a triple advertisement (*i.e.* 3 packets of 39 bytes) at all different transmission power levels. The current profile of the advertisement event was captured with a series $10\,\Omega$ resistor. The energy is then derived by estimating the integral of the current profile and multiplying it by the supply voltage. Figure 3 demonstrates that SPW-1 is 20% more energy-efficient than the reference design when using $4\,dBm$ transmission power and a $3\,V$ battery. The figure also shows how the energy consumption scales with the transmission power level, indicating that significant energy savings can be achieved by turning the power level down to $0\,dBm$ and $-4\,dBm$.

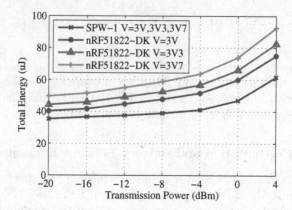

Fig. 3. Energy consumption for the transmission of a BLE triple advertisement.

To facilitate realistic battery lifetime estimations, we also provide the power consumption of the peripherals. Each accelerometer adds an extra constant power consumption of approximately $3\,\mu\text{W}$. Transferring the data from the FIFO buffer of ADXL362 to the memory of the MCU takes approximately $13\,\text{ms}$ (SPI clock at $4\,\text{MHz}$), resulting to a consumption of approximately $135.5\,\mu\text{J}$. Transferring a single acceleration sample from the accelerometer to the MCU consumes approximately $1.9\,\mu\text{J}$ (in contrast to $3.6\,\mu\text{J}$ for nRF51822-DK). The LED consumes $1.6\,\text{mW}$ when turned on.

Next, we combine the consumption measurements in an attempt to provide realistic battery lifetime estimations, based on an indicative scenario. Such estimations demonstrate how the lifetime of the battery scales with the configuration of different parameters, such as the number of accelerometers, the resolution and the sampling frequency. The battery lifetime estimations are based on the following equation:

$$T = \frac{E_{BAT}}{P_I + P_{XL} \times N + (E_{SPI} + E_{BLE}) \times f_s \times N}, \tag{1}$$

where E_{BAT} is the total energy of the battery; P_I is the idle power consumption; P_{XL} is the power consumption of a single accelerometer; E_{SPI} is the energy consumed for transferring a single acceleration sample over SPI from the accelerometer to the MCU; E_{BLE} is the energy consumed for the transmission of a single sample over BLE given by Fig. 3 and divided by the number of samples inside a packet; f_s is the sampling frequency; and N is the number of accelerometers.

In particular, we consider a scenario where SPW-1 streams raw accelerometer data using the undirected connectionless BLE advertisements (similarly to [10]). Although data reliability can be addressed at the receiver [22], this communication approach does not provide delivery guarantees and, thus, can be only applied to applications that can tolerate data loss or make use of specific missing data techniques [13]. We also assume the following. We assume that for resilience to interference all three advertisement packets are populated with the

Table 1. Battery Lifetime Approximations in Days

Tx Power	Freq. (Hz)	1 Accelerometer		2 Accelerometers	
		8-bit	12-bit	8-bit	12-bit
4 dBm	1	1174	873	750	520
	10	240	140	125	72
	20	127	72	65	36
	50	53	29	26	14
−4 dBm	1	1328	1054	879	654
	10	314	194	167	101
	20	170	102	87	52
	50	71	42	36	21

same payload. We further assume the maximum BLE packet size of 39 bytes (24 bytes of payload), which provides necessary space for either 4 triaxial samples of 12-bit resolution or 8 triaxial samples of 8-bit resolution; and that the SPI bus between the accelerometers and the MCU is clocked at 4 MHz. Lastly, we assume that the system is powered by a 210 mAh coin cell battery (3 V).

Table 1 shows the battery lifetime estimations, in days, assuming different configuration scenarios. The frequency column represents the sampling frequency of the accelerometer(s). Notice that the battery lifetime ranges from few weeks to few years, depending on the configuration. Observe that at high sampling frequencies the energy consumption is dominated by frequent duty cycles. At low sampling frequencies, instead, the idle consumption becomes increasingly more important. In [16], the authors use accelerometers with 8-bit resolution to perform activity classification. Experimenting with different sampling frequencies, the authors show that the performance of the classifier reaches a high level at approximately 10 Hz with only marginal improvement at higher frequencies. In this configuration, the battery lifetime of SPW-1 is approximated at 240 days. For comparison, using the same methodology, the reference design yields a battery lifetime of approximately 172 days for the same configuration (an improvement of 40%).

4.2 Wireless Performance

In this section, we evaluate SPW-1's wireless performance. We, first, benchmark it against the reference design (nRF51822-DK employs a PCB monopole antenna) in an anechoic chamber. In particular, both wearable sensor units were mounted on a ground plane. At the other side of the room, at a distance of 4.4 m, a receiver unit with two orthogonally polarised patch antennas was used [10]. In both cases, the transmitter was programmed to transmit advertisement packets at a period of 100 ms (4 dBm transmission power). The receiver unit was programmed to log the RSSI of all the received packets. In both experiments, the position of the receiver was fixed while two motors rotated the wearable device

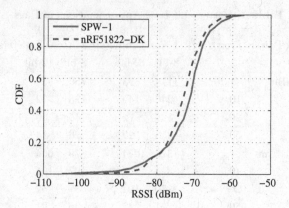

Fig. 4. Comparison of the wireless performance of SPW-1 to nRF51822-DK in the anechoic chamber.

through all angles in 3D space. Figure 4 plots the CDF (cumulative distributed function) of the RSSI of all the packets received for SPW-1 and the reference kit. Observe that, in a controlled environment, SPW-1 performs 2 dB better than nRF51822 in the median case. Overall, despite the significantly lower size (*i.e.* less ground plane, and less isolation between the antenna and surrounding components), SPW-1 maintains the same level of wireless performance.

We, next, evaluate the wireless performance of SPW-1 in a residential environment. Specifically, the following experiments were conducted in a typical house in the city of Bristol, UK. In each one of two adjacent rooms, we deployed a receiver unit identical to the ones used in the previous experiment. SPW-1, also programmed as in the previous experiment (*i.e.* 4 dBm transmission power), was mounted on the wrist of a human, who was performing random walks and random activities within the room for approximately 10 min (room size: 3×3 m). Therefore, the measurements capture the effect of body shadowing and multipath propagation in a wide variety of situations. Figure 5 shows the CDF of the RSSI of all the received packets, as measured from the receivers located in the same room and the adjacent room respectively. At the maximum transmission power setting, observe that in the case of the same room, the median is at -68 dBm; whereas, in the adjacent room, the median is at -84 dBm. In the same figure, we also plot the packet error rate (PER) of a nRF51822 receiver for different RSSI values. Assuming an acceptable PER threshold of 5%, we observe that SPW-1 can fully cover a single room (99.9% of the cases) and 87.2% of the cases of the adjacent room. The wireless performance at lower transmission power levels can be approximated by shifting the CDFs in the x-axis accordingly. For instance, if single room coverage is sufficient for a given application, the transmission power could be set to -4 dBm. This configuration yields 33% less energy consumption for transmission (see Fig. 3 and Table 1), covering 98.6% of the single room cases with a PER of less than 5%.

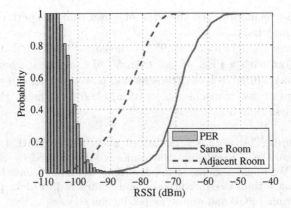

Fig. 5. Wireless performance in the a residential environment.

For reference, a performance comparison study of other antennas in the same environment can be found in our previous work [1].

5 Conclusion

SPW-1 is a wearable activity monitor that is based on two accelerometers for activity sensing and BLE for wireless communication. As a research platform, SPW-1 has multiple purposes with different requirements. Primarily, it is meant to be used as a lightweight and low-profile data collection tool for long-term activity monitoring outside the laboratory. To decrease the dependency on user maintenance, long battery lifetimes are required. Furthermore, access to the raw data and to the accelerometer configuration settings is also fundamental. Moreover, SPW-1 supports external sensors and external antennas to facilitate research on wearable computing and body-centric communications.

Ultra low energy consumption is a primary design goal. SPW-1 embeds two accelerometers that may function as an energy-efficient alternative to a gyroscope. We measured the consumption of SPW-1 and benchmarked it against the off-the-shelf nRF51822-DK. The comparison demonstrates significant improvements. Assuming the use of a coin cell battery, SPW-1 consumes approximately 45% less power for processing and in idle mode, and 20% less energy for wireless transmission. Battery lifetime estimations in a indicative scenario demonstrate the dependency of the battery lifetime to the configuration settings of the accelerometers (estimations range from weeks to years). For example, a configuration used in [16] yields a battery lifetime estimation of 240 days.

Wireless performance is also fundamental, especially in residential monitoring. Controlled measurements, in an anechoic chamber, benchmark the wireless performance of SPW-1, demonstrating a 2 dB marginal improvement with regards to the reference design, despite its significantly smaller size. In addition, we performed measurements in a residential environment with thick brick walls, in which SPW-1 was mounted on the wrist of a user that was performing random activities and random walks within a $9\,m^2$ room. In this scenario, SPW-1 was able to fully cover a single room (99.9% of the cases) and 87.2% of the cases of the adjacent room with a PER of less than 5%. In scenarios where only single room coverage is required, a lower transmission power setting can yield 33% less energy consumption for transmission, covering 98.6% of the single room cases with a PER of less than 5%.

Acknowledgment. This work was performed under the SPHERE (a Sensor Platform for Healthcare in a Residential Environment) IRC funded by EPSRC, Grant EP/K031910/1. We would also like to thank Altium Ltd and Premier EDA Solutions Ltd for sponsoring Altium Designer licenses, and Simtek EMS Ltd for partially sponsoring and performing PCB and prototype production services.

References

1. Abdullah, M.W., Fafoutis, X., Mellios, E., Klemm, M., Hilton, G.: Investigation into off-body links for wrist mounted antennas in bluetooth systems. In: Proceedings of the Loughborough Antennas and Propagation Conference (LAPC) (2015)
2. Analod Devices: ADXL362 - Micropower, 3-Axis, ±2 g / ±4 g / ±8 g, Digital Output MEMS Accelerometer, Rev. B (2013)
3. Bergmann, J., McGregor, A.: Body-worn sensor design: What do patients and clinicians want? Ann. Biomed. Eng. **39**(9), 2299 (2011)
4. Bluetooth SIG.: Specification of the Bluetooth System - Covered Core Package version: 4.0 (2010)
5. Chan, M., Estève, D., Fourniols, J.Y., Escriba, C., Campo, E.: Smart wearable systems: current status and future challenges. Artif. Intell. Med. **56**(3), 137–156 (2012)
6. Cheng, J., Chen, X., Shen, M.: A framework for daily activity monitoring and fall detection based on surface electromyography and accelerometer signals. IEEE J. Biomed. Health Inf. **17**(1), 38–45 (2013)
7. Cruz-Jentoft, A.J., Franco, A., Sommer, P., Baeyens, J.P., Jankowska, E., Maggi, A., Ponikowski, P., Rys, A., Szczerbinska, K., Michel, J.P., Milewicz, A.: Silver paper: the future of health promotion and preventive actions, basic research, and clinical aspects of age-related disease-a report of the European Summit on Age-Related Disease. Aging Clin. Exp. Res. **21**(6), 376–385 (2009)
8. Department of Economic and Social Affairs - United Nations: World Population Ageing: 1950–2050. Technical report (2011)
9. Fafoutis, X., Di Mauro, A., Dragoni, N.: Sustainable medium access control: Implementation and evaluation of odmac. In: Proceedings of the IEEE International Conference on Communications Workshops (ICC), pp. 407–412, June 2013
10. Fafoutis, X., Tsimbalo, E., Mellios, E., Hilton, G., Piechocki, R., Craddock, I.: A residential maintenance-free long-term activity monitoring system for healthcare applications. EURASIP J. Wirel. Commun. Netw. **2016**(31), 1 (2016)
11. Gupta, P., Dallas, T.: Feature selection and activity recognition system using a single triaxial accelerometer. IEEE Trans. Biomed. Eng. **61**(6), 1780–1786 (2014)
12. Kan, Y.C., Chen, C.K.: A wearable inertial sensor node for body motion analysis. IEEE Sens. J. **12**(3), 651–657 (2012)

13. Karadogan, S., Marchegiani, L., Hansen, L., Larsen, J.: How efficient is estimation with missing data? In: Proceedings of the 2011 IEEE International Conference on Acoustics, Speech and Signal Processing (ICASSP), pp. 2260–2263. IEEE (2011)
14. Kooiman, T.J.M., Dontje, M.L., Sprenger, S.R., Krijnen, W.P., van der Schans, C.P., de Groot, M.: Reliability and validity of ten consumer activity trackers. BMC Sports Sci. Med. Rehabil. **7**(1), 24 (2015)
15. Lee, S., Polito, S., Agell, C., Mitra, S., Firat Yazicioglu, R., Riistama, J., Habetha, J., Penders, J.: A low-power and compact-sized wearable bio-impedance monitor with wireless connectivity. J. Phys. Conf. Ser. **434**(1), 012013 (2013)
16. Maurer, U., Smailagic, A., Siewiorek, D., Deisher, M.: Activity recognition and monitoring using multiple sensors on different body positions. In: International Workshop on Wearable and Implantable Body Sensor Networks (BSN) (2006)
17. Nordic Semi: nRF51822 Development Kit - User Guide v1.4 (2013)
18. Oletic, D., Arsenali, B., Bilas, V.: Low-power wearable respiratory sound sensing. Sensors (Basel) **14**(4), 6535–6566 (2014)
19. Pearson, H.: Children of the 90s: coming of age. Nature **484**, 155–158 (2012)
20. Siekkinen, M., Hiienkari, M., Nurminen, J., Nieminen, J.: How low energy is bluetooth low energy? Comparative measurements with ZigBee/802.15.4. In: Proceedings of the IEEE Wireless Communications and Networking Conference Workshops (WCNCW), pp. 232–237 (2012)
21. Tsai, Y.L., Tu, T.T., Bae, H., Chou, P.: Ecoimu: a dual triaxial-accelerometer inertial measurement unit for wearable applications. In: Proceedings of the International Conference on Body Sensor Networks (BSN), pp. 207–212, June 2010
22. Tsimbalo, E., Fafoutis, X., Piechocki, R.: Fix it, Dont bin it! - CRC error correction in bluetooth low energy. In: Proceedings of the 2nd IEEE World Forum on Internet of Things (WF-IoT) (2015)
23. Ullah, S., Higgins, H., Braem, B., Latre, B., Blondia, C., Moerman, I., Saleem, S., Rahman, Z., Kwak, K.: A comprehensive survey of wireless body area networks. J. Med. Syst. **36**(3), 1065–1094 (2012)
24. Winkley, J., Jiang, P., Jiang, W.: Verity: an ambient assisted living platform. IEEE Trans. Consum. Electron. **58**(2), 364–373 (2012)
25. Woznowski, P., Fafoutis, X., Song, T., Hannuna, S., Camplani, M., Tao, L., Paiement, A., Mellios, E., Haghighi, M., Zhu, N., Hilton, G., Damen, D., Burghardt, T., Mirmehdi, M., Piechocki, R., Kaleshi, D., Craddock, I.: A multi-modal sensor infrastructure for healthcare in a residential environment. In: Proceedings of the International Conference on Communications (ICC) Workshops (2015)
26. Zhang, Y., Markovic, S., Sapir, I., Wagenaar, R., Little, T.: Continuous functional activity monitoring based on wearable tri-axial accelerometer and gyroscope. In: Proceedings of the 5th International Conference on Pervasive Computing Technologies for Healthcare (PervasiveHealth), pp. 370–373 (2011)
27. Ziefle, M., Rocker, C.: Acceptance of pervasive healthcare systems: a comparison of different implementation concepts. In: Proceedings of the 4th International Conference on Pervasive Computing Technologies for Healthcare (PervasiveHealth), pp. 1–6 (2010)

Inertial Sensor Based Modelling of Human Activity Classes: Feature Extraction and Multi-sensor Data Fusion Using Machine Learning Algorithms

Tahmina Zębin[1(✉)], Patricia J. Scully[2], and Krikor B. Ozanyan[1,2]

[1] School of Electrical and Electronic Engineering, University of Manchester,
Manchester M13 9PL, UK
{tahmina.zebin,k.ozanyan}@manchester.ac.uk
[2] Photon Science Institute, University of Manchester, Manchester M13 9PL, UK
patricia.scully@manchester.ac.uk

Abstract. Wearable inertial sensors are currently receiving pronounced interest due to applications in unconstrained daily life settings, ambulatory monitoring and pervasive computing systems. This research focuses on human activity recognition problem, in which inputs are multichannel time series signals acquired from a set of body-worn inertial sensors and outputs are automatically classified human activities. A general-purpose framework has been presented for designing and evaluating activity recognition system with six different activities using machine learning algorithms such as support vector machine (SVM) and artificial neural networks (ANN). Several feature selection methods were explored to make the recognition process faster by experimenting on the features extracted from the accelerometer and gyroscope time series data collected from a number of volunteers. In addition, a detailed discussion is presented to explore how different design parameters, for example, the number of features and data fusion from multiple sensor locations - impact on overall recognition performance.

Keywords: Inertial measurement unit · Accelerometer data · Feature extraction · Data-fusion · Machine learning algorithms · Human Activity Recognition

1 Introduction

Despite significant research efforts over the past few decades, activity recognition still remains a challenging problem. Wearable sensor based Human Activity Recognition (HAR) is currently playing a key role in the development of innovative human-machine interfaces and assistive technologies [2]. The information obtained from human physical activity is valuable in the long-term assessment of biomechanical parameters and physiological variables, which can then be used to support care of the elderly, the chronically ill and people with special needs [3]. Moreover, for accurate monitoring of physical activity, information on the type, intensity, and duration of the activities is of substantial interest to the research community [4].

© ICST Institute for Computer Sciences, Social Informatics and Telecommunications Engineering 2017
K. Giokas et al. (Eds.): eHealth 2016, LNICST 181, pp. 306–314, 2017.
DOI: 10.1007/978-3-319-49655-9_38

Over several years, studies of gestures and activity recognition have been confined to clinical settings and conventional lab-based equipment, such as stationary and expensive 3D motion capturing systems and force plates [5]. For studying activities in unconstrained daily life settings, body-worn inertial sensors are emerging as a preferable research option in many cases [6, 7]. In addition, these systems are portable, more affordable than their laboratory counterparts. Hence, in this paper, we have developed an off-the-shelf lower body inertial sensor system. The system is designed and built as a set of 5 sensor units initially, each with an integrated MPU-9150 IMU to capture motion data. The system is specifically designed to study lower body motion. The sensors are connected via ribbon cables to a single control hub based on an Arduino board and an XBee transmitter. The data from the sensor (accelerometer and gyroscope) is post-processed to facilitate an automatic classification of the activities performed.

For modelling and evaluating physical activity, a general-purpose machine learning framework is presented in this paper. The framework comprises components for data acquisition and pre-processing, data segmentation, feature extraction and selection [1, 8], training and classification, decision fusion [9], and performance evaluation. It should be noted that, machine learning based algorithms for recognition of gestures and activities is a relatively new application area, and we provide a systematic insight on the use of classification algorithms (e.g. SVM, ANN) in MATLAB for some common physical activities.

2   Design of the Human Activity Recognition Chain

A typical Human Activity Recognition (HAR) system contains a stream of sensor data at the input stage acquired using multiple sensors worn on the body. The sensor data is then pre-processed to filter out signal variability or artefacts. The processed data is then segmented to isolate the region of interest of the activity or gesture. Afterwards, features that capture the activity characteristics are extracted from the signals within each segment [8]. In the training stage, the extracted features and corresponding ground truth class labels are used as input to train a classifier model in the training stage. In classification stage, the features and a previously trained model are used to calculate a score for each activity class and to map these scores into a single class label in the classification stage. If multiple sensors or classifiers are considered, the output of

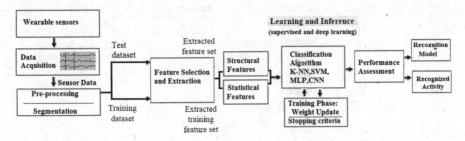

Fig. 1. Components of the human activity recognition chain [1]

several classifiers may subsequently be fused. In addition, a performance evaluation stage allows the assessment of the performance of the recognition system [1]. In the rest of the paper, significant stages (shown in Fig. 1) are used and the design decisions we made for the activity recognition task in hand is presented in detail.

2.1 Sensor Data Collection and Preprocessing

In the first stage of a typical activity recognition system, raw data is acquired using several sensors attached to different locations on the body. In our research the activities were tracked using five sensing units (model: MPU-9150) placed at (a) Sensor 1: Pelvis/waist region, (b) Sensor 2 and 3: Left and right thigh, (c) Sensor 4 and 5: Left and right shank of the volunteer. A schematic diagram of the Inertial Measurement System used for this research is shown in Fig. 2.

A single sensing unit is comprised of a 3-axis accelerometer and a 3-axis gyroscope recording timestamped motion data at a sampling rate of 50 Hz. All the recorded data was sent via XBee to a laptop placed in close proximity to the participant. Five volunteers performed a continuous sequence of six generic ambulatory activities [7] listed in Table 1. The activity was repeated 10 times for each participant, resulting in a dataset of about 120 min.

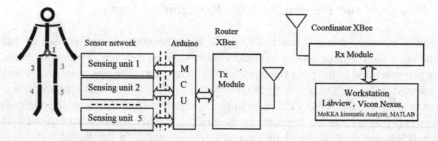

Fig. 2. Schematic of the wearable inertial sensor system and orientation of the sensing unit.

Table 1. Categorical physical activity and Activity ID for the activity recognition task

Activity	Activity ID
Walking	1
Walking_upstairs	2
Walking_downstairs	3
Sitting	4
Standing	5
Lying down	6

2.2   Extraction and Selection of Features

Manual selection of features is a difficult task. The higher the dimensionality of the feature space, the more training data is needed for model parameter estimation and the system becomes more computationally intensive. For real-time processing on embedded systems the objective is to minimize memory, computational power and bandwidth requirement. It is therefore important to use an optimum number of features that will still allow the system to achieve the desired target performance. Current literature uses a wide range of features such as signal based features [10] (e.g. mean, variance, FFT – coefficients, spectral entropy, and overall energy.). Other than that, body model based parameters (calculated from a 3D skeleton using multiple on body sensors) incorporating prior knowledge can lead to higher performance and increase robustness from person to person [3, 6].

By identifying the most salient features for learning, the most useful aspects of the data is used for analysis and future prediction. The hypothesis explored in this research is that feature selection for classification tasks can be accomplished on the basis of convolution [11] and pooling of features, and that such a feature selection process can be beneficial to a variety of common machine learning algorithms. Here, we have utilized the statistical and spectral features from segmented time series data as the features to be processed by the classification algorithm. The 66 features computed from the inertial sensor's accelerometer data are listed in Table 2.

Table 2. List of extracted features from accelerometer data for each activity for the activity recognition scenario

Feature name	Feature number	Additional information
Average value (1 each)	feature (1) feature (2) feature (3)	For all three acceleration components (x,y,z direction)
RMS value (1 each)	feature (4) feature (5) feature (6)	All three acceleration components
Autocorrelation features (3 each)	feature (7:9) feature (10:12) feature (13:15)	Height of main peak; height and position of second peak
Spectral peak features (12 each)	feature (16:27) feature (28:39) feature (40:51)	Height and position of first 6 peaks
Spectral power features (5 each)	feature (52:56) feature (57:61) feature (62:66)	Total power in 5 adjacent and pre-defined frequency bands

3 Training and Classification Using Machine Learning Algorithms

The classifier itself influences the recognition performance of an activity recognition system. The decision for or against different classifier can be made either by having lower computational complexity or simply by superior performance. In our research, we have investigated the performance of several classifiers used in activity recognition to suggest an automated and alternative approach to hand-crafted feature extraction and classification techniques.

Classification techniques such as Nearest Neighbors, Naïve Bayes (NB), Support Vector machine (SVM) and Multi-layer Perceptron (MLP) based neural networks has been tested in this research. In the following sections, we will explore the capabilities and efficiency of two machine learning algorithms: Support vector Machine and multi-layer perception on inertial sensor based human activity recognition data. It should be noted that, machine Learning approaches such as SVM and MLP includes kernel based and random forest feature selection mechanism ensuring the generalization of the relevant features.

3.1 Neural Network Based Classification

Neural networks are capable of performing pattern-recognition techniques useful in the analysis of gait dynamics [12]. In this section activity classification was performed with a MATLAB based multilayer perceptron (MLP) model as a neural network. The multilayer perceptron consists of three or more layers (an input and an output layer with one or more hidden layers) of nonlinearly-activating nodes. Since an MLP is a Fully Connected Network, each node in one layer connects with a certain weight w_{ij} to every node in the following layer. The weight of each node is adjusted in a manner so that minimize the error in the entire output.

Learning occurs in the perceptron by changing connection weights after each piece of data is processed, based on the amount of error in the output compared to the expected result. The learning is carried out through backpropagation, a generalization of the least mean squares algorithm in the linear perceptron. To quantitatively assess the performance of a classification algorithm we have predicted the activities for a small test dataset, and compared them against the known class values. To visually represent the accuracy, a confusion matrix is used in this paper. The confusion matrix is a square matrix that summarizes the cumulative prediction results for all couplings between actual and predicted classes, respectively. As indicated in Fig. 3, it was observed that there has been above 12% misclassification of walking downstairs and sitting activity based on the accelerometer signal based features. Whether features from the gyroscope improve the accuracy, is yet to be explored. In addition, training the network with a bigger database from more volunteers is planned as a part of future research.

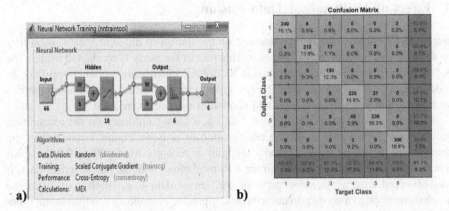

a)   b)

Fig. 3. (a) MATLAB neural network Train tool has been utilized to train the neural network. (b) The confusion matrix shows an accuracy rate of 91.7% for activity recognition for neural network based activity classification.

3.2 Support Vector Machine Based Classification

The Support Vector Machine (SVM) technique is a powerful machine-learning algorithm based on its ability to find non-linear patterns. The classifier is trained at the first stage with a specific activity and their known classes. A MATLAB based 'Classification Learner' App [13] has been used here to auto generate functions to train a classifier based on the dataset. The returned arguments include information of how the dataset is partitioned during the training phase. The remaining samples of the dataset can be used for testing the accuracy of the classifier. The prediction result is visualized in a confusion matrix. Figure 4 shows the Confusion Matrix when the data is classified and tested using support vector machine. During this initial stage of testing 96.7% of the activities were classified correctly. The accelerometer based feature for walking downstairs and sitting down caused 7.4% of false hits which need further specification in classifying that activity. As can be observed from the results the best performance was obtained for SVM classifier because of the suitability of the kernels to the activities we chose to classify.

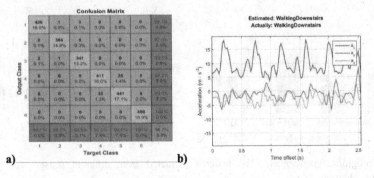

a)   b)

Fig. 4. (a) Confusion Matrix when the data is classified using support vector machine; (b) Screenshot of an activity classified correctly by the recognition system.

4 Effect of Multi-sensor Data Fusion

During our studies, we also experimented on the impact of different sensor modalities on the activity recognition performance. This part of the study is conducted using a the K-NN (nearest neighbor) classifier using MATLAB classification learner app [11]. In order to quantitatively understand the recognition performance, some standard metrics such as accuracy, recall, precision and confusion matrices were used.

From the results presented in Figs. 5 and 6, a strong influence on the recognition accuracy can be observed with the combination of sensors. Figure 5 shows that, the precision of person dependent activity recognition changes from 90% to 94.1% when sensor data from the shank and thigh are also used along with the pelvic sensor data. It was observed that while some parts of the sensor data (e.g. single axis from the accelerometer or gyroscope) do contribute to a precise classification whilst some other axial data might introduce noise. Other than that, the classification performance is found to be 65.7% precision for a person independent scenario (where the classifier is trained with activities from multiple volunteers).

Figure 6 shows the impact of features processed from accelerometer and gyroscope separately and it is observed that even for the person dependent scenario, the gyroscope data contained far less useful features than the accelerometer data. However, features from a gyroscope improve the accuracy in the case where the activities are constrained and distinguished by translation and rotation of the joint angles. A combined accelerometer and gyroscope feature processing is a planned part of our future research.

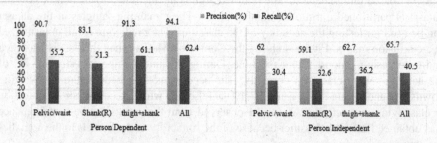

Fig. 5. Activity recognition performance for different sensor position combinations.

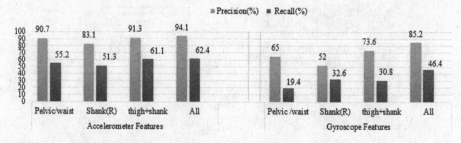

Fig. 6. Recognition performance for features extracted from different sensors for person dependent evaluation

5 Conclusion

The present work described the development of an IMU-based measurement system and investigated the feasibility of its use in human activity recognition and classification scenario. The activities of the system were selected to be of low complexity, which allowed us to compare algorithms in terms of overall recognition performance. For designing more complex activity recognition system, the procedural stages involved and studied in this research will infer some intuitive decisions. In addition, accurate information on the sensor model, positioning and orientation of sensors during different activities will provide generalization and will contribute to a open dataset for human activity recognition based research. Future research will include Composite activities, Concurrent and overlapping activities and also some multi-attribute classification approaches and deep learning approaches for activity recognition in a multi-sensor scenario.

Acknowledgments. Tahmina Zebin would like to thank the Presidents Doctoral Scholar award scheme, University of Manchester for funding her PhD.

References

1. Bulling, A., Blanke, U., Schiele, B.: A tutorial on human activity recognition using body-worn inertial sensors. ACM Comput. Surv. **46**(3), 1–33 (2014)
2. Ugulino, W., Cardador, D., Vega, K., Velloso, E., Milidiú, R., Fuks, H.: Wearable computing: accelerometers' data classification of body postures and movements. In: Barros, L.N., Finger, M., Pozo, A.T., Gimenénez-Lugo, G.A., Castilho, M. (eds.) SBIA 2012. LNCS, vol. 7589, pp. 52–61. Springer, Heidelberg (2012)
3. Mannini, A., Sabatini, A.M.: Machine learning methods for classifying human physical activity from on-body accelerometers. Sensors **10**(2), 1154–1175 (2010)
4. Shaopeng, L., Gao, R.X., John, D., Staudenmayer, J.W., Freedson, P.S.: Multisensor data fusion for physical activity assessment. IEEE Trans. Biomed. Eng. **59**(3), 687–696 (2012)
5. Bettini, C., et al.: A survey of context modelling and reasoning techniques. Pervasive Mob. Comput. **6**(2), 161–180 (2010)
6. Lara, O.D., Labrador, M.A.: A survey on human activity recognition using wearable sensors. IEEE Commun. Surv. Tutorials **15**(3), 1192–1209 (2013)
7. Ronao, C.A., Sung-Bae, C.: Human activity recognition using smartphone sensors with two-stage continuous hidden Markov models. In: 10th International Conference on Natural Computation (ICNC-2014), pp. 681–686 (2014)
8. Turaga, P., et al.: Machine recognition of human activities: a survey. IEEE Trans. Circ. Syst. Video Technol. **18**(11), 1473–1488 (2008)
9. Fourati, H. (ed.): Multisensor Data Fusion: From Algorithms and Architectural Design to Applications, pp. 509–517. CRC Press, Taylor & Francis Group LLC, United States (2015)
10. Bao, L., Intille, Stephen, S.: Activity recognition from user-annotated acceleration data. In: Ferscha, A., Mattern, F. (eds.) Pervasive 2004. LNCS, vol. 3001, pp. 1–17. Springer, Heidelberg (2004). doi:10.1007/978-3-540-24646-6_1

11. Zeng, M., et al.: Convolutional neural networks for human activity recognition using mobile sensors. In: 6th International Conference on Mobile Computing, Applications and Services (MobiCASE) 2014, pp. 197–205 (2014)
12. Kaufman, K.R.: Future directions in gait analysis. In: RRDS Gait Analysis in the Science of Rehabilitation, pp. 85–112 (2011)
13. Classification learner app for supervised machine learning. http://uk.mathworks.com/help/stats/classificationlearner-app.html

Questioning the Reflection Paradigm for Diabetes Mobile Apps

Dmitri Katz[1(✉)], Nick Dalton[2], Simon Holland[1], Aisling O'Kane[3],
and Blaine A. Price[1]

[1] Open University, Milton Keynes, UK
dmitrikatz23@gmail.com, {simon.holland,
b.a.price}@open.ac.uk
[2] Northumbria University, Newcastle upon Tyne, UK
nick.dalton@northumbria.ac.uk
[3] University College London, London, UK
a.okane@cs.ucl.ac.uk

Abstract. Hundreds of diabetes self-management apps are available for smart phones, typically using a diary or logging methodology. This paper investigates how well such approaches help participants to make sense of collected data. We found that, while such systems typically support data and trend review, they are ill suited to helping users understand complex correlations in the data. The cognitively demanding user interfaces (UI's) of these apps are poorly adapted both to the restricted real estate of smartphone displays and to the daily needs of users. Many participants expressed the desire for intelligent, personalized and contextually aware near-term advice. By contrast, users did not see tools for reflection on prior data and behavior, seen as indispensable by many researchers, as a priority. We argue that while designers of future mobile health (mHealth) systems need to take advantage of automation through connected sensors, and the increasing subtlety of intelligent processing, it is also necessary to evolve current graphs and dashboards UI paradigms to assist users in long-term self-management health practices.

Keywords: User Interface (UI) · Diabetes apps · mHealth

1 Introduction

Among major health conditions, diabetes is one of the most common and costly. It is believed to affect 380 million people worldwide, and numbers are rising. Type 1 diabetes (T1D), which affects roughly 5–10% of people with diabetes, is an autoimmune disease that necessitates daily injections of the hormone insulin in order to control blood glucose levels. While short and long-term complications can be severe, diabetes can be successfully managed with careful attention to lifestyle and the correct use of medications. Self-monitoring and self-management practices are essential for good diabetes outcomes, as the majority of care is by necessity self-care [1]. However, glycemic control can be challenging, as it is a multivariate task affected not only by diet, exercise, and insulin dosages, but also hard to control factors such as stress,

© ICST Institute for Computer Sciences, Social Informatics and Telecommunications Engineering 2017
K. Giokas et al. (Eds.): eHealth 2016, LNICST 181, pp. 315–326, 2017.
DOI: 10.1007/978-3-319-49655-9_39

illness, and natural variability. Diabetes with its strong reliance on diverse data, dynamic treatment, and ability to quantify effects through blood glucose (BG) values, can also be viewed as an edge case that can give insights into the design of similar assistive mHealth technologies.

The paper-based daily diabetes logbook has long been a method of assisting the diabetes management process. The received wisdom is that by patients recording, reviewing, and analyzing tracked factors such as diet, medication dosages, exercise, and location, the patient will be more engaged, form better habits, recognize patterns, and thereby optimize their treatment decisions. This self-management approach has been updated for the ubiquitous smartphone, with hundreds of products allowing not only recording of diverse personal data, but also adding data visualization, data export, social support, food databases, and other functionalities.

However, in an earlier pilot study [2], we found relatively low adoption and retention rates of these diabetes related apps. Many participants were generally positive in assessment, but many viewed the apps as too much work for the benefits delivered. In principle, automation of data streams has the potential to reduce this effort; however, there is little research on the extent to which users are able to extract meaningful insights from this collected data.

Through analysis of user interaction sessions, we present findings that contribute to an increased understanding of: benefits and limitations of the use of data visualizations within diabetes apps; what users want from mobile diabetes apps; potential directions for research into future user interface paradigms and features to better serve user needs in the self-management of chronic conditions.

2 Related Work

The human computer interaction (HCI) community has long investigated the ability of digital technologies to encourage healthier behaviors. The UbiFit garden attempted to foster physical activity using a graphical garden metaphor on a mobile device [3], while Fish'n'Steps used a social mechanism, showing not only the owner's pedometer movements but automatically sharing this information as a motivator [4]. Intille et al. [5] focused on the ability of precisely timed reminders to support healthful behavior change, while King et al. [6] promoted physical activity with early mobile device based exercise programs. The Quantified Self (QS) movement has led to much interest in the role of personal data for life optimization through personal informatics [7]. Li et al. [8] investigated which sorts of questions users seek to answer with collected data, and the shifting nature of their needs. Mamykina et al. [9–11] have written extensively on the use of computer-based systems to aid People with Diabetes (PWD). This work largely focuses on sensemaking, which Mamykina et al. define as the *"perception of new information related to health and wellness, development of inferences that inform selection of actions, and carrying out daily activities in response to new information."* [11]. Kanstrup et al. [12] looked at the situational infrastructure of diabetes management in the home in order to enable participatory design of IT based systems for supporting daily life [13]. The Bant project [14] set out to iteratively develop a smartphone app which variously incorporated diverse elements into a single system:

wireless data transfer from a blood glucose (BG) meter; gamification; decision support; and social elements. Storni [15] introduced an iPhone App TiY (Tag-it-yourself) which attempted to encourage reflective capabilities of diabetes monitoring. And Smith [16] investigated the use of digital photography to aid and augment memory as a method to facilitate visualization, interpretation and reflection.

Much of this research has followed a 'collect and reflect' approach to behavior change, seeking to create tools to assist the user in greater self-knowledge. Many users desire automation of data recording [17]; however, this has the potential to reduce data engagement [8], leaving the *insights derived from the collected data* as the principal opportunity or intervention for self-management. However, successful multivariate data analysis is not a given [18], requiring what Kahneman [19] calls system 2 thinking, which is reflective and requires greater effort as opposed to system 1, which can be thought of as reflexive, intuitive and low effort. This is potentially problematic on a smartphone which is supplementing and changing human thought processes, to allow for people to avoid *"effortful analytic thinking in lieu of fast and easy intuition"* [20]. This suggests that smartphones, due to their size, public use, and portability could be thought of as primarily a System 1 device, with users expecting largely intuitive interactions.

The present paper describes a study undertaken to evaluate the effectiveness of current data visualizations used in popular commercial apps in order to assess their value in communicating diabetes specific information, and to better understand how this might impact long-term use, an area under-represented in current literature.

3   Methodology

There were n = 13 participants in this user interaction study, with an age range from 25–45 years with a mean age of 34 years (SD ± 7.8). Time since diagnosis ranged from 2–26 years, with a mean of 13.5 (SD ± 8.1). Three participants were female. Recruitment of people with T1D willing to undertake user studies proved to be challenging, resulting in recruitment taking longer than initially expected. Participants were primarily located through a Berlin-based diabetes and technology Meetup. We expected that this approach to selection would lead to a potential bias towards a technically literate and early-adopter test group, possibly biasing the findings towards the success of the technology. Overall, 11 of the 13 participants worked or studied in an area connected to an aspect of the study: diabetes; technology; graphic design or software design. All but one participant rated themselves highly comfortable with smartphones and 11/13 had previous experience with diabetes diary apps. Ethical approval was granted by the University Ethics Committee. All respondents were guaranteed confidentiality, and their faces were at no time recorded on video. There were no financial incentives offered.

The sessions began with a short profile questionnaire on personal characteristics, product choices, and previous and current patterns of diabetes app usage. This was followed by a semi-structured interview conducted while the participant reviewed a two-week data set, pre-entered into a range of diabetes apps. To provide authenticity and comparability, this was actual diabetes data from the lead author. This set was comprised of blood glucose levels, carbohydrate intake, exercise, and insulin dosages, for a total of 173 matched entries in each of the various apps. The exception among the apps was the Bant app, due to the restricted nature of this app, designed primarily for the recording of BG levels. The interactions with the apps were captured with a fixed tethered camera attached to an iPhone 5s. This recorded the complete interaction of each participant with each app, along with an audio recording of the interviewer's questions and their answers. We posit that this approach, while subject to some limitations, simulates a near future scenario of automated data entry, as well as giving methodological uniformity across apps and users.

The diabetes apps used in the study were chosen from several sources, as follows. Firstly, the study included the three diabetes logging apps most frequently mentioned by participants in a preceding pilot study: MySugr; SiDiary; and iBGStar. Three other apps were chosen from heterogeneous sources as follows: firstly an app called Bant [14], which was cited in an earlier study in an HCI context; secondly an app Roche, which has potential to be a part of an ecosystem of connected diabetes technologies; and thirdly Diabetik - a representative of a crowd funded, open source, patient initiated project. While this is a small sample of diabetes logging apps, and there are considerable variations in user interfaces, this selection is broadly representative (Figs. 1, 2, 3, 4, 5 and 6).

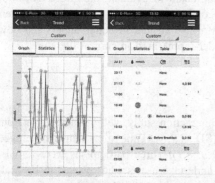

Fig. 1. Accu-Chek Graph showing 14-day graph (left) and Daily diary (right)

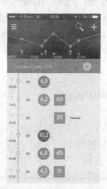

Fig. 2. mySugr diary

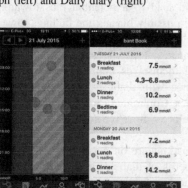

Fig. 3. Bant app showing daily diary

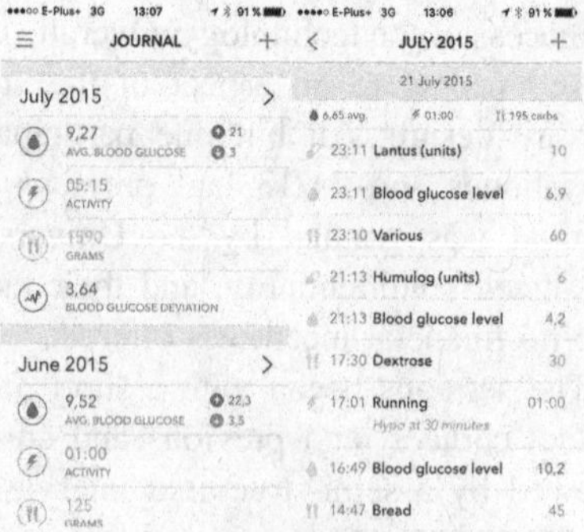

Fig. 4. Diabetik Journal and daily diary

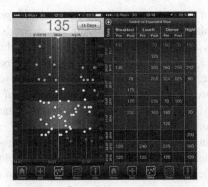

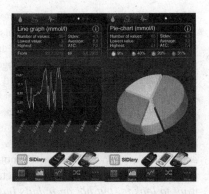

Fig. 5. iBGStar showing 14-day graph and table

Fig. 6. SiDiary showing 14-day graph and Pie Chart

4   Results

From the transcriptions of the recorded user interaction sessions, we analyzed the user's comments to find dominant themes. We found that these apps did support broad overviews of BG management. However, this positive was tempered by, difficulties of in-depth understanding, the need for more actionable data, and in some cases, negative user-experiences related to interaction with sensitive health data.

Before the user interaction session, participants were asked on a 5-point Likert scale questions (1 for "strongly agree" to 5 for "strongly disagree") to assess self-described attitudes towards data reflection and diabetes self-management. Participants rated themselves as generally friendly towards graphics, with a mean of 2.0 (SD 1.0) on "I like graphs and charts", and 1.9 (SD 1.0) on "I enjoy solving puzzles". Users rated themselves as confident on smartphone app usage with a mean rating of 1.25 (SD .6) on the statement "I am comfortable using smartphone apps in general." While participants were reasonably positive on self-management skills, with a 2.1 mean rating (SD .7) on the statement "I am confident that I can troubleshoot my diabetes logs to understand problems." There was a tendency toward dissatisfaction with personal control, with a 3.3 mean rating (SD .9) for the statement "I am in general satisfied with the level of my diabetes control." Only P3 was a habitual daily user of a diabetes logging app at the time of the study, an app that he himself was developing. An additional two out of 13 participants used a logging app on occasion, one largely related to his work as a diabetes patient spokesman.

4.1   App-Based Visualizations Offer Value for General Overviews

The graph functions of these apps were useful for assisting participants in obtaining an overview of glycemic control. Participants P9 and P12 both noted that a pie chart was useful for understanding the relative proportion of elevated BG value. P5 noted that the MySugr graph *"...gives me a very quick graphic feedback on if am I doing good or not.*

If it's flat, if it's green... also by the steepness of the curve, (it) tells me if it's a bad hypo or just a small hypo..." Participants were also capable of observing basic trends. Graphs were useful in this regard, and users were able to note details such as the general frequency of elevated, in range and below normal measurements. P6 reviewed the SiDiary pie chart noting elevated BG levels: *"... this tells me I have to improve something, if every third test is really high blood sugar, I have to do something... only 37% is ok, and I think it should be much more."* P7 noted while viewing the iBGStar graph some elevated levels, and was able to compare them to the rest to conclude, *"... they are doing alright, they have had some quite high points in some days, but generally they are ok."* However, P7 noted graphs are not useful as a daily tool to gain insights but rather to get a bigger picture of the data, *"this stuff (graphs)... you would want to look at, but not on a daily basis... you want to reflect on the last week, or the last month."*

These graphs and their related diaries were seen to support an understanding of direct cause and effect, with all but one (12/13) participant readily reviewing data and engaging in basic cause and effect interpretation. For example, P3 was able to note a hypoglycemia event, leading to hyperglycemia, *"... so it went down really low, then you corrected it with 45 g of carbohydrates, then the next morning the sugar was really high."* P6, when looking at the Diabetik log, was asked what he would have done differently at night, suggested a solution based on this data representation: *"... I would give (myself) more humulog, to get my blood sugar down...(then) I would test it two hours later... to control that everything is working."* P36 was able to trace through the course of a day using the Bant graph stating, *"... the morning at 9:00 it starts with 14.7, its very high for a morning, then 12:00 9.0, it's ok, 18:00 5.0 it's very good, and in the evening 9.1 it's a little high, but there are only four points... I think it's not enough (measurements)."*

4.2   The Challenge of In-depth Understanding on the Smartphone Platform

Given the small dimensions of the smartphone, only limited information can be legibly shown on one screen. At the same time, displaying related information across multiple screens can be overly demanding. Many participants (7/13), noted difficulty comparing data across multiple days, as this often required viewing data on different screens or scrolling. P3 noted: *"It's not easy to compare two days, you always need to scroll up and down."* P3 was overwhelmed with the data during this comparison: *"It's really hard to compare two days.... too much information, too many numbers."* All participants found identifying meaningful connections and patterns between events challenging. For example, P10 while viewing MySugr was unable to recognize that an early meal was eaten without insulin, which caused elevated BG later. P10 reported understanding a pie chart displaying cumulative BG measurement, but couldn't state how this data could be applied in a meaningful way, noting *"One can see that values are bad, but not why."* P7 when asked to make a recommendation on what could have been done better on a specific day said that individual data points were not sufficient to answer this: *"Again I have to look at each one individually... really individual measurements don't tell you anything much because you have to look at them in aggregate, to make any decision, because there are so many variables at play."* One app, Accu-Chek, has a logbook with relatively large and easy to read data entries, but this limits viewing to only one day per screen and does not support in-depth understanding, with P4 stating, *"it's very confusing, you check one day, but you don't see the relations."*

Having excessive information on one screen can also inhibit understanding. When asked to correlate events on the iBGStar app, P2 noted *"I'm not a doctor... I wouldn't use this program... it's too complicated."* Many participants found tables that simply listed data as especially hard to analyze, with P5 stating about Diabetik *"I wouldn't even consider using this, I would dismiss the whole app immediately."* However, seeking to reduce screen clutter by not having all essential information simultaneously visible also increases cognitive load, by overtaxing memory. P6 noted, *"...it's a bit confusing to not see it all at the same time, you always have to check what it is... if I ate something, or if I gave myself insulin, or if it's my blood sugar."*

Five participants had clear difficulties processing all the needed information on the limited space of a smartphone screen. P9 noting how difficult it was to understand the Accu-Check graph data on such a small screen, stated, *"... I think it would be more useful on a computer than on a smartphone."* P11 did not like the interaction requirements to access more information: *"I have to swipe left and right...it's just a bit too much..."* Some participants were frustrated with the app's capabilities on the smartphone as they had preferable experiences with the increased functionalities and display sizes supported by desktop applications. P5 explained, *"Only by entering that data for a while, then importing it to the desktop version, then putting every day on top of the other, then realizing that 80% of mornings are too high, then your realize you really have a problem. So that makes sense, but this app doesn't do it."*

4.3 Insufficient Contextual Information

Diabetes self-management requires rich knowledge of contextual information to inform everyday decisions. Many participants noted that the data did not have enough context to be useful, with P6 reporting *"... here I see my high blood sugar, and... heavy exercise ... what does it tell me... I am doing heavy exercise, or did I do some before, what did I do before at 2:00 p.m.... it was after lunch, and I had another 45 g of (carbs)... it's not helping me why my blood sugar was high in the evening, because I think I did everything right."* P11 said he couldn't really understand data without knowing more about the situations that this data was embedded in, *"...I would need to remember what I did that day, how the weather was... I would need more context."*

4.4 Need for Actionable Information

While looking over collected data, 8/13 participants expressed the desire for help in understanding their collected data, and suggested that these methods of data visualization within these apps were not offering that assistance. For example P7 noted that the limited assistance from these apps still required manual effort comparable to their experiences with paper logbooks, saying, *"I would have to work out everything manually myself. It is a good way of keeping my data to browse through it, but in terms of my ability to make decisions, it isn't much better than writing it down on paper."* A common emergent theme was that reviewing of previous data had limited application to current situations, a key concern of participants. For example, P5 stated, *"Yesterday was yesterday, I don't care, I care about today."* P5 continued about his need for intuitive advice in situ, *"If this app would tell me why this value was too high, and what I did wrong, it would be really great, but it doesn't. It tells me I had a high value here, and even after [...] What I want is a very intuitive interface, that tells me what I did right... and graphically tells me what I did wrong."*

Some participants emphasized that what they really needed from a smartphone app was not the ability to review data, but rather the ability to understand how their choices would affect *"what I can do better in the future"* (P12). P5 acknowledged this lack of functionality and commented *"Most apps haven't helped me in looking forward because it is too complicated."* P7 gave a specific example of how the app could support decision making, but currently does not provide actionable information: *"... the kind of things that are useful (are) over the last month you have consistently gone high in the morning, and then you might realize then you have to take more insulin, because it is the time of day that affects it."* When asked about how this data on this graph would help with better decisions, P7 noted the inability to translate this visualization into action: *"... I would be pretty confused about how to improve it, to be honest. There is not really any indication about what to do to improve the situation. I definitely see its bad, but..."* P12 when assessing the SiDiary Modal day graph said the app *"... tells me you have to look bétter after your diabetes therapy, you have to be better."* But, when questioned as to whether it told her anything about what she had to do better stated, *"No, nothing."*

4.5   Reflecting with Apps can be Emotional

Diabetes management can be frustrating, and interacting with undesired data can increase stress. P7 reflected on the Bant app, *"this interface would stress me out, the red just makes you feel like oh s**t, this isn't a good feeling when you are out [of ideal range]."* P10 on being asked to reflect on the data in the SiDiary app, had a visibly negative experience with the app: *"I don't like it (the interface)...it's so negative... these red dots... demotivating... I didn't do a good job... because maybe I tried to have more green dots, but I failed...I think I just wouldn't use it anymore...too much reflection of the job I did..."* P9 went further and said it could be discouraging to be faced with bad numbers: *"finding out that you are not doing as good a job as you can is always discouraging. It sucks finding out that over time you haven't been doing what's best for you."* P5 also had a negative experience with seeing the number of elevated BG levels, and replied on being asked how he would feel if the values shown were his own data stated, *"S**t, I did s**t. Man you were bad. What have you done?"*

5   Discussion

We have presented findings from a user study that, while limited in its scope, suggests that current generation diabetes diary apps are not adequately meeting user needs for understanding personal data. We argue that this failure is due at least partially to an essential misunderstanding of the smartphone medium, as mobile device users could be expecting low cognitive load [20]. We propose that for diabetes diary apps to successfully integrate into people's lives, these apps should stop trying to convince users to work more, and accept that users want systems that reduce effortful thought about their diabetes management. Perhaps as the IoT infrastructure matures and as apps take advantage of the richer data streams, apps could move away from a basis of retrospection and reflection, and evolve into easy to understand real-time decision support systems, with clearly stated suggestions for actions.

5.1   Limitations and Future Work

As noted earlier, both the recruitment phase and methodology could have introduced bias into some of our findings. In this section we explore some of the limitations of this work as well as areas we have identified for future work.

Limitations: This study used only a limited number of apps. There may exist apps that better support the issues raised. The focus of this study was on logging apps: other paradigms might be beneficial in other ways not directly related to the user understanding personal data - for example encouraging motivation. This study used pre-entered data, whose context was therefore unfamiliar to participants. If participants had been using their own data, it is possible that the memories attached to data entry as well as increased familiarity with the respective apps, would have allowed for improved sensemaking. On the other hand, we argue that the move towards automating data streams could also reduce this familiarity. Lack of previous experience with the apps may have influenced this study, as it is likely that with extended use, participants would become more proficient.

How To Filter Multivariate Data: Health is determined by the interaction of many interrelated factors. Ever-cheaper sensors and connectivity will lead to increasing data streams from many potential sources. However, systems that rely on tables or graph of such data risk overloading the user. UIs could help to meet this challenge by supporting the user in focusing on the most pressing and essential factors, and promoting understanding of the most important correlations between them.

Glanceable Information for Short Interactions: T1D demands frequent attention. Therefore, the user should be able to obtain the desired data or advice as quickly as possible. The UI should decrease the need for attention when the user does not need help. While for many apps the duration of interaction could be a metric for product success, in the case of health systems it might be a sign of failure: evidence of a tendency to disrupt the daily routine.

Immediately Actionable Information, Not Reflection on Data: Many participants indicated desire for health systems that assist with in-the-moment decision-making. It is unclear from our participants to what degree retrospective displaying of data is helpful for immediate decision making. Many users stated they wanted access to information that was relevant to their current situation, not historical events to reflect on. It might be of interest to explore the concealing or even elimination of past data, and emphasize the best course of action for present situations by leveraging advances in data analytics and machine learning. Historic data might be visible on demand, or to illustrate a specific pattern, but otherwise largely hidden by default.

Contextually and Emotionally Sensitive UIs for Everyday Self-Care: As context is important for decision-making in healthcare self-management, systems could integrate location, time, and past patterns and events to get closer to predicting the current needs of the user. Sensitive situations where privacy might be a concern, such as at work, on public transit, or on a date, could affect how users interact with personal data and therefore UI design could dynamically adjust to such situations.

This paper contributes to understanding the strength, weaknesses and challenges of current generation smartphone app UI's designed to support self-management of diabetes. This paper questions whether current paradigms for such apps match the everyday needs of the mobile user. In general, we found that expecting the user to engage in multivariate problem solving through displaying graphs and tables of collected data, was not well suited to the limitations of the smartphone. Mamykina [11] among others, have proposed that PWDs go through cycles of discovery and maintenance: it is not clear that these apps are adequate to support either phase. While much of current literature has focused on building tools to encourage and support the process of reflection and self-knowledge [9–11, 15, 21], it is unclear how much work users are willing to invest in such an approach on a routine basis. The need for understanding context to make sense of data has been previously highlighted [21]. And while this need could be supported by systems that encourage the recording of additional contextual clues, such as photos or tags, this could also increase workload and cognitive overload, creating additional barriers to habitual usage. We theorize that these apps fail to engage users, at least partially, because they fundamentally misunderstand the mobile user's desire to reduce the need for cognitive effort [20, 22]. These diabetes management apps are primarily designed as System 2 systems, requiring careful precise logging and extensive time-consuming reflection, placing these products in direct conflict with the expectations and desires of the mobile user. Reflective, or System 2, thinking is also inherently effortful which when combined with stress provoking diabetes data, could create a major barrier to adoption.

6 Conclusions

We initiated and documented user interaction sessions to study how effectively diabetes logging apps helped participants understand diabetes related personal data. This was achieved by asking them to review diabetes related data, and share their observations and feelings. It appears that these apps would be well served by significant further development. Current diabetes apps offer some real benefits for data review and general overview of glycemic control and some users reported using diabetes diary apps for periodic specific problem solving. In the majority of cases, users were quite comfortable reviewing and engaging with logged data and were aware of its significance in diabetes management. However, participants struggled to find useful correlations in collected data. We speculate that this is partially due to the limited screen dimensions of mobile devices in relation to the complexity of collected data, and that users expect that interaction with a smart phone app will not be cognitively demanding, but rather a smooth and intuitive experience. Health data can have emotional impact. Such potentially negative interactions might be especially challenging in the uncontrolled environment of public use. Automation by way of connected sensors could provide us with the tools to assemble higher quality data, but the gap between data collection and better decision-making is still large. Additionally, as there is reduced data engagement that comes with automation [8], new tools may need to be developed to bolster engagement.

Our interpretation of our participants' responses suggests that rather than tools for interpreting and learning from past events, as the reflection paradigm implies, users want personalized and easy to understand advice for the near term. Such advice should be easily and quickly accessible. The smartphone, due to its screen size and mobile nature, seems ill suited for cognitively demanding analysis. We conclude that the emphasis should be placed on systems that largely remove the demands of reflection, and instead deliver meaningful analysis of collected data with clear suggestions for action.

References

1. AADE guidelines for the practice of diabetes self-management education and training (DSME/T). Diab. Educ. **35**, 85S–107S (2009)
2. Katz, D., Dalton, N., Price, B.: Failing the challenge: diabetes apps & long-term daily adoption. In: International Conference on Advanced Technologies & Treatments for Diabetes ATTD 2015, 18–21 February 2015, Paris (2015)
3. Consolvo, S., McDonald, D.W., Toscos, T., Chen, M.Y., Froehlich, J., Harrison, B., Klasnja, P., LaMarca, A., LeGrand, L., Libby, R., et al.: Activity sensing in the wild: a field trial of ubifit garden. In: Proceedings of the SIGCHI Conference on Human Factors in Computing Systems, pp. 1797–1806. ACM (2008)
4. Lin, J.J., Mamykina, L., Lindtner, S., Delajoux, G., Strub, H.B.: Fish'n'Steps: encouraging physical activity with an interactive computer game. In: Dourish, P., Friday, A. (eds.) UbiComp 2006. LNCS, vol. 4206, pp. 261–278. Springer, Heidelberg (2006). doi:10.1007/11853565_16
5. Intille, S.S.: Ubiquitous computing technology for just-in-time motivation of behavior change. Stud. Health Technol. Inf. **107**, 1434–1437 (2004)
6. King, A.C., Ahn, D.K., Oliveira, B.M., Atienza, A.A., Castro, C.M., Gardner, C.D.: Promoting physical activity through hand-held computer technology. Am. J. Prev. Med. **34**, 138–142 (2008)

7. Ruckenstein, M.: Visualized and interacted life: personal analytics and engagements, with data doubles. Societies **4**, 68–84 (2014)
8. Li, I., Dey, A.K., Forlizzi, J.: Understanding my data, myself: supporting self-reflection with ubicomp technologies. In: Proceedings of the 13th International Conference on Ubiquitous Computing, pp. 405–414. ACM (2011)
9. Mamykina, L., Mynatt, E.D.: Investigating and supporting health management practices of individuals with diabetes. In: Proceedings of the 1st ACM SIGMOBILE International Workshop on Systems and Networking Support for Healthcare and Assisted Living Environments, pp. 49–54. ACM, New York (2007)
10. Mamykina, L., Mynatt, E., Davidson, P., Greenblatt, D.: MAHI: investigation of social scaffolding for reflective thinking in diabetes management. In: Proceedings of the SIGCHI Conference on Human Factors in Computing Systems, pp. 477–486. ACM (2008)
11. Mamykina, L., Smaldone, A.M., Bakken, S.R.: Adopting the sensemaking perspective for chronic disease self-management. J. Biomed. Inf. **56**, 406–417 (2015)
12. Kanstrup, A.M., Bertelsen, P., Glasemann, M., Boye, N.: Design for more: an ambient perspective on diabetes. In: Proceedings of the Tenth Anniversary Conference on Participatory Design 2008, pp. 118–127. Indiana University (2008)
13. Kanstrup, A.M., Glasemann, M., Nielsby, O.: IT-services for everyday life with diabetes: learning design, community design, inclusive design. In: Proceedings of the 8th ACM Conference on Designing Interactive Systems, pp. 404–407. ACM (2010)
14. Cafazzo, J.A., Casselman, M., Hamming, N., Katzman, D.K., Palmert, M.R.: Design of an mHealth app for the self-management of adolescent type 1 diabetes: a pilot study. J. Med. Internet Res. **14**, e70 (2012)
15. Storni, C.: Design challenges for ubiquitous and personal computing in chronic disease care and patient empowerment: a case study rethinking diabetes self-monitoring. Pers. Ubiquit. Comput. **18**, 1277–1290 (2014)
16. Smith, B.K., Frost, J., Albayrak, M., Sudhakar, R.: Integrating glucometers and digital photography as experience capture tools to enhance patient understanding and communication of diabetes self-management practices. Pers. Ubiquit. Comput. **11**, 273–286 (2007)
17. Arsand, E., Frøisland, D.H., Skrøvseth, S.O., Chomutare, T., Tatara, N., Hartvigsen, G., Tufano, J.T.: Mobile health applications to assist patients with diabetes: lessons learned and design implications. J. Diab. Sci. Technol. **6**, 1197–1206 (2012)
18. Choe, E.K., Lee, N.B., Lee, B., Pratt, W., Kientz, J.A.: Understanding quantified-selfers' practices in collecting and exploring personal data (2014)
19. Kahneman, D.: Thinking, Fast and Slow. Macmillan, New York (2011)
20. Barr, N., Pennycook, G., Stolz, J.A., Fugelsang, J.A.: The brain in your pocket: evidence that smartphones are used to supplant thinking. Comput. Hum. Behav. **48**, 473–480 (2015)
21. Owen, T.: Don't let me down: using contextual information to aid diabetics. In: Proceedings of the 13th International Conference on Ubiquitous Computing, pp. 523–526. ACM (2011)
22. Adams, A.T., Costa, J., Jung, M.F., Choudhury, T.: Mindless computing: designing technologies to subtly influence behavior. In: Proceedings of the 2015 ACM International Joint Conference on Pervasive and Ubiquitous Computing, pp. 719–730. ACM (2015)

Questioning Classic Patient Classification Techniques in Gait Rehabilitation: Insights from Wearable Haptic Technology

Theodoros Georgiou[1]([⊠]), Simon Holland[1], Janet van der Linden[1], and Glenis Donaldson[2]

[1] Centre for Research in Computing, The Open University,
Milton Keynes MK7 6AA, UK
Theodoros.Georgiou@open.ac.uk
[2] Faculty of Health, Psychology and Social Care,
Manchester Metropolitan University, Manchester M15 6GX, UK

Abstract. Classifying stroke survivors based on their walking abilities is an important part of the gait rehabilitation process. It can act as powerful indicator of function and prognosis in both the early days after a stroke and long after a survivor receives rehabilitation. This classification often relies solely on walking speed; a quick and easy measure, with only a stopwatch needed. However, walking speed may not be the most accurate way of judging individual's walking ability. Advances in technology mean we are now in a position where ubiquitous and wearable technologies can be used to elicit much richer measures to characterise gait. In this paper we present a case study from one of our studies, where within a homogenous group of stroke survivors (based on walking speed classification) important differences in individual results and the way they responded to rhythmic haptic cueing were identified during the piloting of a novel gait rehabilitation technique.

Keywords: Stroke · Classification · Rhythmic haptic cueing · Haptic Bracelets

1 Introduction

Stroke is a sudden and devastating illness, affecting approximately seventeen million people worldwide each year [1], making it the second single most common cause of death. Four out of five stroke victims survive their stroke [1] but over half stroke survivors are left with a disability, making stroke one of the leading causes of complex adult disabilities [2]. Post-stroke disabilities have a higher impact on an individual than any other chronic disease [2] with more than half of all stroke survivors left dependent on others for everyday activities.

Current research has shown that walking to a rhythm can lead to significant improvements in various aspects of gait for stroke survivors, such as temporal and spatial asymmetries [3–6]. The benefits of walking to a rhythm, as a form of therapy for such conditions, are well established. However, most studies fail to identify individual differences between participants and tend to treat them as a homogenous group.

© ICST Institute for Computer Sciences, Social Informatics and Telecommunications Engineering 2017
K. Giokas et al. (Eds.): eHealth 2016, LNICST 181, pp. 327–339, 2017.
DOI: 10.1007/978-3-319-49655-9_40

The primary aim of our study was to explore the concept of rhythmic haptic (touch based) cueing as an alternative to the more established audio rhythm used for gait rehabilitation. This study enabled us to gather the views of stroke survivors and health professionals through hands-on involvement with a new technology. In particular, we were exploring the possibility of using a small wearable prototype device we designed, called *The Haptic Bracelets*, to deliver haptic cueing in an appropriate rhythm for walking. The Haptic Bracelets are lightweight devices wearable on both limbs at ankle level, that are capable of monitoring and analysing gait and delivering rhythmic haptic cueing via low latency vibrators on alternating legs [7].

During our study, motion capture data was collected and analysed to help identify design questions, characterise issues relevant to the future design and operation of the technology and to refine our understanding of the context of use and the theoretical background. A previous paper [8] considered data from questionnaires, interviews, and from dialogues between stroke survivors, health professionals and interaction designers that were carried out during sessions. In this paper we consider the issues and questions raised in the context of the analysis of the motion capture data.

Using traditional grouping measurements, based on gait velocity measured with a stopwatch, all our participants were classified as having the same ambulatory capability. However, the kinematic data we collected showed some major individual differences and we argue that such differences can play an important role during rhythm based gait rehabilitation interventions.

New technologies like the Haptic Bracelets can help establish other measures that might play a useful role in physiotherapy practice. Amongst other applications for diagnosis, monitoring and therapy, the Haptic Bracelets can provide richer data for a more accurate classification of stroke survivors based on their walking capabilities. It is this particular application that we explore in this paper.

2 Background

2.1 Post Stroke Gait Impairments

Gait coordination is often compromised after stroke with survivors experiencing what is known as "hemiparetic gait"; a condition commonly characterised by reduced walking speed [9], stride time variability [10], increased step length variability [10], and temporal and spatial gait asymmetry [11].

Many health problems are associated with this condition. The non-paretic (stronger) limb may be exposed to higher vertical forces [12] which can in turn lead to joint pains due to increased repetitive loading [13], bone degeneration [14], and increased risk of fractures. Hemiparetic gait is also directly linked to an increased risk of falling observed after stroke, doubling the risk of hip fracture [15]. Besides physical health issues, gait rehabilitation is also of paramount importance for the restoration of independence and thus an overall better quality of life [16].

Chronic stroke survivors (6+ months after their stroke incident) generally exhibit hemiparetic gait, which limits function and can restrict participation in society. However, due to neuroplasticity, even at this later stage motor relearning is still a possibility [17].

Gait recovery is one of the major goals in post-stroke rehabilitation [18]. Therefore, for many decades, hemiparetic gait has been the object of study for the development of methods for gait analysis and rehabilitation [19].

2.2   Rhythmic Cueing for Gait Rehabilitation

Use of an auditory rhythm provided by a metronome has been investigated and successfully demonstrated as a means of improving hemiparetic gait with immediate, though not necessarily lasting, effects [3] – although studies for other neurological conditions that affect gait suggest that with extended training, effects can last for weeks [20].

Studies where participants were asked to walk on a treadmill showed that they could synchronise their steps to a rhythmic audio metronome [21]. Audio cues also helped participants with post-stroke gait impairments to show improvements in spatial [22] and temporal symmetry [21]. The step time asymmetry and the paretic (affected leg) step time variability of participants also improved significantly [23], as did the ability to make gait adjustments in response to changes in the cue [24]. Rhythmic cueing is therefore a promising approach, but the use of audio may not be the best medium for in-home or out-and-about scenarios for rehabilitation, where it is important to keep the audio channel clear for reasons of safety, sociability, and to remain aware of the environment. With audio cues alone it is difficult to differentiate which cue is for which leg [23], thus missing out on some potentially beneficial aspects of attention and proprioception in gait rehabilitation.

2.3   The Role of Entrainment

Rhythmic cueing is based on entrainment models. In physics, entrainment is a natural phenomenon where two or more periodic processes interact with each other to adjust to a common or related period. However, it was only recently (early 1990s) that the human capacity for biological entrainment became better understood and applications for movement rehabilitation of neurological conditions were studied. As discussed above, applications included the use of auditory cues to synchronise human motor responses into stable time relationships. In such cases, biological entrainment mechanisms act between the external rhythm and the motor response to stabilise and regulate gait patterns [3].

When considering cues for movement, it is important to distinguish between stimulus response models and the biological entrainment model. With the stimulus-response model, as the name suggests, the user responds directly to each stimulus. By contrast, after hearing a few initial beats, most people can generally tap along to a regular pulse in more or less exact synchronisation. Consequently, entrainment is the common foundation for the various applications of metronomic rhythmic sensory stimulation in any modality.

2.4   Patient/Participant Ambulatory Classification

Classifying stroke survivors based on 'ambulation capability' is an important aspect of rehabilitation treatment. Historically, gait velocity is shown to have predictive validity for rehabilitative outcome. After reviewing gait related classification techniques, ranging from stroke survivors' self-assessment questionnaires to motor control tests performed by health professionals, Perry et al. [25] concluded that when treated as an independent measure, gait velocity has strong potential for classifying people based on what is referred to as their 'community walking status'. Less than 0.4 m/s predicts household walking; 0.4 to 0.8 m/s predicts limited community walking; and more than 0.8 m/s predicts unlimited community walking [25].

However, there is also an argument *against* the use of gait velocity as the sole metric for classification of people suffering from gait related impairments. Olney et al. [26], for example, argue that using gait velocity figures alone can neither assist in understanding the nature of gait deficits nor support direct treatment. They suggest that while gait velocity is reflective of gait performance it does not have "explicative capacity", and is often insufficient in discriminating among post-stroke ambulators. Taylor et al. [27] noted that gait velocity as measured in the clinic can predict the walking speed of a person in the community only if it is greater than 0.8 m/s. Considering that stroke survivors tend to walk more slowly than 0.8 m/s, and the classification starts with 0.4 m/s for "household capability", followed by 0.4 to 0.8 m/s for limited community capability, and more than 0.8 m/s for full community capability [25], velocity based classification systems are of limited scope.

Temporal symmetry, on the other hand, may be an additional and valuable measure that can be used when trying to classify stroke survivors into ambulation groups. Temporal symmetry is defined as the ratio of time between each leg swing and stance time of the gait cycle (see the Results section and Fig. 1.). Patterson et al. [28] suggest that temporal symmetry may assist in further discrimination of post-stroke ambulators; more specifically those with gait speeds less than 0.6 m/s.

The main reason for widespread use of velocity data alone for patient classification is not so much its accuracy of gait capability prediction, but the ease by which it can be recorded and applied in the clinical setting. After all, all a clinician needs to record and calculate someone's gait velocity is a stopwatch. However, small affordable technologies are increasingly available that open up the possibility of other measures that might begin to play a role in physiotherapy practice.

3   Aim of the Study

As outlined above, stroke survivors are often classified in different categories based on their walking speeds. These categories are then for some purposes treated as homogenous groups. Even though this classification system has some uses within the clinic, and helps clinicians and health professionals establish a benchmark for quantifying and comparing the progress of individuals during gait rehabilitation and physiotherapy sessions, it has limited diagnostic and predictive value.

The aim of this paper is to highlight individual differences found in participants of gait related studies within otherwise homogenous groups and investigate the potential of lightweight wearable devices for exploring such differences.

4 Research Approach and Technology Used

The present preliminary study is part of wider exploratory programme to explore the potential of new technologies, the kinds of data that they offer and their analytic use. The study involved a repeated measure design, with stroke survivors walking both with and without haptic cues. During the course of the study we talked in depth with participating stroke survivors and the physiotherapist who was directing sessions. This gave us rich qualitative data to help better understand the needs of stroke survivors and health professionals, and to help improve future design prototypes.

We also collected quantitative data from a state of the art motion capturing system. These quantitative data, the way they are analysed and the questions they raise are discussed in the sections below.

4.1 Data Gathering – Technologies

Data were recorded using a Qualisys Motion Capturing System, whose high spatial and temporal resolution allowed for precise motion of leg and hipbone joints to be captured. The system consists of eight optoelectronic cameras, with a sampling frequency of 100 Hz. The trajectories of 20 markers placed on anatomical lower limb landmarks, and 4 additional tracking clusters placed on the right and left shank and thigh, were collected and filtered using a fourth–order zero lag Butterworth low-pass filters, with a 6 Hz cut off frequency.

The rhythmic haptic cue was controlled using a pair of Haptic Bracelets. The Haptic Bracelets are a lightweight, wearable wireless technology developed at the Open University, able to collect motion data and provide precise haptic cueing via vibro-tactiles. Generally, one bracelet is worn on each leg near the ankle. Haptic cues are delivered via high precision low-latency vibrotactiles with wide dynamic range. The metronomic delivery of cues to alternate legs is co-ordinated via a laptop, but this is being ported to smartphone for applications outside the lab.

A methodology of repeated measures ensured that participants acted as their own controls, so that any variability in the two conditions could be attributed solely to the device and the rhythmic haptic cueing, rather than to errors induced by the re-attachment of markers or to day-to-day gait variability.

4.2 Participants

Participants were included in the study if they had sustained a unilateral stroke (haemorrhagic or ischemic) more than 6 months ago; if they could walk independently for 5 min; and were able to walk for a minimum of 20 m without the use of a walking aid.

Four adults were recruited (see Table 1). Three were males and one female, and all of the participants had a right hemiparesis. Three participants exhibited aphasia but all had recovered the ability to speak and express themselves in a coherent manner. The mean age was 58.5 ($\pm$9.47) years. The relatively wide age range does not play a significant role in gait symmetry ratios [29]. The time since the onset of stroke varied from 6–43 years. All four subjects completed a minimum of five gait trials whilst wearing normal-wear footwear. None of the participant wore splints.

Exclusion criteria included: neurological, orthopaedic, respiratory, cardiovascular or musculoskeletal problems that would prevent safe participation in testing, and any skin conditions that might be aggravated by wearing the haptic bracelet or movement analysis markers. Ethical approval for the study was gained from the Open University and the Manchester Metropolitan University ethics committee.

Table 1. Participants' demographics

	Age	Gender	Side of stroke	Year of stroke
P1	46	Female	Right	2001
P2	57	Male	Right	2004
P3	68	Male	Right	1972
P4	63	Male	Right	2009

5 Procedure

The sessions took part over three days. The first day included a familiarisation session, where participants visited the gait laboratory and were tested using the inclusion criteria by a team of expert physiotherapists. We also introduced participants to the Haptic Bracelets.

Each participant then completed a minimum of five walks on a ten-metre walkway at their natural walking pace, without haptic cueing. This allowed them to familiarise themselves with the procedure and the environment, and allowed for recording of base-line kinematic and kinetic data. Participants' preferred own pace was used for metronomic cueing, as this is considered to be the most beneficial cueing rate when used within the context of gait rehabilitation to improve symmetry [5].

On the second day, the first two participants took part in hands-on sessions in which kinematic and kinetic data was recorded without, and then with haptic cueing. On day three, this was repeated with the remaining two participants.

In general, the device was fitted to both lower limbs with the vibrotactiles fitted over the medial border of the tibia where the haptic pulse could be felt (one exception to this is noted later in the paper). The tempo of the haptic cue was calculated individually from each participant's step cycle/cadence (mean time taken from heel strike to heel strike of the same leg) during the baseline measurements on day one.

The intensity of the haptic cue was then adjusted to a comfortable level. The participants had approximately ten minutes for familiarisation with the device (either walking on the spot or sitting and marking time to the beat). Once ready, the participants were asked to 'follow the rhythm' as they performed a minimum of five walks.

All four participants were classified as community ambulators in the higher level of the classification scale (gait velocity > 0.8 m/s). Being community ambulators means they are *"capable of independent mobility outside the home, including the ability to confidently negotiate uneven terrain, private venues, shopping centres and other public venues"* [30]. This relatively high walking speed put all participants in the same upper level of community ambulators. However, aspects of P2's condition merit particular consideration as follows.

P2 had symptoms of aphasia that were found to hinder him in switching attention from one leg to the other fast enough to follow the rhythmic haptic cue delivered on alternating legs. Also, his stroke incident left him with severe loss of sensitivity on his left leg. The aphasia and sensitivity loss led P2 to prefer the use of a single Haptic Bracelet strapped on his left (paretic) leg, with its vibration intensity set to the maximum. All of the other participants could readily switch attention between their limbs and their perceptual sensitivity levels were higher. These participants preferred the vibration intensity to be set at 40%.

6 Measures of Gait Asymmetry

For clarity in interpreting the results, it may help to briefly review key measures of gait, in particular swing and stance times, and how these are used to characterise various kinds of gait asymmetry. When walking from a standing start, one starts by swinging one leg while the other supports the weight of the body. Figure 1 shows the stages a leg passes through during a single step. The toes of one leg are lifted up (at the point labelled TO in Fig. 1 below), initialising the swing time of that leg. The leg then moves forward and the heel strikes the ground (labelled HS in Fig. 1). At this point the swing time ends and the stance time begins. Stance time ends when the toes of that foot lift off from the ground again. These stages define the swing and stance time of each leg individually.

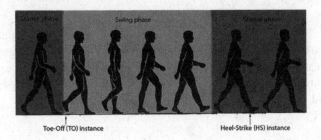

Fig. 1. The gait cycle from toe off to heel strike of one leg.

In the case of stroke survivors suffering from hemiparesis, one leg is affected more than the other. This affected leg is known as the "paretic" leg. The research literature cites several methods of calculating gait symmetry, but the ratio measure (Eq. (1)) is relatively simple and easy and easy to interpret [31].

$$ratio = V_{Paretic\ limb}/V_{non-Paretic\ limb}. \tag{1}$$

Using this formula, we can calculate the *stance time ratio*, the *swing time ratio*, the *swing-stance time ratio* and the *overall temporal symmetry ratio*.

The *stance time ratio*, as the name suggests, is the ratio of time spent during the stance phase between both limbs. If, for example, a person spent on average 0.5 a second on the paretic limb and 0.8 s on the non-paretic limb, the stance time ratio would be $0.5/0.8 = 0.625$. The *swing time ratio* is calculated in the same way, but using the swing time instead. The *swing-stance time ratio*, again, as the name suggests, can be calculated by dividing the swing time by the stance time of each limb. This gives a swing-stance time ratio value *for each* leg. The *overall temporal symmetry* can then be calculated by dividing the paretic swing-stance ratio by the non-paretic swing-stance ratio value. A summary of how these terms are defined is provided in Table 2.

Table 2. Summary on how swing time ratio, stance time ratio, swing-stance time ratio and temporal asymmetry ratio are calculated.

	Right Leg (R)	Left Leg (L)
Example patient	Paretic	Non-Paretic
Swing time	R_{swing_time}	L_{swing_time}
Swing time ratio	$R_{swing\_time}/L_{swing\_time}$	
Stance time	R_{stance_time}	L_{stance_time}
Stance time ratio	$R_{stance\_time}/L_{stance\_time}$	
Swing /stance time ratio	$R_{ss\_ratio} = R_{swing\_time}/R_{stance\_time}$	$L_{ss\_ratio} = L_{swing\_time}/L_{stance\_time}$
Temporal asymmetry ratio	$R_{ss\_ratio}/L_{ss\_ratio}$	

As previously noted, overuse of the non-paretic leg (i.e. temporal gait symmetry ratio value greater than one) exposes it to higher vertical forces, leading to joint pains, bone degeneration, and increased risk of fractures – thus gait asymmetry is something to identify and try to reduce.

7   Results

Using the measures of gait asymmetry characterised above, let us now consider the results.

Table 3. Individual Stance and Swing time ratios, with and without cueing. Stance time ratio with value less than 1.0 means that more time is spent on the non-paretic leg [28]. Swing time ratio with value greater than 1.0 means that the paretic leg takes longer to swing (leaving the body supported on only the non-paretic leg for longer).

	Stance time ratio		Swing time ratio	
	Haptic cue off	Haptic cue on	Haptic cue off	Haptic cue on
P1	0.76	0.74	1.58	1.64
P2	0.88	0.87	1.30	1.20
P3	0.90	0.90	1.20	1.20
P4	0.95	0.95	1.10	1.10

Table 4. Individual swing/stance time ratios and temporal asymmetry ratios, with and without cueing. The temporal asymmetry ratio was calculated by dividing the paretic by the non-paretic value for each of the two conditions. For example, for P1's Haptic off condition: $0.85/0.44 = 1.93$.

		Haptic cue off		Haptic cue on	
	Leg	Swing - stance ratio	Temporal asymmetry ratio	Swing - stance ratio	Temporal asymmetry ratio
P1	Paretic	0.85	1.93	0.90	2.20
	Non-paretic	0.44		0.41	
P2	Paretic	0.66	1.53	0.60	1.20
	Non-paretic	0.43		0.50	
P3	Paretic	0.62	·1.27	0.62	1.38
	Non-paretic	0.49		0.45	
P4	Paretic	0.60	1.20	0.60	1.05
	Non-paretic	0.50		0.57	

Comparing the results in Table 3, we can see that in the context of the study, the cueing appeared to improve swing time ratio for P2, but to make worse the swing time ratio for P1. No change was observed in either the stance or the swing time ratio for P3 and P4. Similarly, in Table 4, cueing appeared to improve the temporal asymmetry ratio for P2 and P4, but to make it worse for P1 and P3.

Thus, both swing time ratio (Table 3) and temporal asymmetry ratio (Table 4) measurements suggest that P2 and P4's symmetry was improved (from 1.53 to 1.20 and 1.20 to 1.05 respectively) while P1 and P3's symmetry got worse (from 1.93 to 2.20 and 1.27 to 1.38).

8 Discussion

Clearly the results raise many questions about how wearable haptics should be best used for Rhythmic Sensory Stimulation (RSS). As discussed in Sect. 2.2, RSS is known in general to be a successful approach to gait rehabilitation. However, the above results (and the discussion below) demonstrate that individual differences in stroke survivors need to be better understood to help determine appropriate therapy in individual cases. In this paper, we leave this wider issue for further research: for now we focus on the more restricted point that despite conventional classification methods treating our participants as broadly homogeneous, the results clearly demonstrate major individual differences. Thus, these results have implications for reconsidering classification methods. More specifically, all participants in this study were classified as community ambulators based on their baseline walking velocity (>0.8 m/s). When hypothetically considering averaged kinematic data for all participants, changes for the better and worse balance out. However, looking at individual participants, the approach worked well for two participants, but not for the two others.

Interesting detail emerges when we look at the individual data of each participant. By looking at the data in Table 3, it is clear that some participants were more symmetric than others at the start of the study (as shown by uncued baselines with ratios closer to 1.0). This is even clearer from Table 4, where temporal symmetries are calculated using measurements from *both* legs. Here, the walking symmetries between participants have a wide margin of variation; varying from 1.93 to 1.20. According to these data, P1 spent almost twice the time on her affected leg, while P4 spent almost equal amount of time on both legs.

The results demonstrate that the homogeneity of the participant group as judged by conventional measures is misleading: they draw detailed attention to limitations in the use of velocity as a measure of gait performance. Such an overall conclusion is not new, but the results add considerable detail in characterising the nature and extent of the problem [13, 28].

More generally, the results were interesting and unexpected. In this small case study, Rhythmic Haptic Cueing (RHC) had little or no effect on either the stance or swing time ratio (Table 3) for participants whose ratio was good to start with (P3 and P4). However, for those who were more asymmetric without the cue (P1 and P2), the RHC did have an effect; with one getting worse, and the other improving. As regards the temporal asymmetry ratio (Table 4), the most asymmetric participant appeared to become less symmetric and the most symmetric participant appeared to approach perfect symmetry.

9   Conclusion

This study introduced rhythmic haptic cueing to a small group of stroke survivors and health professionals. The rhythmic haptic cueing was delivered through our prototype wearable device, the Haptic Bracelets, which acted as a technology probe [32]; where a new technology is placed and used in the environment it was designed for and observing how users interact with it. As part of this technology probe approach, complete motion capture data was collected and analysed, not to test any particular hypothesis, but for observing the participant's reaction to the rhythmic haptic cueing and its effect on their gait, and to help frame future research questions.

After analysing the kinematic data collected by a Qualisys Motion Capture System, we saw that for two participants (P2 and P4), rhythmic cueing had a potential benefit with their gait becoming more symmetric, whereas P1's data indicated tendencies of destabilisation (becoming more asymmetric). This raises many questions, but as a minimum brings into question the way patients are classified on their ambulation capability. In this study, within an otherwise homogenous group (based on the gait velocity test), motion capture results suggest widely different reactions to rhythm-based intervention on gait rehabilitation.

This demonstrates that group homogeneity cannot be assumed based solely on velocity. Our findings give detailed confirmation to the criticism of velocity alone as a classification metric [13, 28]. As a result of the varying responses to rhythmic cueing revealed in this study, we propose in future work to study individual differences in sensory, motor, attention, and rhythm perception capabilities (for example, probing the ability to tap along with steady beats) so as to correlate these with varying changes in gait symmetry elicited by rhythmic cueing.

References

1. Stroke Association. https://www.stroke.org.uk/sites/default/files/stroke_statistics_2015.pdf
2. Adamson, J., Beswick, A., Ebrahim, S.: Is stroke the most common cause of disability? J. Stroke Cerebrovasc. Dis. 13(4), 171–177 (2004)
3. Thaut, M.H., Leins, A.K., Rice, R.R., Argstatter, H., Kenyon, G.P., McIntosh, G.C., et al.: Rhythmic auditory stimulation improves gait more than NDT/Bobath training in near-ambulatory patients early poststroke: a single-blind, randomized trial. Neurorehabil. Neural Repair 21(5), 455–459 (2007)
4. Thaut, M.H., Kenyon, G.P., Schauer, M.L., McIntosh, G.C.: The connection between rhythmicity and brain function - Implications for therapy of movement disorders. IEEE Eng. Med. Biol. 18(2), 101–108 (1999)
5. Roerdink, M., Bank, P.J., Peper, C., Beek, P.J.: Walking to the beat of different drums: practical implications for the use of acoustic rhythms in gait rehabilitation. Gait Posture 33(4), 690–694 (2011)
6. Holland, S., Wright, R.L., Wing, A., Crevoisier, T., Hödl, O., Canelli, M.: A pilot study using tactile cueing for gait rehabilitation following stroke. In: Fardoun, H.M., Penichet, V. M.R., Alghazzawi, D.M. (eds.) REHAB 2014. CCIS, vol. 515, pp. 222–233. Springer, Heidelberg (2015). doi:10.1007/978-3-662-48645-0_19
7. Georgiou, T., Holland, S., van der Linden, J.: Rhythmic haptic cueing for entrainment: assisting post-stroke gait rehabilitation. In: 8th Cambridge workshop on Universal Access and Assistive Technology, Cambridge (2016)
8. Georgiou, T., Holland, S., van der Linden, J., Tetley, J., Stockley, R.C., Donaldson, G., et al.: A blended user centred design study for wearable haptic gait rehabilitation following hemiparetic stroke. In: Proceedings of the 9th International Conference on Pervasive Computing Technologies for Healthcare, Istanbul (2015)
9. Olney, S.J.: Hemiparetic gait following stroke. Part I: characteristics. Gait Posture 4(2), 136–148 (1996)
10. Balasubramanian, C.K., Neptune, R.R., Kautz, S.A.: Variability in spatiotemporal step characteristics and its relationship to walking performance post-stroke. Gait Posture 29(3), 408–414 (2009)

11. Chen, G., Patten, C., Kothari, D.H., Zajac, F.E.: Gait differences between individuals with post-stroke hemiparesis and non-disabled controls at matched speeds. Gait Posture **22**(1), 51–56 (2005)

12. Kim, C.M., Eng, J.J.: The relationship of lower-extremity muscle torque to locomotor performance in people with stroke. Phys. Ther. **83**(1), 49–57 (2003)

13. Norvell, D.C., Czerniecki, J.M., Reiber, G.E., Maynard, C., Pecoraro, J.A., Weiss, N.S.: The prevalence of knee pain and symptomatic knee osteoarthritis among veteran traumatic amputees and nonamputees. Archiv. Phys. Med. Rehabil. **86**(3), 487–493 (2005)

14. Nolan, L., Wit, A., Dudziñski, K., Lees, A., Lake, M., Wychowañski, M.: Adjustments in gait symmetry with walking speed in trans-femoral and trans-tibial amputees. Gait Posture **17**(2), 142–151 (2003)

15. Pouwels, S., Lalmohamed, A., Souverein, P., Cooper, C., Veldt, B., Leufkens, H., et al.: Use of proton pump inhibitors and risk of hip/femur fracture: population-based case-control study. Osteoporos. Int. **22**(3), 903–910 (2011)

16. Richards, C.L., Malouin, F., Wood-Dauphinee, S., Williams, J.I., Bouchard, J.P., Brunet, D.: Task-specific physical therapy for optimization of gait recovery in acute stroke patients. Archiv. Phys. Med. Rehabil. **74**(6), 612–620 (1993)

17. Alexander, L.D., Black, S.E., Patterson, K.K., Gao, F., Danells, C.J., McIlroy, W.E.: Association between gait asymmetry and brain lesion location in stroke patients. Stroke **40**, 537–544 (2009)

18. Lindquist, A.R., Prado, C.L., Barros, R.M., Mattioli, R., da Costa, P.H., Salvini, T.F.: Gait training combining partial body-weight support, a treadmill, and functional electrical stimulation: effects on poststroke gait. Phys. Ther. **87**(9), 1144–1155 (2007)

19. Olney, S.J., Richards, C.: Hemiparetic gait following stroke. Part I: characteristics. Gait Posture **4**(2), 136–148 (1996)

20. Benoit, C.E., Dalla, B.S., Farrugia, N., Obrig, H., Mainka, S., Kotz, S.A.: Musically cued gait-training improves both perceptual and motor timing in Parkinson's disease. Front. Hum. Neurosci. **8**, 494 (2014)

21. Roerdink, M., Lamoth, C.J., Kwakkel, G., Wieringen, P.C., Beek, P.J.: Gait coordination after stroke: benefits of acoustically paced treadmill walking. Phys. Ther. **87**(8), 1009–1022 (2007)

22. Prassas, S., Thaut, M., McIntosh, G., Rice, R.: Effect of auditory rhythmic cueing on gait kinematic parameters of stroke patients. Gait Posture **6**(3), 218–223 (1997)

23. Wright, R.L., Masood, A., MacCormac, E.S., Pratt, D., Sackley, C., Wing, A.: Metronome-cued stepping in place after hemiparetic stroke: comparison of a one - and two-tone beat. ISRN Rehabil. (2013)

24. Pelton, T.A., Johannsen, L., Chen, H.Y., Wing, A.M.: Hemiparetic stepping to the beat: asymmetric response to metronome phase shift during treadmill gait. Neurorehabil. Neural Repair **24**(5), 428–434 (2010)

25. Perry, J., Garrett, M., Gronley, J.K., Mulroy, S.J.: Classification of walking handicap in the stroke population. Stroke **26**(6), 982–989 (1995)

26. Olney, S.J., Griffin, M.P., McBride, I.D.: Temporal, kinematic, and kinetic variables related to gait speed in subjects with hemiplegia: a regression approach. Phys. Ther. **74**(9), 872–885 (1994)

27. Taylor, D., Stretton, C.M., Mudge, S., Garrett, N.: Does clinic-measured gait speed differ from gait speed measured in the community in people with stroke? Clinic. Rehabil. **20**(5), 438–444 (2006)

28. Patterson, K.K., Parafianowicz, I., Danells, C.J., Closson, V., Verrier, M.C., Staines, W.R., et al.: Gait asymmetry in community-ambulating stroke survivors. Archiv. Phys. Med. Rehabil. **89**(2), 304–310 (2008)

29. Patterson, K.K., Nadkarni, N.K., Black, S.E., McIlroy, W.E.: Temporal gait symmetry and velocity differ in their relationship to age. Gait Posture **35**(4), 590–594 (2012)
30. Lord, S.E., Rochester, L.: Measurement of community ambulation after stroke. Stroke **36**, 1457–1461 (2005)
31. Patterson, K.K., Gage, W.H., Brooks, D., Black, S.E., McIlroy, W.E.: Evaluation of gait symmetry after stroke: a comparison of current methods and recommendations for standardization. Gait Posture **31**(2), 241–246 (2010)
32. Hutchinson, H., Mackay, W., Westerlund, B., Bederson, B.B., Druin, A., Plaisant, C., et al.: Technology probes: inspiring design for and with families. In: Proceedings of the SIGCHI Conference on Human Factors in Computing Systems, New York, pp. 17–24 (2003)

Stress Detection Using Smart Phone Data

Panagiotis Kostopoulos$^{(\boxtimes)}$, Athanasios I. Kyritsis,
Michel Deriaz, and Dimitri Konstantas

Information Science Institute, GSEM/CUI,
University of Geneva, Geneva, Switzerland
{panagiotis.kostopoulos,athanasios.kyritsis,michel.deriaz,
dimitri.konstantas}@unige.ch

Abstract. In today's society, working environments are becoming more stressful. The problem of occupational stress is generally recognized as one of the major factors leading to a wide spectrum of health problems. However work should, ideally, be a source of health, pride and happiness, in the sense of enhancing motivation and strengthening personal development. In this work, we present StayActive, a system which aims to detect stress and burn-out risks by analyzing the behaviour of the users via their smartphone. The main purpose of StayActive is the use of the mobile sensor technology for detecting stress. Then a mobile service can recommend and present various relaxation activities "just in time" in order to allow users to carry out and solve everyday tasks and problems at work. In particular, we collect data from people's daily phone usage gathering information about the sleeping pattern, the social interaction and the physical activity of the user. We assign a weight factor to each of these three dimensions of wellbeing according to the user's personal perception and build a stress detection system. We evaluate our system in a real world environment with young adults and people working in the transportation company of Geneva. This paper highlights the architecture and model of this innovative stress detection system. The main innovation of this work is addressed in the fact that the way the stress level is computed is as less invasive as possible for the users.

Keywords: Stress detection · Smartphone · Sleeping pattern · Social interaction · Physical activity

1 Introduction

Stress is a mental condition that everybody experiences in his life, sometimes even daily. Today stress is omnipresent as never before and it is one of the major problems in modern society. Stress symptoms may be affecting people's health, even though they might not realize it. People may think illness is to blame for

This work was co-funded by the State Secretariat for Education, Research and Innovation of the Swiss federal government and the European Union, in the frame of the EU AAL project StayActive (aal-2013-6-126).

© ICST Institute for Computer Sciences, Social Informatics and Telecommunications Engineering 2017
K. Giokas et al. (Eds.): eHealth 2016, LNICST 181, pp. 340–351, 2017.
DOI: 10.1007/978-3-319-49655-9_41

that nagging headache, their frequent insomnia or their decreased productivity at work. But stress may actually be the culprit. Due to all these negative effects, it can be assumed that early assessment of stress condition, and early suggestions on how to reduce it, may reduce its overall impact and lead to improved health state of individuals. Stress detection technology could help people better understand and relieve stress by increasing their awareness of heightened levels of stress that would otherwise go undetected [1]. Detecting stress in natural environments is beneficial to avoid developing burn-out situations and illnesses.

The most common method to quantify stress is to simply ask people about their mood using questionnaires. There are standard methods for doing so like the Perceived Stress Scale questionnaire (PSS) [2]. Questions in the PSS assess to what degree a subject feels stressed in a given situation.

Nowadays wearable devices such as mobile phones and wearable sensors are ubiquitous in our lives. Several researchers have tried to understand personality from mobile phone usage [1,10]. Our stress detection system aims to use technology to recognize stress levels using data from the devices that users always carry and wear.

Sleeping patterns, social life and physical activity are connected with the presence of stress in people's lives [3]. We take into account these three dimensions for building our stress detection system. The motivation for creating a solution based only on the daily phone usage of people is based on the idea to be as less invasive as possible for the end-user.

The rest of this paper is organized as follows. In Sect. 2, our designed stress detection system is described in detail. Experimental results using real data are reported and discussed in Sect. 3. Future work to be done on StayActive is presented in Sect. 4. Finally, a brief conclusion is drawn in Sect. 5.

2   System Design

The StayActive system [15] provides an Android application running on a smartphone. We have chosen the Android based solution because it is an open source framework designed for mobile devices. The Android Software Development Kit (SDK) provides the Application Programming Interface (API) libraries and developer tools necessary to build, test and debug applications for Android. We implemented the prototype in Java using the Android SDK API 23. The idea of the full StayActive system is the following. There is a combination of a mathematical model and a Machine Learning (ML) approach which work independently in order to compute the stress level of the users. The mathematical model is running on the phone of the user being a light application with minimized battery consumption. The reason is that we want to make the users able to use the application for the biggest possible amount of time without needing to recharge their phone. This application will be synchronized with the ML approach running on the server of the StayActive system. The results of the two individual models will be combined and give a final stress level to the users. In this paper the mathematical approach running on the phone is explained in detail and the ML approach and the integration procedure is introduced.

2.1 System Overview

In this study we aim to find physiological or behavioral markers for stress. Although there are still several open questions regarding the links between the behaviour of a person and their stress level, in StayActive we take a pragmatic approach and build an initial stress detection system which can be extended and refined. The general architecture of our stress detection system is given in Fig. 1.

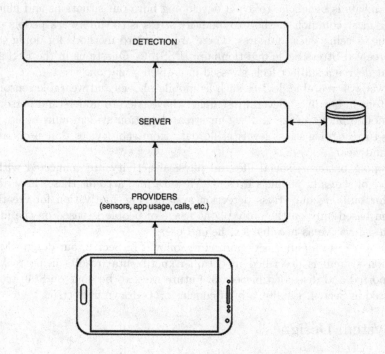

Fig. 1. StayActive system architecture overview.

Providers. The first layer is the one that collects and provides the data to upper layers. The provider module contains all the implemented data providers, which are responsible for collecting a specific type of data from the device. They are free to implement the data monitoring behaviour as they wish. The currently implemented providers collect the following type of data: type of physical activity, calls and SMS, ambient light and temperature, location, battery level, screen on/off intervals, Wi-Fi, step counter, number of screen touches and finally type of applications launched. We give some examples of the results of these providers in Figs. 2, 3, 4 and 5.

Server. The server module is responsible for receiving data from the mobile devices and storing it in a database. We aggregate all the data and we process

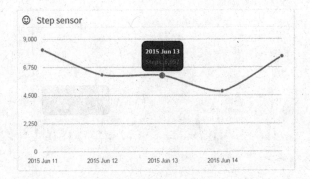

Fig. 2. Visualization of data from the step counter provider.

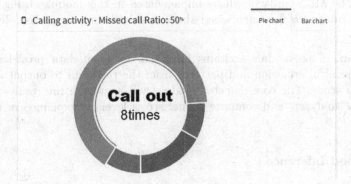

Fig. 3. Visualization of data from the call provider.

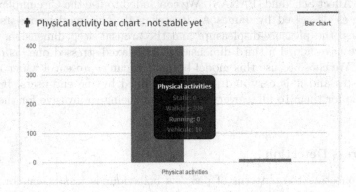

Fig. 4. Visualization of data from the physical activity provider.

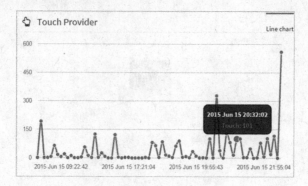

Fig. 5. Visualization of data from the screen touch provider.

it in order to extract a relaxation score for each user as explained in the next section. The ML approach will be implemented in this module, using features produced from providers mentioned above, and will compute a stress level.

Detection. This module contains analyzers for each data provider, which extract useful information and patterns from the raw data to output a partial relaxation score. The core detector module will aggregate the results of these individual analyzers and compute a final stress level, as explained in the next section.

2.2   Mood Inference

Aside from gathering as many data as possible from the smartphone, the system will prompt the user to fill in a questionnaire with his subjective self-perception of his mood. First we researched several validated models that psychologists have proposed to measure and describe affect and emotion, including the Positive and Negative Affect Schedule (PANAS). We concluded to use the Circumplex Model of Affect as described by James A. Russell [14]. This model consists of two dimensions: the pleasure-displeasure and the arousal-sleep dimension. On top of this we have added a third dimension, the relaxed-stressed one, as depicted in Fig. 6. We chose to use this model because it can represent a wider range of mood states and it is easy and quick to be filled by the end-users. It will be acceptable for them to fill it every day without being so invasive for their daily life.

2.3   Stress Detection

Simply collecting the patterns of people's behaviour is insufficient for helping them improve their personal wellbeing. It is important to use different dimensions of people's wellbeing and compute their stress level. That way, we will be able to help them by giving advice for reducing their stress level and therefore improving

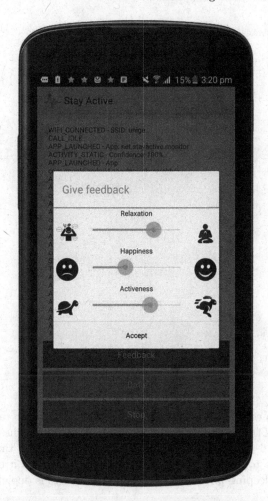

Fig. 6. User interface for the mood inference.

their quality of life. Our stress detection module takes into account three main dimensions of wellbeing: the sleeping pattern of the users, their social interaction and their physical activity.

Sleeping Pattern. There is a large body of research work which analyzes the link between sleep hygiene and the mood of people [11, 12]. People usually exchange sleep for additional working hours as a coping mechanism for busy lifestyles. In our stress detection module we take into account the user's duration of sleep. We set the number of normal sleeping hours at 8 and penalize insufficient sleep and oversleeping. We set the lower threshold of normal sleeping hours at 7 and the upper threshold at 9 h according to [4]. For any extra missing or more hours of sleep we penalize the behaviour of the user with a weight factor per

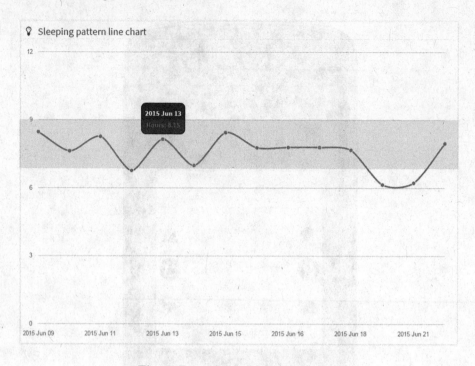

Fig. 7. Example of a sleeping pattern.

hour. In order to compute the sleeping pattern of the user we take into account the interaction of the user with his phone, by monitoring touches on the device's screen. Between 6 p.m. and 10 a.m. we compute the biggest time interval that the user did not touch his screen and we infer the duration of his sleep. An example of the sleeping pattern of a user for some days is depicted in Fig. 7.

Social Interaction. The daily social interaction of people has a serious impact on many dimensions of wellbeing [12]. People who maintain dense social connections are more likely to have resilient mental health. They tend to be able to cope with stress and often are better able to manage chronic illness.

On the other hand regarding communication, researchers are hypothesizing that perhaps people become so used to and even dependent on receiving constant messages, emails, and tweets, that the moment they do not receive one, their anxiety increases. People feel compelled to check their phone constantly, which can then lead to disappointment when there are no new messages, and increased stress about why no one is messaging them, or when the next message might come.

However, repetitive checking of mobile phones is considered a compulsive behaviour [9]. People who are highly dependent on the Internet for interaction act impulsively, avoid emotions, and fail to keep up a proper planning or time management [8]. We identify features which are relevant for detecting problematic phone usage and therefore increase the stress level of the user.

In our system we take into account the number of touches of the screen (quantifying the usage of applications on the phone), the number of calls and the number of SMSs as factors for the social interaction of the users using their smartphones. The accumulated result per day is multiplied with the corresponding weight factor and therefore it is accumulated in the total relaxation score. The accumulated result of the social interaction dimension is computed using weights. These weights of the subdimensions of the social pattern are computed by asking the users in the beginning of the experiment to prioritize the ways of social interaction. The idea of the scoring procedure is the following. We assign a weight factor to each of the three subdimensions of social interaction. This factor is based on the response of the participants to the following question which was asked in the beginning of the experiment. Which of the three subdimensions do they personally consider as the most important for their communication with other people? To the most important dimension we assign a weight of $w_1 = 0.4$ and to the rest we assign a weight of 0.3 respectively ($w_2 = w_3 = 0.3$), so that $w_1 + w_2 + w_3 = 1$.

Physical Activity. Physical activity plays a key role in the control of neuroendocrine, autonomic, and behavioral responses to physical and phychosocial stress. Physical activity is commonly regarded as beneficial to both physical and psychological health, and is seen as an effective preventive measure and treatment for stress-related diseases. Physically active people show reduced reactivity to physical stressors as well as reduced susceptibility to the adverse influences of life stress [13]. Several studies have linked exercise to improved depression, self-esteem and stress [5,6]. Our system monitors the physical activity of the user, making the distinction between the type of activity (e.g. walking, running, bicycling). We have also implemented a step counter which gives us the opportunity to find the number of steps that each user took per day. The American Heart Association uses the 10,000 steps metric as a guideline to follow for improving health and decreasing risk of heart disease, the leading cause of death in America. 10,000 steps a day is a rough equivalent to the Surgeon Generals recommendation to accumulate 30 min of activity most days of the week.

At first, in our model we assign the maximum value of wellbeing, and therefore the lowest stress level, when reaching the goal of 10,000 steps per day. If someone reaches less than this number we penalize (decrease relaxation score) with a weight factor per 1,000 steps. After the reception of the data for one month and based on the answers of the users to the Circumplex Model of Affect, we extract the pattern between the ideal physical activity of each individual user and his daily steps. Therefore extracting the personal pattern of the user we assign this value to the maximum value of wellbeing for this user. Then the comparison and the behavior of the user is compared with this personalized new value.

3   Evaluation with Real Data

For the evaluation of our data, we followed an empirical mathematical model. We monitored the behaviour of the user in the above mentioned three dimensions (sleeping pattern, social interaction and physical activity) collecting data for a month. Therefore we take this data as the basis for extracting the personalized stress level of each individual user that uses the StayActive application.

3.1   Relaxation Score

At first we compute a relaxation score for each individual user for every day of the monitoring month. The relaxation score is in the scale of [0–10] where the more stressed you are, the lower your score will be (so the more relaxed you are the higher your relaxation score). The idea of the scoring procedure is the same with the score assignment of the subdimensions of the social interaction. We assign a weight factor to each of the three dimensions of wellbeing that we have taken into account in our study. This factor is based on the response of the participants to the following question which was asked in the beginning of the experiment. Which of the three dimensions do they personally consider as the most important for their wellbeing? To the most important dimension we assign a weight of $w_1 = 0.4$ and to the rest we assign a weight of 0.3 respectively ($w_2 = w_3 = 0.3$), so that $w_1 + w_2 + w_3 = 1$. Based on these factors we are able to calculate the per day relaxation level of each person as depicted in Figs. 8 and 9 according to the Eqs. 1 and 2. Therefore we compute a result per dimension and adding them we calculate the final daily relaxation score of the user. For each of the three dimensions we normalize the results in the scale of [0–10] and then multiply each of them with the respective factor. Adding the three results per user, per day we extract the daily relaxation level of each user.

We should highlight that the values of the three dimensions are in three different scales. Therefore, in order to compute the result in one common scale we respect the following procedure:

1. Firstly we compute the standardized values of the items. This value is also called the normal deviate and it represents the distance of one data point from the mean, divided by the standard deviation of the distribution.

$$std\_vl = (unstd\_vl - mean)/\sigma \qquad (1)$$

   where std_vl is the standardized value and σ is the standard deviation.
2. Secondly we use factor weights to compute the unstandardized score.

$$unstd\_sc = w_1 * dm_1 + w_2 * dm_2 + w_3 * dm_3 \qquad (2)$$

   where $unstd\_sc$ is the unstandardized score, w_i is the weight score of the item i and dm_i is the standardized value of the item i.

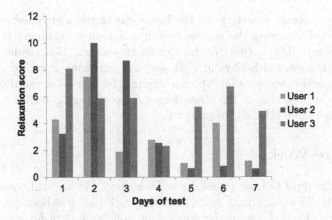

Fig. 8. Relaxation score evolution for three users.

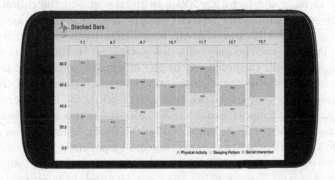

Fig. 9. Relaxation score as represented by each dimension.

3. We find the minimum and the maximum of the scores and accordingly we translate everything in the scale of [0–10] by normalizing the results. Following the above mentioned procedure even if we have dimensions which are measured in different scales we produce a relaxation score in the scale of [0–10].

3.2   Preliminary Results

The five participants of our tests were young adult members from our research group. The evaluation of the results takes place by asking the people who participated in the experiment how they felt on each day corresponding to the monitoring month when data was collected, without knowing the outcome. Then, we compare their personal perception with the relaxation score that we have computed using the StayActive application for each individual day. The more score you have the less stressed you are. This is the first step of evaluating the accuracy of the relaxation score that we produced through our empirical model.

Secondly, we extract a pattern for the behaviour of the user based on the data that we collected during the testing month and then we compare this pattern with the average daily activity of the user for this month. We calculate the deviation from the normal behaviour that we have extracted from the one-month experiment and based on that we characterize the user as stressed or not. We also calculate the mean of the stress factor for each person during a month in order to have more relevant information.

4   Future Work

This is a first model of our stress detection system. We are still enhancing and improving it. The immediate steps after the work that has been presented are the following. Further use of the application collecting data for a month from people outside our lab. We have already started the trials with the transportation company of Geneva and factory workers in Bucharest and the collected results will be more representative for real life working scenarios. In the long term, we are targeting a final ML approach which will take more features into account in order to improve the accuracy of stress detection. Having collected a set of initial data, these will be processed in the statistical software R in order to build a workflow with the aim to acquire a first understanding of the data as well as prepare them as much as possible for the initial modeling phase. Having concluded to the best model under the given dataset, this along with the data preprocessing workflow, will be employed on the Spark framework on the server side, so as to take advantage of the real time data assessment modules along with the Big Data processing capabilities. For the improvement of our algorithm we will analyze data from biosensors like the heart rate and the heart rate variability of the user adding them as extra dimensions to our system. The long term idea of StayActive is to provide adults with a personalized, adaptable tool which can also monitor some changes to biological signals like skin conductance and heart rate, using wearable sensors and link them to a low relaxation score (increased stress level). Then it will recommend and present various relaxation activities just-in-time in order to allow the users to carry out and solve everyday tasks and problems at work.

5   Conclusions

Stress detection is a research field that can have a big impact on the improvement of people's daily life. In this paper we presented a stress detection system which takes into account three main dimensions of wellbeing. The sleeping pattern, the physical activity of the users and their social interaction were accumulated with different weight factors and give an estimation of the daily stress level of the user. To the best of our knowledge, this is the first system that computes a stress score based on different dimensions of human wellbeing. The main innovation of this work is addressed in the fact that the way the stress level is computed is as less invasive as possible. Our solution relies only on the daily phone usage of people. Also we acquire the ground truth for the importance of each dimension of wellbeing for each individual by asking the users. This leads us to a personalized model which focuses on the personality of each individual user.

References

1. Sano, A., Picard, R.W.: Stress recognition using wearable sensors and mobile phones. In: Humaine Association Conference on Affective Computing and Intelligent Interaction, pp. 671–676 (2013)
2. Cohen, S., Kamarck, T.W., Mermelstein, R.: A global measure of perceived stress. J. Health Soc. Behav. **24**, 385–396 (1983)
3. Norris, R., Carroll, D., Cochrane, R.: The effects of physical activity and exercise training on psychological stress and well-being in an adolescent population. J. Psychosom. Res. **36**, 55–65 (1992)
4. Alvarez, G., Ayas, N.T.: The impact of daily sleep duration on health: a review of the literature. Prog. Cardiovasc. Nurs. **19**, 56–59 (2004)
5. Fox, K.R.: The influence of physical activity on mental well-being. Public Health Nutr. **2**, 411–418 (1999)
6. Paffenbarger, R.S., Hyde, R., Wing, A.L., Hsieh, C.: Physical activity, all-cause mortality, and longevity of college alumni. New England J. Med. **314**, 605–613 (1986)
7. Nevit, M.C., Cummings, S.R., Kidd, S., Black, D.: Risk factors for recurrent non-syncopal fall. A prospective study. J. Am. Med. Assoc. **261**, 2663–2668 (1986)
8. Li, S., Chung, T.: Internet function and Internet addictive behavior. Comput. Hum. Behav. **22**, 1067–1071 (2006)
9. Oulasvirta, A., Rattenbury, T., Ma, L., Raita, E.: Habits make smartphone use more pervasive. Pers. Ubiquit. Comput. **16**, 105–114 (2012)
10. Muaremi, A., Arnrich, B., Trster, G.: Towards measuring stress with smartphones and wearable devices during workday and sleep. BioNanoScience **3**, 172–183 (2013)
11. Moturu, S., Khayal, I., Aharony, N., Pan, W., Pentland, A.: Sleep, mood and sociability in a healthy population. In: 33rd Annual International Conference of the IEEE EMBS, pp. 5267–5270 (2011)
12. Lane, N.D., et al.: BeWell: a smartphone application to monitor, model and promote wellbeing. In: 5th ICST/IEEE Conference on Pervasive Computing Technologies for Healthcare, pp. 23–26. IEEE Press (2011)
13. Rimmele, U., Seiler, R., Wirtz, P.H., Ehlert, U., Heinrichs, M.: The level of physical activity affects adrenal and cardiovascular reactivity to phychosocial stress. Psychoneuroendocrinology **34**, 190–198 (2009)
14. Rusell, A.J.: A circumplex model of affect. J. Pers. Soc. Psychol. **39**, 1161–1178 (1980)
15. Kostopoulos, P., Nunes, T., Salvi, M., Togneri, D., M.: StayActive: an application for Detecting Stress. In: INNOV 2015: The fourth International Conference on Communications, Computation, Networks and Technologies (2015)

SenseCare: Using Affective Computing to Manage and Care for the Emotional Wellbeing of Older People

Raymond R. Bond[1(✉)], Huiru Zheng[1], Haiying Wang[1],
Maurice D. Mulvenna[1], Patrick McAllister[1], Kieran Delaney[2],
Paul Walsh[2], Alphonsus Keary[2], Rubén Riestra[3], Sabina Guaylupo[3],
Matthias Hemmje[4], Jana Becker[4], and Felix Engel[5]

[1] University of Ulster, Coleraine, UK
{rb.bond,h.zheng,hy.wang,md.mulvenna}@ulster.ac.uk
[2] Cork Institute of Technology, Cork, Ireland
[3] Inmark Group, Madrid, Spain
[4] Research Institute for Telecommunication and Cooperation (FTK),
Dortmund, Germany
[5] Fernuni Hagen, Hagen, Germany

Abstract. This paper discusses an opportunity for using *affective computing* modalities to support the monitoring of emotional wellbeing of older people. The ageing population is escalating and is associated with an increase in the number of persons with dementia. It is also reported that older people can suffer from social isolation and that people with dementia can experience a range of negative emotions such as anxiety and depression. We present a model to care for a person's emotional wellbeing in the home using multiple-modalities such as video, audio, electrodermal activity and photoplethysmography.

Keywords: Affective computing · Emotion · Older people · Ageing · Dementia

1 Introduction

The number of persons exceeding 85 years of age has almost doubled in the past decade and it is well documented that the entire ageing population will at least double by the year 2050 [1]. This will result in escalating health care costs and chronic diseases such as dementia. Healthcare institutions and researchers have been investigating potential solutions and new healthcare paradigms to alleviate this burden. These paradigms have included a number of connected health solutions. Whilst connected health research has received special attention in recent years, there is no agreed definition for this concept. Nevertheless, according to Caulfield et al. [2] *"Connected Health is where all stakeholders in the process are 'connected' by means of timely sharing and presentation of accurate and pertinent information regarding patient status through smarter use of data, devices, communication platforms and people"*. Connected health research has had a focus on the use of smart environments, home

© ICST Institute for Computer Sciences, Social Informatics and Telecommunications Engineering 2017
K. Giokas et al. (Eds.): eHealth 2016, LNICST 181, pp. 352–356, 2017.
DOI: 10.1007/978-3-319-49655-9_42

automation, ambient intelligence, telehealth and mHealth and has involved the use of sensors in the home coupled with algorithms to detect certain events such as activities of daily living and events such as falls. Whilst these are important areas of research, there is also a need to provide solutions for monitoring and caring for the emotional wellbeing of older people and in particularly people with dementia. This is needed given that an increasing proportion of the ageing population often suffer from social isolation or social exclusion [3]. Social isolation has an obvious effect on emotional wellbeing and can yield negative emotions such as depression, sadness and fear and people with dementia can have periods of agitation and aggression [3]. Others have suggested the use of social media networks that are tailored for the demographic of older people [4]. Nevertheless, the emerging area of affective computing has provided the opportunity to monitor and care for the emotional wellbeing of older people and in particular people with dementia.

2   SenseCare Model

Affective computing is the study of how machines can understand and respond to human 'affect' and emotions [5]. Paul Ekman, a pioneer in emotion research, stated that there are six universal emotions, i.e. anger, fear, disgust, surprise, joy, sadness [5]. Affective computing is inter-disciplinary in nature and spans computer science and psychology. If the affective computing vision is to be realised, it will bring about a revolution in artificial intelligence, which will have an impact on how humans interact with machines. Researchers in this discipline experiment using a range of modalities to determine human emotions. This includes 2 Dimensional (2D) and 3 Dimensional (3D) video (to classify facial expressions and body gestures), audio (to classify voice intonations and prosody), electroencephalography (EEG - brain signals), photo-plethysmography (PPG - for measuring pulse rate/valence), Electrodermal Activity (EDA - for measuring skin conductance/arousal) and facial electromyography (EMG - for measuring facial muscles). A requirement for the SenseCare project is to monitor emotion via non-invasive sensors using a platform that does not require excessive interaction or cognitive effort from the user. Consequently, since EEG and EMG require considerable resource to setup and are not regarded as convenient wearable technologies, we have initially decided not to consider these modalities in the Sense-Care platform. However, the modalities we are considering have been presented in Table 1 along with a number of strengths and weaknesses for each sensor. These strengths and weaknesses are pertinent to the context of the SenseCare project. Figure 1 also illustrates the current SenseCare model where sensor data (video, audio, EDA and PPG signals) are streamed to a server for feature extraction and emotion classification via machine learning algorithms. To protect privacy, video/audio features can be extracted outside the cloud. If there is a deviation from positive emotions, a next of kin or carer is automatically notified to intervene personally or provide appropriate digital content via the home entertainment system (this can involve a voice-over-IP conversation, streaming the person's favourite television programmes or family videos/photos from social media). Alternatively, a next of kin or carer can access the system's dashboard at any time. By default the system will indicate which days, times

Table 1. Relevant strengths/weaknesses of each selected modality in SenseCare model.

Mode	Strengths	Weaknesses
EDA	Validated for measuring arousal Conveniently measured from the wrist using a wristband Not infringing on privacy	Relies on a person wearing a device and thus is dependent on a person with dementia remembering to wear it daily and to recharge it
PPG	Measures pulse rate and can be used to infer heart rate variability. It also complements EDA in using the arousal-valence space Can be conveniently measured from the wrist using a wristband or from the ear lobe Not infringing on privacy	Not always an accurate measure of heart rate and accuracy is affected by activity Relies on a person wearing a device and thus is dependent on a person with dementia remembering to wear it daily and to recharge it
Video	Established science for classifying emotions from facial expressions An inexpensive sensor that can be easily placed around the home, e.g. above mirrors, TVs and kitchen sinks	Not all emotions are expressed facially No data is collected if the user is not in the frame Infringing on privacy
Audio	An inexpensive sensor that can be easily placed around the home, e.g. near telephones and in social areas such as the longue and kitchen	Not all emotions are expressed verbally No data is collected if the user is not speaking Infringing on privacy

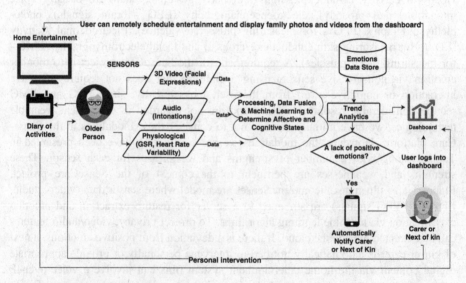

Fig. 1. Framework for monitoring and caring for the emotional wellbeing of older people.

Table 2. Vignettes illustrating potential use case scenarios of the SenseCare platform.

SenseCare use case scenarios
1. Sonia is an elderly lady who has dementia and lives on her own. She gets frequent phone calls from family members and often receives a call from her nephew Ben. The SenseCare platform has computed that Sonia's emotional wellbeing has been declining over a short period of time and the carer has been notified of this. The carer logs onto the dashboard and observes some trends. It highlights that Sonia's positive emotions peak during a periodic phone call she receives once a month on a Tuesday afternoon. The carer visits Sonia and carries out a mental health assessment. Sonia's health seems to be fine but after gaining permission, the carer phones Ben to reinforce that his phone calls have a positive effect on Sonia's emotional wellbeing and he is encouraged to phone more often, perhaps weekly. Ben is delighted to be notified of this and calls Sonia once a week. A few months later, the SenseCare platform shows that this weekly phone call has had a significant effect on Sonia's emotional wellbeing
2. Jim is an elderly man with dementia and lives on his own. He is normally happy throughout the week but still gets a visit from a carer once a month. The SenseCare system detects that Jim has been feeling down during the start of each week because of a lack of visits and he feels isolated on Mondays especially. The system notifies his daughter Susan via SMS. Susan is a busy professional and can't physically intervene early in the week as she travels for business meetings and needs to provide for her young family. Susan logs onto the dashboard the following Monday and has a video Skype conversation with her Dad. She then sets up a TV schedule for her Dad and selects recent family videos and photos from her Facebook to be streamed to her Dad's home entertainment throughout the day. During mid-week, Susan logs back onto the dashboard and selects the emotion analysis feature and is reassured that her Dad was much happier during Monday and decides to set up a programme for every Monday

and activities (recorded from a diary) provide the periods of 'happiness' or 'unhappiness'. For example, the system will indicate which personal visit, phone call, television programme or any other activity correlated with various emotional episodes. Table 2 provides two vignettes that illustrate potential use case scenarios for the SenseCare model.

3 Conclusion

We present a model that uses affective computing to help care for the emotional wellbeing of older people and specifically those people with dementia. The project team are currently developing this model and will test it in a number of scenarios.

Acknowledgements. Funded by Marie Skłodowska-Curie Actions in Horizon 2020.

References

1. Lutz, W., Sanderson, W., Scherbov, S.: The coming acceleration of global population ageing. Nature **451**, 716–719 (2008)
2. Caulfield, B.M., Donnelly, S.C.: What is connected health and why will it change your practice? QJM **106**(8), 703–707 (2013)

3. Moore, P., Xhafa, F., Barolli, L., Thomas, A.: Monitoring and detection of agitation in dementia: towards real-time and big-data solutions. In: Proceedings of the 8th IEEE International Conference on P2P, Parallel, Grid, Cloud and Internet Computing (3PGCIC), pp. 128–135 (2013)
4. Boyd, K., Nugent, C., Donnelly, M., Sterritt, R., Bond, R., Lavery-Bowen, L.: EasiSocial: an innovative way of increasing adoption of social media in older people. In: Bodine, C., Helal, S., Gu, T., Mokhtari, M. (eds.) ICOST 2014. LNCS, vol. 8456, pp. 21–28. Springer, Switzerland (2014)
5. Picard, R.W.: Affective Computing, vol. 252. MIT Press, Cambridge (1997)

PPmH 2016

Patient's Empowerment and Behaviour Change: Complementary Approaches in EU Projects PALANTE and PEGASO

Maria Renata Guarneri[1(✉)], Marco Decandia Brocca[2], and Luca Piras[2]

[1] Dept. Design, Politecnico di Milano, Via Durando 38A, Milan, Italy
mariarenata.guarneri@polimi.it
[2] Lombardia Informatica SpA, Via Taramelli, Milan, Italy
{marco.decandia,luca.piras}@cnt.lispa.it

Abstract. Patient empowerment is widely considered a key component of an effective Health-care system. Empowerment, by effective communication, information and education and thanks to innovative ICT solutions, enables patients to be more active players in their own health, improving the quality of patient/physician relationship and, as a consequence, helping the physician to be more effective as well. However, a patient cannot be properly empowered unless he wants to. He has to be an active part of the empowerment process. Hence, we can say that empowerment requires the patient to have the right attitude, which, often and for various reasons, it is not the case. Proactive initiatives need to be undertaken to develop the correct attitude towards patient empowerment.

This paper provides an overview of key concepts in relation to *patient empowerment* and illustrates the approach of two EU-funded projects tackling empowerment from different perspectives. PALANTE project (http://www.palante-project.eu) has worked extensively on empowerment and many different way of fostering empowerment in different kind of patients. PEGASO Fit 4 Future project (www.pegasof4f.eu), on the other side, is working on the development of a Behaviour Change Platform, a system, which may be an effective complement of any empowerment effort.

The results of PALANTE have shown that empowerment can only be achieved by developing an attitude of better attention to lifestyle and self-monitoring and care. This can be developed through information and education and with the support of instruments that can foster behaviour change.

Keywords: Patient empowerment · Engagement · Chronic conditions · Prevention · Behaviour change · Healthcare · Motivation · Healthy lifestyle

1 Introduction

Starting from the experience and the results from two EU-funded projects – PALANTE and PEGASO Fit 4 Future - this paper provides an overview of key concepts with regards to patient empowerment.

© ICST Institute for Computer Sciences, Social Informatics and Telecommunications Engineering 2017
K. Giokas et al. (Eds.): eHealth 2016, LNICST 181, pp. 359–369, 2017.
DOI: 10.1007/978-3-319-49655-9_43

Patient empowerment enables patients to take an active role in their own healthcare provision, which allows them to stay easily informed and 'self-manage' their own health services. In the context of an ageing population and increasing number of chronic patients, patient empowerment is a key tool to reduce healthcare costs and improve quality and efficiency of the health delivery process.

With this objective, PALANTE has sought (through a number of specific field trials in different countries) to empower patients so they are able to make informed decisions about their health, take an active role in their care and collaborate effectively with their healthcare team through the use of information and communication technologies. The project is now in its completion phase and the results are illustrated in this paper, however one of the key finding has been also that "empowerment" requires the right attitude and needs to be developed.

PEGASO Fit 4 Future is a project that addresses prevention and is oriented to the younger population. Objective of PEGASO is to develop the right attitude towards healthy lifestyles by fostering and supporting motivation for behaviour change.

It is the opinion of the authors that the work of the two projects is complementary and while patient empowerment today mostly focuses on individuals in need of care and it is particularly relevant for chronic patients (which is the focus of PALANTE), an early education in understanding "health" in wide sense and the development of awareness towards healthy behaviours (which is the focus of PEGASO) is fundamental in developing the "future" empowered patient.

The paper is organised in three main sections covering respectively:

- the concept of patient empowerment, illustrating the principles of successful patients empowerment and the main approaches;
- an overview of the PALANTE project and its main findings from the; and
- an overview of the project PEGASO Fit 4 Future, illustrating how awareness about health and motivation can be developed through an approach oriented to behaviour change.

Some conclusions and acknowledgments are then provided.

2 The Concept of Patient Empowerment

Any care process is built around a relationship between patient and doctor. Any doctor has a better chance of achieving maximum result by engaging in a productive relationship with a collaborative patient. The doctor has to be good at his job, of course, but the patient as well, needs to have the right attitude, knowledge and tools to provide his carers with appropriate information, feedback and event hints. Patient's empowerment aims at creating the best possible conditions for that to happen.

The concept of patient empowerment is not new; it dates back to the 1960s when "social action and self-help ideologies have placed an emphasis on the rights and abilities of individuals and communities rather than deficits or needs" [1].

Over the decades the issue has attracted growing interest and, now, patient empowerment is considered a potential tool to reduce healthcare costs and improve efficiency of the health systems, reinforcing healthcare quality. Patient empowerment has become an element of high priority in the EU health strategy, supported by national and regional health authorities.

"Chronic diseases are now the biggest cause of death and disability worldwide – including cardiovascular diseases (CVD), cancer, diabetes, obesity, and chronic respiratory diseases – account for an estimated 86% of deaths and 77% of the disease burden in the European Region, as measured by disability-adjusted life years (WHO 2009). This development has brought about a fundamental shift in health systems and healthcare, and as a consequence, in the roles and responsibilities of patients.

In line with this health transition the focus on patient responsibilities and their role in managing their health has grown substantially and is an increasing focus of health policy. With this, has come a shift towards care and treatment moving out of the hospitals and into the community and the home, leaving patients and family with a greater responsibility for their own health [2].

Even if the concept of patient's empowerment is widely known, it is difficult to find a commonly agreed definition of empowerment both in literature and among practitioners. A common element to many existing definitions of Patient Empowerment is that it is considered a means of improving health care effectiveness, increasing the efficacy of chronic conditions treatment as well as transforming the relationship between healthcare providers and patients.

During the early phase of the research conducted within the framework of the PALANTE project (EU funded project, ICT PSP 5th call 2011, grant n° 297260), after a thorough literature review, the following definition has been adopted.

"[Empowerment] is the situation where an individual is an active member of his/her own disease management team. Patient empowerment integrates multiple concepts that allow a patient to effectively self-manage his/her disease. In a context of aging population and increasing number of chronic patients, it is considered a key tool to reduce healthcare costs and to improve quality and efficiency of the health delivery process. ICT applications already help to empower patients (...)".

In consideration of the definition given above, it becomes clear that empowerment involves several subjects and requires actions at different levels in the Healthcare Systems. Back in 1999, Edward Wagner, working with his team at the Mac Coll Institute for Healthcare Innovation [3], developed the Chronic Care Model (CCM) [4] with the goal of designing a framework where all subjects involved in the care of chronic patients were considered and areas of improvement could be easily identified.

The CCM provides a structure for organisation/practice change and encompasses six elements, or areas, for improvement, namely: Health Care Organisation, Community Resources, Self-Management Support, Delivery System Design, Decision Support, and Clinical Information Systems.

More recently, the World Health Organisation (WHO) has expanded the CCM framework, designing a model called Innovative Care for Chronic Conditions (ICCC). The new "framework, recognizes a broader policy environment that envelops patients and their families, health care organizations, and communities" [5].

Going deep into these models is out of the scope of this paper. What is relevant is that they both point out clearly how properly addressing the care of chronic patients requires a joint effort of different people in different contexts and organizations.

Orchestration of these efforts is impossible to achieve unless all players are committed and properly empowered.

The patient is, by definition, at the centre of care process and, in the next paragraphs, we will take a better look at patient's empowerment, trying to highlight the key success factors by having the patient as our focus point.

There are a few distinctive elements that can be considered as pre-conditions for effective empowerment policies and approaches [1]:

Engagement: the patient actively participates in accessing appropriate care, attending and preparing for appointments and using additional resources to maintain a high level of continued involvement in their care.

Knowledge: the patient understands his or her condition, is aware of treatment options but also has a basic understanding of their health care system including benefits, available resources and health care consumer rights.

Collaboration: there is a perceived partnership in care and the patient seeks to participate in shared decision-making about their care. He or she can practice assertive communication and active listening and has a reasonable level of trust in their health care provider and the system.

Commitment: the patient is committed to goals/expectations of his/her own treatment approach.

Tolerance of Uncertainty: the patient's ability to balance the probabilities and risks of treatment paths for instance through shared decision-making processes.

These five points may be considered as foundation stones. Any empowerment approach, to be effective, has to deal with them and, of course, there are many different ways for doing so.

2.1   Approaches to Empowerment

The old models of care, where physicians tell patients what to do and try to motivate them to change, are no longer adequate because patients must be active and informed participants in the health care processes.

There are several ways to put the patient at the heart of the process with an active role. The following paragraphs shortly describe the most common.

Education. It is difficult for patients to do what they don't understand, so the first step to improve patients to take on a more active role in their health care is to educate them. Start by communicating to patients that education is perhaps as important to their health as getting their prescriptions filled. They need to know all they can about their disease [6].

Information. Even an educated patient is helpless without proper information. Information gathering is not an easy task and being an active information seeker is helpful in shaping the right mind-set. The issue for the patient is, on one side, not to be misled by wrong or inaccurate information and, on the other side, not to be overwhelmed by information overload. In the past, gathering information was not easy at all, nowadays, thanks to the Net, finding information is easy, what s difficult is finding the relevant one. Education provides good grounding for that, as it is harder misleading an educated patient then a not educated one. The role of the caregiver as a guide is of paramount relevance.

Motivation. Keeping motivation high is another key success factor. Motivation depends on many things. Inevitably, motivation has ups and downs but there are approaches and techniques that can hep to keep it high. To keep going, clear and reachable goals are a must, and people need to have a good level of confidence about themselves and in the system. On the contrary, when motivation is low, people are likely to stop gathering information, keeping themselves properly documented about their health and they are likely to be less compliance with their set care path.

Communication. Proper communication is essential but often, looking at care processes and at the communication flow among the involved players, deficiencies can be spotted in several cases. Good communication requires all players to have the right information easily accessible otherwise the care process may be harmed or even compromised. Improving communication is not only a matter of providing players with the right tools, it also require keen attention to the process, which sometimes calls for process reengineering, including the development of tools that better fit and are tailored to the process. When proper communication protocol and processes are not in place, even the best tools may turn out to be ineffective, at best.

In the following two sections the approaches followed by the two projects are illustrated.

3   PALANTE

PALANTE (PAtients Leading and mANaging their healThcare through EHealth) is an eHealth implementation project with 21 partners aiming to reach 70,000 new users of electronically-fuelled health services. Users from most pilots have a chronic disease.

The main goal of PALANTE is to improve eHealth services that empower patients so that they make informed decisions about their health, take an active role in their care and collaborate effectively with their healthcare team of professionals through the use of information and communication technologies. The project has pursued its objectives through the implementation, scaling up and optimization of 9 pilot studies, of which 7 are new pilots – developed within PALANTE. Two pilots, in Denmark and France, were already running, however their experience was very important for the new pilots. All 9 pilots were evaluated according to a shared protocol.

The project has generated a rich pool of knowledge, experiences, lessons learned, validated approaches and innovation elements for the benefit of its direct and indirect beneficiaries, the members of the implementing consortium itself and a much broader audience. While, it became clear that it was challenging to make the overall PALANTE project more than the sum of the individual pilots; the results achieved are satisfactory and allowed all project partners to learn more about the services provided and process of empowerment, going beyond the mere support of the implementation of the pilots.

While pilots are of heterogeneous nature, it has been possible to classify them according to three clusters:

Healthcare portal: it includes those Pilots that do not address to a specific pathology but enable the sharing of clinical documents and information between healthcare providers and patients. In some cases, pilots can incorporate booking appointment tools and services.

Chronic Disease Management: this cluster intends to group Pilots mainly focused on the care pathway that the healthcare professional establishes for the patient in a chronic condition, rather than his/her remote monitoring.

Telemedicine services: this cluster refers to remote monitoring systems usually adopted for patient affected by a specific pathology.

Some Pilots cannot be associated with just one of the three clusters. Indeed, some Pilots have characteristics that position themselves in an area between two clusters. All pilots focused on a set of services and not necessarily on all the services available to citizens. For instance, Lombardy focuses on the management of a care pathway and on sharing personal health information through a web portal (Fig. 1).

Within the PALANTE project, different services have been assessed against a wide population of users. The results are of great help for the design of new services as well as for re-designing eHealth strategies.

The research has bee designed having in mind, as guiding principles, the following questions:

- Which role might eHealth play for patient empowerment?
- How should eHealth be designed to empower patient?
- Which other variables should be taken into account?

The evaluation work has been carried out using the PAM methodology. The Patient Activation Measure (PAM), licensed by Insignia health [7], is a methodology assessing an individual's knowledge, skill, and confidence for managing one's health and healthcare. Individuals who measure high on this assessment typically understand the

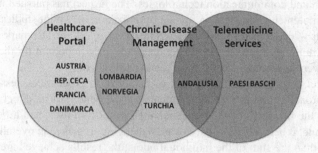

Fig. 1. PALANTE pilots by cluster

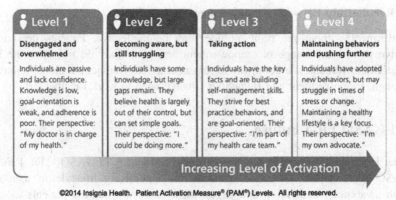

Fig. 2. PAM levels

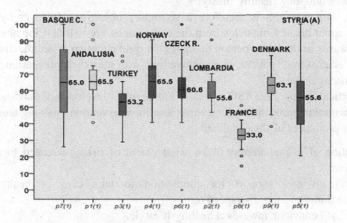

Fig. 3. PAM of PALANTE pilots

importance of taking a pro-active role in managing their health and have the skills and confidence to do so.

PAM was developed using qualitative methods, Rasch analysis, and classical test theory psychometric methods. Developed by Judith Hibbard and colleagues [8] at the University of Oregon, the resulting 13-item measure is a uni-dimensional, interval level, Guttman-like scale (Figs. 2 and 3).

Multiple studies show that PAM scores are predictive of most health behaviours, including:

- preventive behaviours (e.g. obtaining screenings and immunizations);
- healthy behaviours (e.g. healthy diet and regular exercise);
- self-management behaviours (e.g. monitoring and medication management);
- health information seeking. Higher activated individuals also have better health outcomes and lower rates of costly utilization, such as emergency department use and hospitalizations.

3.1 Relationship Between Empowerment and Attitude

Empowerment without the right attitude may be ineffective. Patients need to be proactive to take advantage of empowerment and often they do not have the right attitude. Empowerment is a good way to foster behaviour change, but alone, it may not be enough. Empowerment and Behaviour Change need to work together [9].

4 PEGASO Fit 4 Future

Another EU funded project in the area of empowerment is PEGASO – Fit 4 Future. PEGASO (Personalised Guidance Services for Optimising lifestyle in teen-agers through awareness, motivation and engagement) does not address patients as such; rather it targets healthy people (teen-agers in the case of this project and with a focus on prevention of obesity and lifestyle related diseases) with the objective of "educating" them towards adopting healthy lifestyles.

Patient empowerment is therefore a secondary objective. However by building awareness about healthy lifestyles from the early stages, we will develop also the right attitude towards health, i.e. a person that pays the right attention to health, leading to an informed "empowered" patient, in a positive loop with impact on prevention and better self-care management.

In practical terms PEGASO – Fit 4 Future will develop a Behaviour Change Platform, with an approach based on three level of intervention enabling teen-agers to become co-producers of their wellbeing:

- Generation of self-awareness (acknowledgement of risks associated to unhealthy behaviours);
- Enhancement and support for motivation to take care of health with a short/medium/long term perspective;
- Change of behaviour towards a healthy lifestyle.

4.1 Overview of Approach

The solution proposed by PEGASO comes from the convergence of the need to address the rapidly increasing prevalence of obesity among children and adolescents on one side and the rapid development of ICT, and in particular mobile technologies, on the other side.

The behaviour change solution proposed by PEGASO is based on a **mobile, social and networked gaming platform**, considered as a powerful tool to actively engage the younger population in activities that will stimulate healthier choices in their daily lives. From the technology point of view, cloud computing, and convergence towards mobile are the key enablers.

The PEGASO system framework offers three main functionalities to the users:

1. *Individual & Environmental Monitoring*, through a high level-monitoring platform including wearable sensors and mobile phone as well as multimedia diaries for the acquisition of physical, behavioural and emotional attitude of adolescent.
2. *Feedback System* provides feedback in terms of "health status" changes, required actions to undertake etc. This function will also propose personalized healthy modification of the lifestyle thus promoting active involvement in behaviour change.
3. *Social connectivity and engagement*, social network where users can share experiences with a community of peers concerning e.g. physical activity, food consumptions and everyday habits through different gaming strategies.

4.2   Elements of Behaviour Change

PEGASO considers four levels of engagement towards persuasion for user empowerment in healthcare: awareness of risks, motivation, affective learning and finally behaviour change.

Various types of expertise/knowledge and technologies feed these levels of engagement.

Develop Awareness: teenagers need to be aware of what they are doing; what is right and what is wrong for their healthy living. Some of them are unconsciously and automatically acting, and often under estimate or have no clear notion about information they receive. Monitoring lifestyle of teen's activity, collecting parameters and integrating their own data will enable self-awareness on their current situation. Through developing self-awareness and self-reflection, the user can frame the problem or the opportunity area to act upon or intervene.

Affective learning is the "highest" learning goal. The learner should trust in something that will happen in several years from now. The use of a constructivist learning model and special media like "social games" are appropriate to reach this goal.

Create Motivation: it is important to motivate teenagers to change their behaviour and sustain motivation in the long-term. The actors in the ecosystem are requested to offer "healthy" (or healthier) benefits and services satisfying their needs or desires. This is quite challenging, since motivation depends on many factors as well as emotions, psychological environment and personality. The system needs to provide constant different layouts of motivational activities where experts, technological frame monitoring and stakeholders services come into play.

Enable Behaviour Change: once teenagers have awareness and motivation, it is important to involve experts and use PEGASO to support the behaviour change process and reinforce existing virtuous behaviours. The turn from old unhealthy behaviours into new healthier ones has to be monitored through technology on a longer period.

In order to create prevention, it is important to change or stop old unhealthy habits and develop new healthier habits. In this respect, PEGASO takes a holistic approach involving the teenager's environment and specifically the families, by means of an education process empowered by training that will be provided on location (schools) and on line. The expert team will give feedbacks to the users allowing them to change their behaviour on a long-term basis. The overall system takes advantage of gaming strategies to persuade users to change their behaviour.

5 Conclusions

Empowerment has positive impacts on the whole care process. On one side the patient brings a better contribution to the care process, on the other side, the patient/carer relationship becomes more effective as the empowered patient is more compliant to the care plan and provides the carer with more appropriate and accurate information.

Empowerment may achieve a lot, contributing to:

- Healthier Behaviours;
- Greater Satisfaction that comes from knowing what's going on;
- Better Decisions (well informed decisions are the best ones);
- Sustainable Services;
- Reduced costs.

Indeed the costs of healthcare are an issue in Europe and there is a stringent need to control the level of expenditure in this area, as the European population is growing older and the prevalence of chronic illnesses is increasing.

Key elements that contribute to controlling such costs are prevention on one hand (to avoid the insurgence of pathologies – in particular those related to lifestyle) and patient empowerment on the other hand (to increase the capability of individuals to self manage their health conditions, to reduce hospitalisation and to ensure a more active and healthy aging). In both areas the adoption of ehealth-based tools and procedures can strongly support development of a new culture of self-care where the individual is aware of health-risks and has self-management capabilities. The results of PALANTE have shown that empowerment can only be achieved by developing an attitude of better attention to lifestyle and self-monitoring and care. This can be developed through information and education and with the support of instruments that can foster behaviour change, such as the PEGASO platform.

PEGASO Fit 4 Future will be tested and piloted with a population of about 400 teen-agers in three European countries (Italy - Lombardy, Spain - Catalonia and United Kingdom – England and Scotland). Results of the pilots will be available in mid 2017.

Acknowledgements. This paper is based on the discussions and on the material produced within the research conducted in the project PALANTE and in the project PEGASO Fit 4 Future.

The PALANTE project is co-funded by the European Commission under the ICT PSP Programme, GA 297260. PALANTE has started in February 2012 and has been completed in July 2015.

The PEGASO Fit 4 Future project is co-funded by the European Commission under the 7th Framework Programme, GA 610727. PEGASO is part of the cluster of projects in the ICT for health area; it has started in December 2013 and will run for 42 months.

The authors wish to thank the partners in both projects for their contribution to this work.

References

1. Realising the potential for patient empowerment for tackling chronic disease BUPA
2. Patient Empowerment – Living with Chronic Disease, The European Network on Patient Empowerment. www.enope.eu
3. http://maccollcenter.org/
4. Wagner, E.H., Davis, C., Schaefer, J., Von Korff, M., Austin, B.: A survey of leading chronic disease management programs: are they consistent with the literature? Manag. Care Q. **7**(3), 56–66 (1999)
5. Innovative Care for Chronic Conditions, World Health Organisation (WHO) (2002)
6. Helping patients take charge of their chronic illnesses – Family Practice Management, AAFP. www.aafp.org
7. http://www.insigniahealth.com/
8. Hibbard, J., et al.: Development of the Patient Activation Measure (PAM): conceptualizing and measuring activation in patients and consumers. Health Res. Educ. Trust **39**, 1005–1026 (2004)
9. Spanakis, E.G., Santana, S., Ben-David, B., Marias, K., Tziraki, C.: Persuasive technology for healthy aging and wellbeing. In: 4th International Conference on Wireless Mobile Communication and Healthcare, Athens, 3–5 November 2014

.CAD Patient Classification Using MIMIC-II

Swarnava Dey[1(✉)], Swagata Biswas[1], Arpan Pal[1], Arijit Mukherjee[1],
Utpal Garain[2], and Kayapanda Mandana[3]

[1] Innovation Labs, Tata Consultancy Services Ltd., Kolkata, India
{swarnava.dey,swagata.biswas,arpan.pal,mukherjee.arijit}@tcs.com
[2] Indian Statistical Institute, Kolkata, India
utpal.garain@gmail.com
[3] Cardiothoracic and Vascular Surgery Department,
Fortis Healthcare Limited, Kolkata, India
kmmandana@gmail.com
http://www.tcs.com, http://www.isical.co.in

Abstract. With availability of large volume of collected data from healthcare centers and significant improvement in computation power, evidence based learning is helping in building robust disease diagnostic models.

In this work MIMIC-II database, consisting of physiologic waveforms and clinical Information about ICU patients, is used for patient classification, taking Coronary Artery Disease (CAD) as a use case.

A learning algorithm (wavelet transform + SVM) is trained and evaluated for CAD patient segregation with 89% accuracy on ICD-9 labeled MIMIC-II Photoplethysmogram (PPG) signals. Due to the noisy nature of machine collected MIMIC-II ICU data, the same SVM model was validated on a local hospital dataset containing doctor labeled PPG signals resulting a 5% accuracy gain.

This work is the first attempt of CAD patient classification on MIMIC-II, using heart rates from easily obtainable PPG signal suitable in mobile/wearable setting.

Keywords: Heart rates · HRV · Wavelet transform · SVM · ICD-9 · PPG · Photoplethysmogram · CAD · Coronary Artery Disease · Bigdata

1 Introduction

MIMIC-II [9] is largescale database of medical records for 32000 patients. Among these patients, waveform (physiologic signals sampled at 125 Hz) data for around *2800* patients are matched with clinical records (information about patients including their diseases). The longitudinal physiologic readings when accompanied by a disease related ground truth, form the bases of evidence based learning of disease based patient classification.

For diagnosis/prognosis on MIMIC-II data, ground truth is sourced from hospital billing codes to perform model training using the physiologic signals and

© ICST Institute for Computer Sciences, Social Informatics and Telecommunications Engineering 2017
K. Giokas et al. (Eds.): eHealth 2016, LNICST 181, pp. 370–375, 2017.
DOI: 10.1007/978-3-319-49655-9_44

the patient's disease class. The billing codes stored in MIMIC-II are International Classification of Disease, Ninth Revision, Clinical Modification (ICD-9 -CM) codes. A more accurate field *Diagnosis on admission* is being added to the new MIMIC-III database [5].

Coronary Artery Disease (CAD) [3] can be defined as the blockage of arteries that supply blood to the heart, resulting from atherosclerosis (an accumulation of fatty materials on the inner linings of arteries). MIMIC-II has 600+ CAD patient's waveforms in the matched dataset forming a rich resource for people working on CAD diagnosis. As of now *coronary angiography* [4] is the only reliable way to diagnose CAD. The World Health Organization has marked CAD as a *modern epidemic* and there are not enough facilities available for timely diagnosis, especially in India due to a high patient to doctor ratio. In our Lab, more than one teams are working together to build non-invasive methods using easily available physiologic signals, to help clinicians screen CAD patients and ensure that the access to angiography is available to patients who really need it.

State of the art (SoA) survey revealed that earlier work attempted CAD diagnosis using ECG signal that not realizable in a mobile or wearable setting. A photoplethysmogram (PPG) signal, easily obtainable from fingertip using pulse oximeter or mobile camera, can denote the cardiac cycle [2]. In the current work feature extraction and machine learning methods were applied on the heart rate timeseries (HR) of 611 patients (around 850 Gigabytes waveform) in MIMIC-II dataset. Though MIMIC-II physiological signals were cleaned before using, the noisy nature of machine collected MIMIC-II ICU data was suspected to be the reason behind relatively low classification accuracy. For a second level validation the same model was evaluated on HR signal from a controlled proprietary PPG dataset and there was significant improvement of results.

This work is first attempt of CAD/non CAD patient classification on public dataset like MIMIC-II, using HR signal from easily obtainable PPG signal, using a new set of wavelet transform based features. This paper reports the design and evaluation of CAD patient diagnosis and is structured as follows: Sect. 2 gives a brief overview of SoA, Sect. 3 discusses the methodology, Sect. 4 outlines the classification results and finally the conclusion is drawn in Sect. 5.

2   Related Work

The SoA survey for the current work was undertaken in three areas namely: (1) earlier works on diagnosis of CAD using PPG signals, (2) CAD diagnosis on a large patient dataset and (3) disease diagnosis on large datasets, specifically MIMIC-II using ICD codes.

Though there is no earlier attempt of using PPG signals for diagnosis of CAD, several earlier works attempt non invasive detection of CAD using ECG and HRV from ECG. In [1] authors applied statistical and signal processing to extract features from HRV (from ECG) and applied SVM for classification. The two datasets comprised of 20 CAD, 20 normal subjects and 6 CAD, 6 normal subjects, respectively. Results indicate accurate classification of the subjects.

In [7] Wavelet Package Transform(WPT) is used to analyze HRV signals. Performance evaluation is done using least square support vector machine(LS-SVM) classification algorithm. An average of 90% accuracy is achieved on the test dataset using db4 as the wavelet function. In [6] HR signal is decomposed into frequency sub-bands using wavelet transform and dimensionality reduction are applied on the coefficients to get top features. Selected features are fed into different classifiers. For 10 CAD subjects and 15 normal subjects, accuracy of 96.8%, sensitivity of 100% and specificity of 93.7% is achieved using a combination of Independent Component Analysis-Gaussian Mixture Model.

This work reports the best result for CAD detection, however dataset size on which the experiments were conducted are small. Also, use of ECG as the physiologic signal source is not realizable for mobile or wearable setting. For the same reason we ignore several CAD detection methods using costly technique like Stress Cardiovascular Magnetic Resonance(CMR), Single Photon Emission Computed Tomography(SPECT) etc. In the area of disease diagnosis on large datasets, no attempt was found to use MIMIC-II database for diagnosis of CAD. However, MIMIC-II dataset is used for several other disease diagnosis works.

3   Methodology

The end to end system is represented in Fig. 1 and detailed in later subsections. Total 611 patients in MIMIC-II dataset are having PPG data (CAD:267 and non CAD:344), segregated using SQL queries on the MIMIC-II clinical database.

3.1   Data Acquisition

PPG signal for MIMIC-II, sampled at 125 Hz, is obtained using WFDB tools [10].

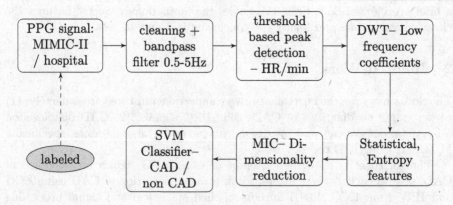

Fig. 1. Processing chain

ICD-9 code 414.01 is taken as CAD and all other patients except patients with any circulatory disease are taken as non CAD, as per doctor's advise.

The PPG waveform is obtained from the patients in a local hospital using a standard pulse oximeter, sampled at 60 Hz. This doctor verified PPG dataset is comprised of files from 14 CAD and 15 non CAD patients. Detected cardiac cycles [11] from PPG waveform, are used to get interpolated $(60 * \frac{1}{RR})$ HR bits/minute timeseries.

3.2 Feature Extraction

CAD or non CAD patients, having associated PPG waveform can be represented as vectors $V_1, V_2, ..., V_n$ for n number of patients. The vector $V_i \in R^{t_i}$ contains PPG signal sample at time t_i. It is observed from literature that patients with CAD have different heart rate variations from normal people, noticed in low frequency ranges [6]. Wavelet analysis helps both time and frequency localization using different sized windows at desired frequencies [11]. The wavelet transform of V_i is given as: $[W_\psi Vi](a,b) = \frac{1}{\sqrt{|a|}} \int_{-\infty}^{\infty} \overline{\psi\left(\frac{t-b}{a}\right)} Vi(t)dt$, where $\psi(t)$ is the transforming function called the mother wavelet. The scaling and translation parameters are a and b respectively. For HR signal, daubachies wavelet db3 [12] is found to be most suitable as mother wavelet after observing the similarities with the HR signals, both visually and using energy and entropy measures. The HR signal from PPG of V_i are wavelet transformed to find coefficients. Statistical and entropy related features like mean, variance, maximum and minimum of energy, amplitude, frequency are computed from each coefficient. Total number of features extracted is dependent on the number of coefficients generated, i.e., level of DWT decomposition and for the current work the level of decomposition used is *four*.

3.3 Feature Selection and Classification

In order to avoid *curse of dimensionality* [13] only the top contributing features (usually 5–10) were selected given by MIC [8] strength. Sample MIC strength of top five parameters for MIMIC-II data are *0.56,0.54, 0.49,0.39, 0.39* and for collected data are *0.72,0.58,0.54,0.49, 0.39*.

The selected features are used to train an SVM classifier [14] and evaluated using 10-fold cross validation. The idea behind SVM is to construct a hyperplane or a set of hyperplanes in a high dimensional space such that the given input gets classified into different classes. For the current work linear SVM did not give good results as it was not possible to construct a maximum-margin hyperplane that divides the training set into two classes. Different kernels were evaluated to map the input space to a high dimensional feature space using non linear transformation and *radial* kernel with tuning gave best results.

4   Experiments and Results

The various accuracy measures used in current context can be expressed as follows: (1) True positive (TP): CAD correctly identified as CAD (2) False positive (FP): Non CAD incorrectly identified as CAD (3) True negative (TN): Non CAD correctly identified as Non CAD (4) False negative (FN): CAD incorrectly identified as Non CAD

$Sensitivity = \frac{TP}{TP+FN}$ i.e., correctly identified CAD out of total CADs
$Specificity = \frac{TN}{TN+FP}$ i.e., correctly identified non CAD out of total non CADs
$Accuracy = \frac{TP+TN}{TP+FP+TN+FN}$ i.e., all correct identifications out of all patients.

The experimental results of two class classification for both MIMIC-II and local hospital datasets (described in Sect. 3.1) is presented in Table 1.

Table 1. Comparative classification results in local hospital and MIMIC-II patients

Dataset	Patient & class labels	Accuracy	Sensitivity	Specificity
MIMIC-II	CAD:267 NCAD:344 Total:611	89%	86%	90%
Local hospital	CAD:14 NCAD:15 Total:29	93%	92%	94%

In summary, for MIMIC-II 14% of CAD patients and 10% of non CAD patients were predicted wrongly and it is suspected that machine noises, motion artifacts etc. in MIMIC-II data (collected automatically at ICU setup), is the reason behind this relatively low classification accuracy Table 1. For the current work signal files of 611 patients were cleaned by visual inspection and some erroneous data may have remained. Thus, for a second level validation, the same model was validated on a controlled dataset of 29 patients collected from a local hospital (Sect. 3.1) and the increase in both sensitivity and specificity was 6% and 4% respectively. Joint analysis with consultant doctor revealed that the two misclassified patient out of 29, were diabetic, which possibly prevented the 100% correct classification.

The efficacy of the feature extraction and learning algorithm developed in the current work proved to be high as the model was trained using ICU data collected at USA and gave good results when evaluated on a hospital dataset in India.

5   Conclusion

In this work the issue of evidence based disease diagnosis is addressed on a large patient database taking CAD as an example disease.

On a set of patients labeled CAD/nonCAD, each having associated PPG waveform, wavelet transform was applied to generate wavelet coefficients at frequency ranges where peaks are often observed for cardiac patients. Statistical and entropy related features were extracted from coefficients and top contributing features were selected using MIC dimensionality reduction. Selected features were used to train SVM classifier and evaluate the classifier Performance. With no prior benchmark of CAD patient classification on MIMIC-II dataset, the above scheme classified MIMIC-II PPG signals labeled by ICD-9 code with 89% accuracy. Due to noisy nature of MIMIC-II data the scheme was re-evaluated on a doctor labeled hospital dataset resulting in 5% accuracy gain. The major contribution of the work is CAD diagnosis using easily obtainable PPG signal suitable in mobile/ wearable setting. The local hospital data does not have many samples and this is probably the scenario for many datasets and therefore, these datasets might not be suitable for training and validating machine learning algorithms. In this context, our present experiment shows that use of a pre-trained network (e.g., trained on MIMIC-II dataset) could be useful for the problem in hand. As significant time was spent in manual feature extraction, use of unsupervised feature extraction and transfer learning from MIMIC-II model will be explored for CAD diagnosis in future endeavors.

References

1. Kampouraki, A., et al.: Heartbeat time series classification with support vector Machines. IEEE Trans. Inf. Technol. Biomed. **13**(4), 512 (2009)
2. Mohamed, E.: On the analysis of fingertip photoplethysmogram signals. Curr. Cardiol. Rev. (2012). doi:10.2174/157340312801215782
3. Coronary artery disease. https://en.wikipedia.org/wiki/Coronary_artery_disease
4. Cardiac catheterisation and coronary angiography. http://www.nhs.uk/conditions/CoronaryAngiography/Pages/Introduction.aspx
5. MIMIC-II vs MIMIC-III. https://mimic.physionet.org/mimicdata/whatsnew/
6. Giri, D., et al.: Automated diagnosis of coronary artery disease affected patients using LDA, PCA, ICA discrete wavelet transform. Knowl. Based Syst. **37**, 274 (2013)
7. Kheder, G., et al.: HRV analysis using wavelet package transform and Least Square Support Vector Machine. Int. J. Circ. Syst. Sig. Process. **2**(1) (2008)
8. Reshef, D.V., et al.: Detecting novel associations in large datasets. Science. **334**(6062), 1518–1524 (2011)
9. Saeed et al.: Multiparameter Intelligent Monitoring in Intensive Care II (MIMIC-II): a public-access intensive care unit database **39**, 952–960 (2011). doi:10.1097/CCM.0b013e31820a92c6
10. The WFDB software package. https://www.physionet.org/physiotools/wfdb.shtml
11. Camm, et al.: Heart rate variability: standards of measurement, physiological interpretation, and clinical use. Circulation **93**, 1043–1065 (1996)
12. Daubechies, I.: Ten Lectures on Wavelets. Society for Industrial and Applied Mathematics, Philadelphia (1992)
13. Verleysen, M., François, D.: The curse of dimensionality in data mining and time series prediction. In: Cabestany, J., Prieto, A., Sandoval, F. (eds.) IWANN 2005. LNCS, vol. 3512, pp. 758–770. Springer, Heidelberg (2005). doi:10.1007/11494669_93
14. Cortes, C., Vapnik, V.: Networks, support-vector networks. Mach. Learn. **20**(3), 273–297 (1995). doi:10.1023/A:1022627411411

Data Mining of Intervention for Children with Autism Spectrum Disorder

Pratibha Vellanki[✉], Thi Duong, Dinh Phung, and Svetha Venkatesh

Pattern Recognition and Data Analytics, Deakin University, Waurn Ponds, Australia
pratibha.vellanki@research.deakin.edu.au

Abstract. Studying progress in children with autism spectrum disorder (ASD) is invaluable to therapists and medical practitioners to further the understanding of learning styles and lay a foundation for building personalised intervention programs. We use data of 283 children from an iPad based comprehensive intervention program for children with ASD. *Entry profiles* - based on characteristics of the children before the onset of intervention, and *performance profiles* - based on performance of the children on the intervention, are crucial to understanding the progress of the child. We present a novel approach toward this data by using mixed-variate restricted Boltzmann machine to discover entry and performance profiles for children with ASD. We then use these profiles to map the progress of the children. Our study is an attempt to address the dataset size and problem of mining and analysis in the field of ASD. The novelty lies in its approach to analysis and findings relevant to ASD.

1 Introduction

Autism Spectrum Disorder (ASD) is a neurodevelopmental disorder that onsets at an early age and limits the child's interaction with the world. It affects about 1% of the population globally [1]. The main areas that are affected due to ASD are cognition, sensory perception, language and communication, social relationships, and repetitive behaviors.

Children with ASD exhibit individual learning abilities and disabilities, resulting in a spectrum nature. This makes clustering children with ASD challenging. The conventional treatments are highly individualized, involve rigorous observation, data collection and analysis to determine and adapt the course of intervention. Moreover, for efficient intervention the children depend on the environmental setting with minimal distractions, and sensory profiles. Applied Behavioral Analysis (ABA) is the most popular conventional method that involves breaking single skills into smaller units and delivering the units in a structured manner till the skill is learnt [2]. While these methods are proven to be effective, they are time consuming and expensive: preparation of material and manual recording of data.

Of more importance are the opportunities wasted between diagnosis and the availability of therapists. It is suggested that the intervention for ASD shows desired effects when it is started at an early age [3]. Hence, there is a need

© ICST Institute for Computer Sciences, Social Informatics and Telecommunications Engineering 2017
K. Giokas et al. (Eds.): eHealth 2016, LNICST 181, pp. 376–383, 2017.
DOI: 10.1007/978-3-319-49655-9_45

for alternate treatment methods that can both fill in the waiting gap between diagnosis and intervention, and later append the one-on-one intervention time with the therapist.

Research suggests that computers may preferably be used to deliver therapy due control on the environment and their data recording capabilities. It has also been observed that children with ASD are likely to prefer computers as social discomfort, often common in ASD, may be avoided [4]. Our research picks up from this path and aims to help analyze and build possible techniques toward personalized intervention for children with ASD.

Data from children with ASD can be used for profiling them before beginning intervention on a computer-based program. Using data from a computer based application, Vellanki *et al.* [5] proposed using the age, the sex, and the performance of the child on a few fundamental skills at the onset of the intervention to determine *entry profiles*. We expand on this by additionally determining their *performance profile* using data from the children once they have progressed along the syllabus of the intervention. We then analyze their progress by observing their performance profiles with respect to where they were before intervention, determined by entry profiles. This is done by mapping the entry profiles onto their performance profiles. Our study not only gives a deeper understanding of the learning profile of children by tracking progress, but also lays the foundation for tailoring personalized syllabus.

In this study, we use the data collected from TOBY Playpad, an iPad-based comprehensive intervention program [6]. Data comprises 283 children who navigated through its structured syllabus consisting of 34 skills in four skill areas. The highly correlated and mixed-variate data also contains missing elements where the child is on the path to completion, making it challenging to deal with. This calls for complex techniques such as the mixed-variate restricted Boltzmann machines to integrate and model the data leading to the discovery of *entry* and *performance* profiles. Our sample size of our dataset is significantly larger than traditional ASD datasets [7] and to the best of our knowledge, such a data-based research is only possible for the first time due to the availability of computer-based applications.

In summary, the aims of this study are: (1) To discover entry profiles of a cohort taking intervention on TOBY Playpad, (2) To discover performance profiles of this cohort after they have made some progress on the syllabus, and (3) To qualitatively analyze and map the progress of the children from entry profiles to performance profiles.

2   Related Background

Patient profiling based on individual characteristics and the diagnosis is crucial in determining the course of medical intervention, especially for children with ASD. Each child with ASD exhibits highly individualised learning patterns and may show different results for standard procedures. It is hence of importance to (a) determine the entry profile for children with ASD and (b) to track their progress so a personalised course of intervention can be recommended. Research on discovering profiles among children with ASD and using them for administering interventions that cater to individual needs is contemporary [8]. We are driven by this novel problem and employ data from TOBY Playpad - an iPad application in implementing our ideas.

One of the main challenges with our data is that it is in a mixed-variate space and does not naturally integrate with traditional techniques for clustering. For example, sex, age, and performance on the skills of TOBY syllabus measured in terms of *Learn Units* (LU). Learn units are similar to count data in a document, thus enabling us to use a topic modelling based approach for discovering latent profiles. Tran *et al.* [9] propose a mixed variate restricted Boltzmann machine (MV.RBM) that integrates this type of data, which was successfully used to model chronic health data, in a similar setting [10].

Replicated Softmax is an undirected, two-layered, generative model of word counts that can be trained using Contrastive Divergence and is modelled using RBM [11]. Replicated Softmax smoothly integrates with the modelling of age and sex and can be modelled together using the mixed-variate RBM model.

3   Data Source and Dataset

TOBY Playpad [6] is a comprehensive iPad program that facilitates intervention for children with ASD, developed by a team of computer scientists and autism experts. It integrates independent learning and caregiver assistance in a regulated environment that allows recording data seamlessly on a structured syllabus. The hierarchical construction of the TOBY syllabus places fundamental skills at the top of the tree and releases complex skills one by one as the child masters skills along the syllabus tree. TOBY follows a predefined algorithmic criteria for prompting, reinforcement and mastering [6]. The structure of TOBY allows us to record learning in a controlled manner by keeping the ways in which the syllabus can be navigated and mastered fixed.

The simple units of teaching in TOBY are stimuli, response, prompt and reinforcement. Within each skill these four units are repeated until the skill is mastered. The TOBY iPad syllabus is divided into four categories: Imitation, Sensory, Expressive Language and Receptive language. Imitation (13 skills) involves video stimuli, and the child responds by emulating the action presented in the video. Sensory (3 skills) involves matching tasks with a visual stimulus (image) and response is selected from a set of three images presented. Expressive Language (9 skills) - learning how to speak words, involves visual stimulus and the child responds by vocalizing the label of the object. Receptive Language (9 skills) - learning the connection between words and visual representations in a reverse manner.

To quantify learning via TOBY, we use a measure called the Learn Unit (LU). A LU indicates number of stimulus - response pairs that the child requires to master each skill; higher number of LUs indicating increased difficulty faced by the child in the skill [5].

Users download TOBY onto their personal iPads and the learning occurs in the child's natural environment. The caretaker uploads the data recorded by TOBY onto a server[1]. This data is accessed and de-identified in a secure manner by the developers. The data consists of 283 children using TOBY for intervention. Children start using TOBY at random entry times and show progress based on their ability, and time spent on intervention. As a result, each child is at a different place in the intervention. The children who are a part of our study have undergone some progress - the child must have mastered at least one entry skill and another skill within the same category as the entry skill. Our data contains information on the age, sex and performance across the syllabus attempted for the child. The inter-quartile range of age of the children in this study is 1.58 to 9.75 years. Our dataset studies performance of 152 male and 44 female children; the caretakers of 87 children chose to withhold information about the child's sex.

We divide our data into two subsets: (1) entry profile data - contains the performance of the child on the entry skills of TOBY (first skill in each of the 4 skill categories) in terms of LU required to master, and the sex and the age of the child; (2) performance data - contains the LUs required to master all the skills in the syllabus attempted so far by the children.

4   Framework

We first discover entry profiles by modeling the sex, age and LUs required to master entry skills of the syllabus using MV.RBM [9]. We then model the LUs required to master all the skills attempted in the syllabus to discover performance profiles. For this study, we identify three data types to the multivariate visible units used in our research: *binary* for sex, *continuous* for age, and *Replicated Softmax* for LUs required to master skills [5].

One of the complexities of real data is that it consists of missing elements. Our data is complete in age but in the cases where the caretakers withheld information about the sex of the child, there are missing instances. Missing data also occurs when a child has not yet mastered certain skills in the syllabus. We deal with data missing in LUs by substituting zero for simplicity. We represent sex by two binary variables, one denoting if the child is male and the another variable denoting if a child female and when the sex of the child is unknown, the both these values take on zero. The latent posterior equation of RBM consists of the product term involving v_n, which results in the model to account for no statistics from the missing elements.

We use CD with a batch size of 100 children for learning the parameters. After 100 data sweeps posterior hidden units are extracted and clustered for similar profiles using K-means. In this manner, we obtain both entry profiles and performance profiles. We then use t-SNE, a dimensionality reduction technique, for visualizing the results in a two-dimensional space.

---

[1] This study is approved by the university ethics committee.

5 Results

We present the results of our experiment in three parts: entry profiles, performance profiles and their description, and mapping of entry profiles to performance. Mapping enables us to study how the members of the cohort diverge after progress on syllabus.

5.1 Entry Profiles

Figure 1 shows the discovered 5 *entry profiles* (EP). We describe the shared characteristics of the entry profiles before listing their specific properties.

Regarding the diversity in skills attempted, children in EP 1 and EP 2 mastered entry skills across most categories: at least 2 and at most from all 4 categories, followed by children in EP 4: at least 1 and at most 4. While children in EP 3 and EP 5 managed to master entry skills up to 3 categories.

With respect to the difficulties among entry skill from all categories, most children found Receptive most challenging (EP 1, EP 2, and EP 4) evident from the highest medians, followed by Sensory (EP 1 and EP 2) or Expressive (EP 4). Children from EP 3 and EP 5 did not master the Receptive and among the remaining 3 categories mastered, they found Sensory most difficult. It is interesting to observe that the discrepancy in the amount of work required (e.g. LUs) to master Sensory is most significant for all groups involved, followed by Receptive.

EP 1 (85 males) and EP 4 (44 females) found Imitation to be the least challenging - lowest LU accumulation. Within EP 4 the entry skills in all categories were found to be mastered by around uniform number of children.

EP 2 (58 children, sex unknown) and EP 3 (29 children, sex unknown) mastered Imitation and Expressive Language entry skills with the equally least efforts (lowest LUs). Within EP 3, the ability to master skills in these two categories is more uniform (evident by small interquartile in their LUs). Compared to EP 1, EP 2 achieved mastery in Receptive with lesser LUs. Distribution of LUs for EP 5 (67 males) bears similarity with that of EP3, however, the medians and the variances are much higher for EP 5, especially for Sensory.

5.2 Performance Profiles

Figure 2 shows the discovered 9 *performance profiles*. We observe that with an increase in complexity of the data the clusters are not well defined and they overlap often. We expect this behavior because ASD is a spectrum and well-defined clustering of the children is challenging. We describe the characteristics of the *performance profiles* (PP).

In a broader view, we observe that the children belonging to PP 1, PP 2, PP 7 and PP 8 have mastered 10 or fewer skills on the entire syllabus; children from PP 4 and PP 5 have mastered almost 20 skills; and children from PP 6 and PP 9 have mastered mostly 20 skills or more.

PP 1, PP 2, PP 7, and PP 8 consist of 30, 35, 47 and 40 children respectively. Sensory skills were mastered by most. The accumulated LU statistics shows a similar distribution for PP1, PP 2 and PP 7, Sensory being the most difficult to master, followed by Receptive Language when attempted. Compared to the other profiles, PP 7 and PP 8 have found Imitation difficult to master.

PP 4 and PP 5 consist of 18 and 35 children. They preferred Imitation and Sensory categories. PP 4 struggled and show little progress in the language skills - comparatively higher LUs in language areas than other skills.

PP 6 and PP 9 consist of 31 and 15 children and have mastered most skills. PP 6 found Receptive most difficult, followed by the Expressive. PP 9, on the other hand, found Receptive and Sensory most difficult. It is also observed that PP 9 struggled with the later skills of Imitation, which consist of learning oral

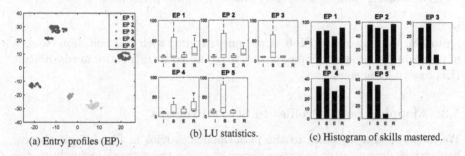

(a) Entry profiles (EP).   (b) LU statistics.   (c) Histogram of skills mastered.

Fig. 1. Entry Profiles and their group characteristics. Here, I - Imitation, S - Sensory, E - Expressive Language and R - Receptive Language are the skill categories. In the sub-figures (b) and (c) the y-axis shows LUs. Sub-fig (b) shows the boxplot of LUs acquired by children in each entry skill. Sub-fig (c) shows the number of children who mastered each entry skill.

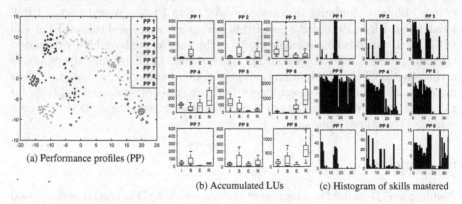

(a) Performance profiles (PP)

(b) Accumulated LUs   (c) Histogram of skills mastered

Fig. 2. Performance profiles and their group characteristics. Sub-fig (b) shows the boxplot of LUs acquired by children in skill category. Here the LUs under each category are accumulated for a category level analysis. Sub-fig (c) shows the number of children who mastered each of the 34 skills (x-axis).

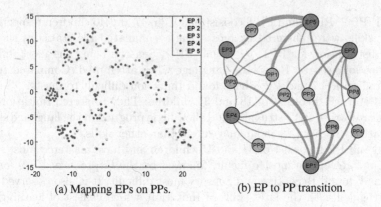

(a) Mapping EPs on PPs.   (b) EP to PP transition.

Fig. 3. Progress tracking using entry profiles (EP) and performance profiles (PP).

imitation, as compared to PP 6. A person struggling with oral imitation (sounds of vowels and consonants) subsequently may find vocalizing entire words difficult (Expressive Language).

5.3   Mapping Entry Profiles to Study Progress

We map the entry profiles to the performance profiles in Fig. 3a and observe how groups diverge after progress. Figure 3b shows the network highlighting the relationship between entry and performance profiles. Here the thickness of the connection denotes the probability of migration between a pair of entry and performance profiles.

We observed groups based on the patterns of migration: group 1 (EP 1 and EP 2), group 2 (EP 4) and group 3 (EP 3 and EP 5). The members of these groups also bore similarity in entry profiles. Group 1 transgressed toward PP 2, PP 3, PP 4, PP 5, PP 6, PP 8 and PP 9. Group 3 transitioned toward PP 1 and PP 7. EP 4, which is an all-female group, is the only one to have highly dispersed after the progress. These observations may be critical to determine the weakness and strengths of the children and adapt the intervention course based on their mapping. Medical practitioners might find this kind of analysis invaluable for gaining a deeper understanding of how different children with ASD behave on a standard structured syllabus.

6   Conclusion

Profiling and tracking the progress of children with ASD is crucial personalized intervention. The nuance in this study is possible due to the dataset we present, but at the same time dealing with heterogeneous, mix-variate, and highly correlated data with missing elements needs complex models. We present entry and performance profiles discovered using MV.RBM on a dataset of 283 children and map their progress after administering intervention. This helps us to observe how groups that are similar at the onset of the intervention react differently to the same syllabus. Our study of progress mediated by the discovery of entry profiles and performance profiles is, to the best of our knowledge, first of its kind. Followed up with predictive analysis, it can help recommend suitable intervention paths for children with ASD. Such an analysis might be invaluable to medical practitioners to furthering the understanding of learning patterns of children with ASD.

References

1. American Psychiatric Association. Diagnostic and statistical manual of mental disorders (DSM-5®). American Psychiatric Pub (2013)
2. Lovaas, O.: Behavioral treatment and normal educational and intellectual functioning in young autistic children. J. Consult. Clin. Psychol. **55**(1), 3–9 (1987)
3. Dawson, G., et al.: Early behavioral intervention, brain plasticity, and the prevention of autism spectrum disorder. Dev. Psychopathol. **20**(3), 775 (2008)
4. Hetzroni, O., Tannous, J.: Effects of a computer-based intervention program on the communicative functions of children with autism. J. Autism Dev. Disord. **34**(2), 95–113 (2004)
5. Vellanki, P., Phung, D., Duong, T., Venkatesh, S.: Learning entry profiles of children with autism from multivariate treatment information using restricted Boltzmann machines. In: Li, X.-L., Cao, T., Lim, E.-P., Zhou, Z.-H., Ho, T.-B., Cheung, D., Motoda, H. (eds.) PAKDD 2015. LNCS (LNAI), vol. 9441, pp. 245–257. Springer, Heidelberg (2015). doi:10.1007/978-3-319-25660-3_21
6. Venkatesh, S., Phung, D., Duong, T., Greenhill, S., Adams, B.: TOBY: early intervention in autism through technology. In: Proceedings of the SIGCHI, pp. 3187–3196. ACM (2013)
7. Peters-Scheffer, N., Didden, R., Korzilius, H., Sturmey, P.: A meta-analytic study on the effectiveness of comprehensive aba-based early intervention programs for children with autism spectrum disorders. Res. Autism Spectr. Disord. **5**(1), 60–69 (2011)
8. Garnett, M.S., Attwood, T., Peterson, C., Kelly, A.B.: Autism spectrum conditions among children and adolescents: a new profiling tool. Aust. J. Psychol. **65**(4), 206–213 (2013)
9. Tran, T., Phung, D., Venkatesh, S.: Mixed-variate restricted Boltzmann machines. In: Proceedings of the 3rd ACML, pp. 213–229 (2011)
10. Nguyen, T.D., Tran, T., Phung, D., Venkatesh, S.: Latent patient profile modelling and applications with mixed-variate restricted Boltzmann machine. In: Pei, J., Tseng, V.S., Cao, L., Motoda, H., Xu, G. (eds.) PAKDD 2013. LNCS (LNAI), vol. 7818, pp. 123–135. Springer, Heidelberg (2013). doi:10.1007/978-3-642-37453-1_11
11. Hinton, G.E., Salakhutdinov, R.: Replicated softmax: an undirected topic model. In: NIPS, pp. 1607–1614 (2009)

From Wellness to Medical Diagnostic Apps: The Parkinson's Disease Case

Stefan Kueppers[1,2]($\boxtimes$), Ioannis Daskalopoulos[1], Ashwani Jha[3],
Nikos F. Fragopanagos[4], Panagiotis Kassavetis[3,6], Effrosyni Nomikou[5],
Tabish Saifee[3], John C. Rothwell[3], Kailash Bhatia[3], Marco U. Luchini[2],
Marco Iannone[4], Theano Moussouri[3,5], and George Roussos[1]

[1] Birkbeck College, University of London, London, UK
stefan@dcs.bbk.ac.uk
[2] Benchmark Performance Ltd., London, UK
[3] University College London, London, UK
[4] re:technica Ltd., London, UK
[5] Audience Focus Ltd., London, UK
[6] Boston University, Boston, USA

Abstract. This paper presents the design and development of the
CloudUPDRS app and supporting system developed as a Class I medical device to assess the severity of motor symptoms for Parkinson's
Disease. We report on lessons learnt towards meeting fidelity and regulatory requirements; effective procedures employed to structure user context and ensure data quality; a robust service provision architecture; a
dependable analytics toolkit; and provisions to meet mobility and social
needs of people with Parkinson's.

1 Introduction

It is well understood that modern smartphones present unique opportunities for
mobile healthcare. Indeed, there are numerous wellness and self-tracking apps
readily available in all major mobile phone platform markets and many more
have been developed to conduct research in various aspects of mobile telecare.
Yet, the vast majority of these apps do not conform to the safety, quality, performance and regulatory requirements set for medical devices and as such they
can only be employed either to encourage a healthy lifestyle or for research purposes correspondingly, but are not tools for medical diagnosis. This fact is often
explicitly reflected in their terms and conditions of use for example, quoting
from a popular Parkinson's Disease app, the developers state that "we cannot,
and thus we do not, guarantee or promise that you will personally receive any
direct benefits." In contrast to this situation, this paper presents the design and
development of the CloudUPDRS app and its associated information management and analytics platform, which meets the standards set for medical devices.
In particular, we describe how CloudUPDRS achieves the accurate, precise, and
repeatable assessment of motor symptoms for people with Parkinson's (PwP),

© ICST Institute for Computer Sciences, Social Informatics and Telecommunications Engineering 2017
K. Giokas et al. (Eds.): eHealth 2016, LNICST 181, pp. 384–389, 2017.
DOI: 10.1007/978-3-319-49655-9_46

which clinicians can use with confidence. The app is currently undergoing examination by the Medicines and Healthcare products Regulatory Agency (MHRA) in the UK towards its full registration as a medical device.

The successful development and operational deployment of the CloudUP-DRS app and its supporting service at the level required to achieve conformal performance to medical device regulations, thus establishing it as a valuable diagnostic tool for clinicians, demanded that we address several key problems. In this paper we present the key contributions of this work towards achieving this goal. Specifically, we describe:

- How to effectively combine a guided data collection procedure imposed by the app to provide structured user context, with a fully automated signal processing pipeline thus making possible the unsupervised but consistent interpretation of sensor data captured during the performance of motor assessment activities.
- The development of a data analytics toolkit for the assessment of tremor, bradykinesia and gait measurements following the MDS Unified Parkinson's Disease Rating Scale, the standard clinical tool for the diagnosis of PD.
- The development of an information management, data mining and dashboard service developed following the concept of microservices and the lambda architecture, incorporating stream and batch processing pathways to ensure scale out performance and responsiveness.

2   Background and Rationale

PD symptoms are typically caused by the loss of neurones that produce dopamine, a key chemical messenger in the brain, decreased levels of which lead to abnormal brain activity (cf. [1] for more details). Care for patients with PD involves the management of both motor and non-motor symptoms as well as palliative care.

Since symptoms vary greatly independent of treatment and PD progresses at different rates in different individuals, it requires regular clinical monitoring and medication adjustment. Monitoring and adjustment however require hospital visits and assessment under the standard Movement Disorders Society's Unified Parkinson's Disease Rating Scale (MDS-UPDRS) [2]. Due to these constraints, such reviews are relatively infrequent, carried out typically only a few times per year. This in turn limits opportunities to precisely quantify PD progression and the effectiveness of patient stratification [8]: the restricted availability of data concerning individual variability and actual symptom trends limit opportunities to adapt care to the needs of a particular individual at a specific time.

Indeed, it is possible to employ certain aspects of movement that are disrupted in Parkinson's as surrogate biomarkers of dopamine levels and in fact this is precisely the purpose of Part III of the MDS-UPDRS. Further pursuing this insight, in [3] we investigated the possibility to precisely quantify and implement the MDS-UPDRS methodology as a smartphone app to enable the assessment of motor performance through tremor, gait and bradykinesia measurements

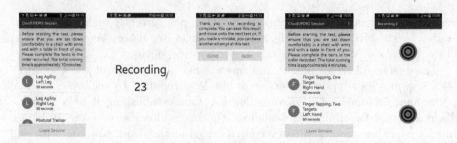

Fig. 1. Views of the user interface of the CloudUPDRS app showing session management, tremor recording and finger tapping activities.

obtained from standard sensors embedded in smartphones within a clinical setting. By adopting this approach, we also intend to capture in-depth medical intelligence supporting the discovery of longitudinal trends, promoting deeper understanding of the patterns of normal daily symptom variations, and predicting the onset of dyskinesias thus facilitating high-precision personalised targeting of treatment.

3   The CloudUPDRS App

As discussed in the previous section, in [3] we demonstrate the feasibility of using smartphones as a means to assess commonly occurring motor symptoms of PD in a clinical setting. Specifically, we designed, developed and validated in a field study a prototype app on Android implementing Part III of the MDS-UPDRS. Using the accelerometer and touch screen sensors commonly available in modern smartphones, we are able to carry out hand and leg tremor measurements, as well as gait and bradykinesia assessments using finger tapping tasks to replicate the majority of these tests. In [3] tests were administered by an experienced clinician in the lab using an HTC Desire device and the collected sensor data were extracted and processed using standard biomedical data analysis software. Participants were also tested in the same areas of motor performance using the standard lab procedure outlined in MDS-UPDRS and using bespoke biomedical data acquisition equipment to obtain a baseline for comparing the performance of the app.

In CloudUPDRS we employ the data collection and analysis techniques described in [3] to develop an app with extended functionality that enables its independent but dependable use by PwP and their carers at home and in their communities. The app implements a comprehensive work-flow partially depicted in Fig. 1, which provides audio, video and textual guidance on how to conduct the actions required by the tests and automatically adapts to match the specifications of its host device. The app is also provisioned with a delay tolerant background service to manage session data that ensures that information is safely submitted for further processing to a supporting online service also developed specifically to provide this function and described in more detail in Sect. 4 below.

Overall, the CloudUPDRS system consists of the following elements:

1. PD patient smartphone apps for Android and iOS that carry out motor performance measurements and wellness self-assessment; conduct session management; securely transfer captured data to the CloudUPDRS service; and, present an interface providing guidance and feedback.
2. Cloud-based scalable data collection engine that safely and securely collects data from patients' smartphones; ensures secure data management; and applies the MDS-UPDRS processing pipeline.
3. Data-mining toolkit for medical intelligence incorporating quantitative and semi-structured data, and longitudinal analyses, clustering and classification; and a clinical user interface incorporating visualisation.

4   The CloudUPDRS Service Platform

The CloudUPDRS service platform enables the secure capture, management and analysis of data collected by the app and provides effective communication of insights generated to clinicians enabling them to explore alternative treatment scenarios. To cater for the diverse needs of the PwP population in the UK, the platform has been engineered to facilitate scalable performance by adopting the microservices architecture [9]. The microservices architectural style is set in contrast to traditional monolithic web applications and aims to maximise opportunities for vertical decomposition and scaling-out, which are critical for high performance and service resilience in data intensive situations.

In CloudUPDRS, microservices are loosely coupled and employ lightweight communication and coordination mechanisms such as the Consumer-Driven Contract pattern and implemented on Apache Thrift (cf. https://thrift.apache.org/) selected due to its highly efficient and compact protocol structure. System componentization follows the design displayed in Fig. 2, enforced via versioning of published RESTful interfaces. CloudUPDRS microservices are deployed as docker containers (cf. https://www.docker.com/) although internal implementation details vary to match the specific preferences and expertise of project partners responsible for their implementation and their suitability for the task in hand. For example, while the data collection and signal processing APIs are implemented using python and django REST within an nginx/gunicorn container, semi-structured longitudinal analytics are implemented as Ruby bundles.

Finally, the service platform has been designed with the expectation that in order to meet performance metrics for its interactive features at full operation scale it will require the on the fly integration of archived information from its longitudinal datastore with real-time streams captured for example during concurrent patient consultations. To facilitate this modus operandi, we have structured workflows implemented through microservices following the lambda architecture [7], which provides an intuitive model for the fusion of both types of data on the fly.

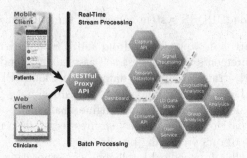

Fig. 2. CloudUPDRS microservices implementing the lambda architecture.

5   Lessons Learnt and Conclusions

Bounded Context. The pervasive computing community has invested significant effort in techniques for modelling and adapting to user context, which is critical for the interpretation of sensor data streams. This role for context was re-confirmed in our work and in the case of the Intel/Fox Foundation project. Yet, when context modelling is not possible or incurs prohibitively high costs, an effective alternative is to bound context by imposing structure and thus predictability to user actions during sensing, an approach that was successfully applied with the CloudUPDRS app. Guided user experiences can contain the degrees of freedom possible and as a consequence the computation of motor performance indicators becomes consistent and repeatable.

Choice of Analytics. Recent years have also witnessed the rapid growth of machine learning methods for sensed data as an active area of research. While there are clearly situations when the development of new algorithms and techniques is required, in other cases there seems to be good reason to opt for a more traditional approach. In CloudUPDRS we discovered that in full-scale operational systems predictability and consistency of algorithmic performance obtained through extensive experience with the tradeoffs related in tuning machine learning techniques, may be more valuable than higher but vacillating performance.

Data Quality. Data quality in pervasive computing has often been investigated by considering specific stages of the processing pipeline in isolation. In CloudUP-DRS rather than optimise individual stages we engineer an end-to-end quality assurance strategy that we find to be more effective. It incorporates features of the user experience, which permit the user to initiate the repeat of tests when an external event has disrupted the session, to increasing the duration of individual tests so as to enable oversampling and cross-validation, to employing heuristics that allow us to quickly identify data quality problems in the captured signal. We find that it is the combination of these features rather than any single one alone that helps ensure a higher quality of data.

Certification. The higher standard of evidence demanded for the registration of an app as a conforming medical device has significant resource implications. Indeed, it is not surprising for development costs to be an order of magnitude higher than those of an equivalent research project. The need for formal quality assurance processes in particular adds considerable overheads. Consequently, it appears judicious to recognise commercial considerations from the earliest stages of the process.

Microservices Architecture. Although our experience in this area is incomplete, claims in favour of architectures build around microservices appear justified, especially for sensor data streaming mobile systems with execution profiles similar to CloudUPDRS. Adoption of this approach has allowed greater flexibility during development, facilitated easy scaling-out of the service, and enabled the development team to gain operational experience and hence effectively evolve system features and performance.

In this paper we presented the design and development of the CloudUPDRS app which has achieved Class I medical device conformity and we presented key findings and techniques that helped us achieve this goal.

Acknowledgments. Project CloudUPDRS: Big Data Analytics for Parkinson's Disease patient stratification is supported by Innovate UK (Project Number 102160). The project partners would also like to thank Parkinson's UK for providing access to their online forums and assisting with the recruitment of survey participants.

References

1. European Brain Council: Parkinson's disease Fact Sheet (2011)
2. Goetz, C.G., et al.: Movement disorder society-sponsored revision of the unified Parkinson's disease rating scale (MDS-UPDRS): scale presentation and clinimetric testing results. Mov. Disorders **23**(15), 2129–2170 (2008)
3. Kassavetis, P., Saifee, T.A., Roussos, G., Drougkas, L., Kojovic, M., Rothwell, J.C., Edwards, M.J., Bhatia, K.P.: Developing a tool for remote digital assessment of Parkinson's disease. Mov. Disorders J. **3**, 59–64 (2015)
4. Martin, E.: Novel method for stride length estimation with body area network accelerometers. In: IEEE Topical Conference in Biomedical Wireless Technologies, Networks, and Sensing Systems (BioWireleSS), pp. 79–82 (2011)
5. Martin, E., Shia, V., Bajcsy, R.: Determination of a patient's speed and stride length minimizing hardware requirements. In: Proceedings of International Conference on Body Sensor Networks, pp. 144–149 (2011)
6. Marx, V.: Human phenotyping on a population scale. Nat. Methods **12**, 711–714 (2015)
7. Marz, N., Warren, J.: Big Data: Principles and Best Practices of Scalable Realtime Data Systems. Manning Publications, New York (2013)
8. Matthews, P.M., Edison, P., Geraghty, O.C., Johnson, M.R.: The emerging agenda of stratified medicine in neurology. Nat. Rev. **10**, 15–27 (2014)
9. Newman, S., Microservices, B.: Designing Fine-Grained Systems. O'Reilly Media, Sebastopol (2015)
10. Schapira, A.H.V., Emre, M., Jenner, P., Poewe, W.: Levodopa in the treatment of Parkinson's disease. Eur. J. Neurol. **16**, 982–989 (2009)

CardioFit: Affordable Cardiac Healthcare Analytics for Clinical Utility Enhancement

Arijit Ukil[1](✉), Soma Bandyopadhyay[1], Chetanya Puri[1],
Rituraj Singh[1], Arpan Pal[1], and K.M. Mandana[2]

[1] Innovation Lab, Tata Consultancy Services,
Ecospace, Rajarahat, Kolkata 700156, India
{arijit.ukil,soma.bandyopadhyay,chetanya.puri,
singh.rituraj,arpan.pal}@tcs.com
[2] Cardiothoracic and Vascular Surgery Department, Fortis Healthcare Limited,
Kolkata, India
kmmandana@gmail.com

Abstract. In this paper, we present CardioFit, a completely noninvasive cardiac condition monitoring system that enhances the clinical utility of health care analytics like lowering false detection of cardiac arrhythmia condition, higher accuracy in heart rate variability (HRV) computation. It performs powerful local analysis to enable accurate as well as easy-to-use, round-the-clock in-house, remote or mobile cardiac health checking. Here, photoplethysmogram (PPG) is the sole physiological signal considered for cardiac health management. It is to be noted that PPG carries significant necessary features what is available from electrocardiogram (ECG) signal. Unlike ECG, extraction of PPG is noninvasive, easy and affordable using smartphone or other low cost sensors. However, PPG is frequently contaminated with various kinds of motion artifacts and noise. Our robust concoction of signal processing and machine learning techniques exhibit higher accuracy in the detection and removal of the corrupt PPG signal segments. The proposed mechanism substantially improves the detection capability of the cardiac condition. Efficacy of our scheme is depicted using publicly available MIT-Physionet database as well as through our own field-collected real-life PPG data.

1 Introduction, Motivation and Contribution

Cardio-vascular disease is one of the biggest killers as per American Heart Association [1]. However, cardio-vascular diseases are preventable and early detection would effectively avert untimely human life loss. There are number of challenges that need to be overcome for delivering less error-prone cardiac condition detection. First of all, PPG extracted through smartphone, pulse oximeter or wearable sensor is often corrupted with ambient noise, motion artifacts and other noise sources. Even the warning systems in hospital ICU (Intensive Care Unit) are prone to transient noise [2], which leads to high number of false alarms [2, 3]. In fact, high false negatives (higher undetected cardiac conditions) would be deadly to the patients [4].

© ICST Institute for Computer Sciences, Social Informatics and Telecommunications Engineering 2017
K. Giokas et al. (Eds.): eHealth 2016, LNICST 181, pp. 390–396, 2017.
DOI: 10.1007/978-3-319-49655-9_47

We claim that our proposed method, CardioFit has the potential to eliminate the corrupt PPG segments with higher accuracy that minimizes the false negatives in the decision process. Another advantage is that the infrastructure requirement of CardioFit is nominal (only smart phone or other smart wearables suffice) and due to its completeness with local analytics, users can check health condition locally and can consult specialists remotely whenever required. Novelty of our proposed scheme is to reduce the number of false alarms in the detection of cardiac anomaly conditions like arrhythmia to a larger extent. Our uniqueness of the proposed scheme is that we analyze only PPG signal to interpret the heart condition whereas most of the state-of-the art solutions consider ECG, arterial blood pressure (ABP), and other pressure signals along with PPG [4–6]. CardioFit enhances the clinical utility significantly through effective corruption removal from PPG. Our method consists of supervised machine learning along with biomedical signal processing and information theoretic techniques. We use Morphologically Adaptable Dynamic Time Warping (MADTW), similarity based morphological pattern analysis for detecting and removing the corrupted signal segments [8]. It helps to detect an efficient and effective cardiac health monitoring like arrhythmia estimation and classification, accurate heart rate variability computation. CardioFit is sufficiently generic for implementing in wearable sensors, smart watches, smart phones, PC workstations, ICU monitors and ambulances; wherever PPG signal is available.

We organize our paper as follows. In Sect. 2, we describe the system architecture and present the CardioFit scheme and algorithms. The results demonstrating the efficacy of our proposed scheme are presented in Sect. 3. Finally, we conclude in Sect. 4.

2 CardioFit: Scheme and Algorithms

CardioFit consists of five main functional blocks: 1. *Raw PPG signal extraction*: It is done using smart phones, pulse oximeter or other sensors, [7] 2. *Multistage decorruption*: Mono-signal PPG corruption detection and elimination, 3. *Cardiac-parameter extraction*: Heart Rate (HR) is extracted using robust signal processing technique [8], 4. *Statistical Analysis*: To investigate the statistical trend of the cardiac-parameters for cardiac abnormality, 5. *Decision*: To decide the normality and abnormality of the heart condition along with detecting arrhythmia aiming low false negative alarms.

PPG signals extracted from smart phones or other wearables contain high amount of corruption particularly due to motion artifacts. Directly processing such noisy and corrupted signal invariably results in false alarms. In order to minimize such false alarms, we propose multi-stage decorruption.

2.1 Multi-stage Decorruption of PPG Signal

We classify the corruption in PPG as: 1. Extremas and 2. Intricates, where extremas are the corruptions due to larger, transient disturbance and intricates are due to smaller, mostly prolonged disturbances as shown in Fig. 1.

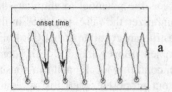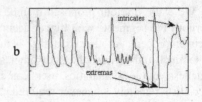

a   b

Fig. 1. PPG signal (a), ideal or expected, (b) as extracted from camera or other sensors

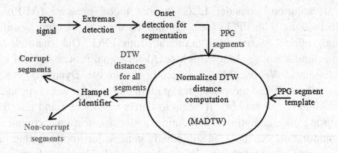

Fig. 2. Complete process of our proposed CardioFit multistage PPG decorruption

Extrema detection. We apply extreme value statistics and consider modified Thompson Tau technique [11, 17], to statistically find the extremas.

Intricate detection. PPG signal consists of series of segments $\Omega_k, k = 1, 2, \ldots K$ and each segment (Fig. 1a) identifies a single complete heart beat. Segmentation or pulse period detection of PPG signal is achieved by identifying the onset times through slope-adjusting and realigning through weighted slope sum function (SSF) [9]. In order to compute the intricate corruptions in each PPG segment Ω_k, Dynamic Time Warping (DTW) with modification (Morphologically Adaptable DTW (MADTW)) is applied. We normalize each segment as $\Omega_k \to \Omega_k \times \frac{max(\mathbb{T})}{max(\Omega_k)}$, where $\mathbb{T}$ is a typical PPG segment template, following the derivation of the most probable segment length [8, 15]. DTW distance $\delta_{\Omega_k, \mathbb{T}}$ is computed between the PPG segment template $\mathbb{T} = \{t_1, t_2, \ldots, t_M\}$ of length M and normalized segments $\Omega_k = \{\omega_1, \omega_2, \ldots, \omega_{l_p}\}_k, k \in K$ of the extracted PPG segments as:

$$\delta_{\Omega_k, \mathbb{T}} = \delta([\omega_1, \omega_2, \ldots, \omega_{l_p}], [t_1, t_2, \ldots, t_M])$$

$$= \mathcal{D}(\omega_{l_p}, t_M) + min \begin{cases} ([\omega_1, \omega_2, \ldots, \omega_{l_{p-1}}], [t_1, t_2, \ldots, t_{M-1}]) \\ \\ ([\omega_1, \omega_2, \ldots, \omega_{l_{p-1}}], [t_1, t_2, \ldots, t_M]) \end{cases}$$

where, $\mathcal{D}(\omega, t) = Eucl(\omega, t) := \sqrt{\sum_{i=1}^{N} (\omega_i - t_i)^2}$, $\delta_{\Omega_k, \mathbb{T}}\big|_{corrupt}(\approx 7.8) \gg$
$\delta_{\Omega_k, \mathbb{T}}\big|_{normal}(\approx 1.5)$.

We apply Hampel filter [10, 14] on the computed DTW distances of each PPG segment $(\delta_{\Omega_k,T}), k = 1, 2, 3, \ldots$. When Hampel identifier declares certain DTW distances among $\delta_{\Omega_k,T}$ outlier, the corresponding PPG segment(s) is declared as corrupt. Proposed multistage decorruption technique of PPG is shown in Fig. 2.

3 Experimental Methodology and Results

We have collected real-field PPG data from 10 healthy subjects with uniform distribution (5 males and 5 females) through pulse-oximeter by controlled experiments like five different motion artifacts (a. finger twist, b. light hand movement, c. medium hand movement, d. hard hand movement, e. body movement) to simulate the near real-life noise and artifacts, which are annotated as shown in Fig. 3. First we validate our proposed corruption removal method on this real-field PPG signal. In Fig. 4, we illustrate an exemplary scenario of corruption detection on real-field data. We have also performed extensive experiments with publicly available MIT-Physionet data [13], where the annotations are made through a majority voting process. In Table 1, we depict the overall average performance merit of both real-field as well as MIT-Physionet data in terms of precision $= \frac{TP}{TP+FP}$, recall $= \frac{TP}{TP+FN}$, and specificity $= \frac{TN}{TN+FP}$, where TP, TN, FN, FP = Total number of true positives, true negatives, false negatives, false positives respectively.

We compare the performance of CardioFit with standard method (SM), the method that does not execute corruption removal as shown in Fig. 5, where PPG signals with 5 types of motion artifacts are considered. First, we show that the computation of HRV (Heart Rate Variability), an important cardiac health marker does not vary much from ground truth (HRV derived from uncorrupted PPG) while comparing CardioFit against standard method (Fig. 6). HRV is calculated by SDNN method which is the standard deviation of NN intervals (beat-to-beat interval) [12]. We observe that Mean Absolute Deviation (MAD) with respect to ground truth of HRV computation for CardioFit = 0.34, whereas for standard method it is =36.5. It is to be noted that standard

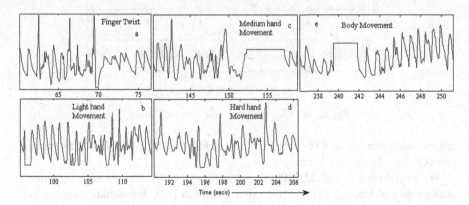

Fig. 3. Different kinds of artifacts (showing five different artifacts) in PPG signal

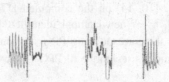

Fig. 4. Corrupt PPG segment (marked red) detection from real field PPG data (Color figure online)

Table 1. Corruption detection performance on MIT-Physionet

Performance metric	Value (%)
Recall	80.4
Specificity	96.4

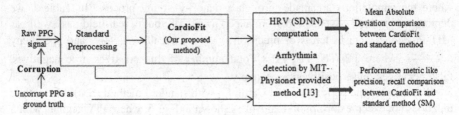

Fig. 5. Performance comparison method between CardioFit and standard method

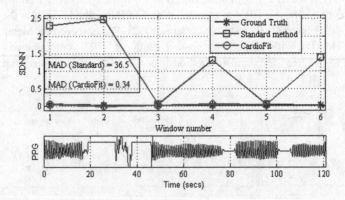

Fig. 6. HRV computation efficacy of CardioFit

preprocessing consists of 1 Hz drift suppression, followed by 30 Hz Low pass filtering with 0.5–4 Hz band pass filtering.

We experimented with MIT-Physionet challenge 2015 datasets with arrhythmia annotations and basic arrhythmia detection algorithm [13]. We demonstrate the performance of detection of bradycardia as shown in Table 2. We find that false negatives

Table 2. Cardiac arrhythmia (bradycardia) detection performance comparison

Performance metric (%)	SM (Bradycardia)	CardioFit (Bradycardia) [8]
Precision	66	62
Recall	97	100

from CardioFit are consistently proved to be very low (i.e. recall is very high → 100%), with comparable precision value [8].

4 Future Works and Conclusion

Our effort is to bring a newer dimension in cardiac-signal analytics with robust machine learning, signal processing, and statistical analysis based algorithms. We endeavor to contribute for minimization of the errors in the diagnosis of cardiac-related diseases that arise owing to the corruption in the physiological signals like PPG derived from smartphone and other affordable sensing devices. We claim that the novel de-corrupting techniques applied on PPG signals have the potential to minimize the false detection of cardiac abnormality conditions that ensures significant clinical utility enhancement. Thus, we establish CardioFit as an affordable, easy-to-use cardiac healthcare analytics tool. We endeavor to extend CardioFit to include other related cardiovascular diseases like angina and myocardial infarction, cardiomyopathy, congenital heart failure etc., along with robust feature detection [16].

References

1. www.heart.org/HEARTORG/General/Cardiac-Arrest-Statistics_UCM_448311_Article.jsp
2. Ganeshapillai, G., Guttag, J.: Real time reconstruction of quasiperiodic multiparameter physiological signals. EURASIP J. Adv.Signal. Process. (2012)
3. Deshmane, A.V.: False arrhythmia alarm suppression using ECG, ABP, and Photoplethysmogram. M.S Thesis, Massachusetts Institute of Technology (2009)
4. Aboukhalil, A., Nielsen, L., Saeed, M., Mark, R.G., Clifford, G.D.: Reducing false alarm rates for critical arrhythmias using the arterial blood pressure waveform. J. Biomed. Inform. **41**(3), 442–451 (2008)
5. Li, Q., Rajagopalan, C., Clifford, G.D.: Ventricular fibrillation and tachycardia classification using a machine learning approach. IEEE TBME **61**(6), 1607–1613 (2014)
6. Lin, W., Zhang, H., Zhang, Y.T.: Investigation on cardiovascular risk prediction using physiological parameters. Hindawi J. Comput. Math. Methods Med. (2013)
7. Banerjee, R., Ghose, A., Choudhury, A.D., Sinha, A., Pal, A.: Noise cleaning and Gaussian modeling of smart phone photoplethysmogram to improve blood pressure estimation. In: IEEE ICASSP, pp. 967–971 (2015)
8. Ukil, A., Bandyopadhyay, S., Puri, C., Pal, A.: Heart-trend: an affordable heart condition monitoring system exploiting morphological pattern. In: ICASSP (2016)
9. Zong, W., Heldt, T., Moody, G.B., Mark, R.G.: An open-source algorithm to detect onset of arterial blood pressure pulses. In: IEEE CINC, pp. 259–262 (2003)

10. Ukil, A., Bandyopadhyay, S., Pal, A.: IoT data compression: sensor-agnostic approach. In: IEEE DCC, pp. 303–312 (2015)
11. Bandyopadhyay, S., Ukil, A., Puri, C., Pal, A., Singh, R. Bose, T.: Demo: IAS: information analytics for sensors. In: 13th ACM Sensys (2015)
12. Misra, A., Banerjee, R., Choudhury, A.D., Sinha, A. Pal, A.: Novel peak detection to estimate HRV using smartphone audio. In: IEEE BSN (2015)
13. http://www.physionet.org/challenge/2015/. Accessed 12 Feb 2016
14. Ukil, A., Bandyopadhyay, S., Pal, A.: Sensitivity inspector: detecting privacy in smart energy applications. In: IEEE Symposium on Computers and Communication (ISCC) (2014)
15. Puri, C., Ukil, A., Bandyopadhyay, S., Singh, R., Pal, A., Mandana, K.M.: iCarMa: inexpensive cardiac arrhythmia management – an IoT healthcare analytics solution. In: IEEE Mobisys Workshop on IoT of Health (2016). (in Press)
16. Bandyopadhyay, S., Ukil, A., Puri, C., Singh, R., Pal, A. Mandana, K.M., Murthy, C.A.: An unsupervised learning for robust cardiac feature derivation from PPG signals. In: IEEE EMBC (2016). (in Press)
17. Bandyopadhyay, S., Ukil, A., Puri, C., Singh, R., Bose, T., Pal, A.: SensIPro: smart sensor analytics for Internet of Things. In: IEEE ISCC (2016). (in Press)

Design Fictions: A Tool for Debating Societal, Legal and Ethical Aspects of Personal and Pervasive Health Systems

Emmanuel Tsekleves[1(✉)], Andy Darby[1], Anna Whicher[2],
and Piotr Swiatek[2]

[1] Lancaster University, The LICA Building, Bailrigg, Lancaster LA1 4YW, UK
{e.tsekleves,a.darby}@lancaster.ac.uk
[2] Cardiff Metropolitan University, Llandaff Campus, Western Ave.,
Cardiff CF5 2YB, UK
{awhicher,pswiatek}@cardiffmet.ac.uk

Abstract. The potential benefits offered by health-related technologies are counterpoised by the societal, legal and ethical challenges concomitant with the pervasive monitoring of people necessitated by such technological interventions. Through the ProtoPolicy research project we explored the production and use of design fictions as a tool for debating the societal, legal and ethical dimensions of personal health systems. Two design fictions were co-created and tested in a series of design workshops with community groups based in Lancashire and Cornwall, UK. A thematic analysis of a debate among older people from the Lancaster group on the Smart Object Therapist design fiction highlighted societal and ethical issues relevant to personal health system design. We conclude that ethics like 'usability' may be usefully based on engagement with directly or indirectly implicated publics and should not be designed into innovation by experts alone.

Keywords: Design fiction · Speculative design · Personal health systems · Legal and ethics · Pervasive healthcare

1 Introduction

As the ageing population of the world is increasing, so is the pace and range of technological innovation to support healthcare in our later lives. In the effort to develop the ageing well agenda, the research and business communities are exploring and developing personal health systems, with the aim of supporting independent and assisted living, and governments are introducing policies that reinforce 'ageing in place' [1]. However, the health-related benefits offered by technology (e.g. independency, better quality care) are counterweighted by the societal, legal and ethical challenges concomitant with the pervasive monitoring of people necessitated by the relevant technologies [2]. There is a need, therefore, for facilitating public engagement and discussion on the social, legal and ethical issues arising from current and, more crucially, emergent technologies in personal and pervasive health systems, and for facilitating an interaction and debate between policy makers and citizens.

© ICST Institute for Computer Sciences, Social Informatics and Telecommunications Engineering 2017
K. Giokas et al. (Eds.): eHealth 2016, LNICST 181, pp. 397–403, 2017.
DOI: 10.1007/978-3-319-49655-9_48

In light of the above we present in this paper the ProtoPolicy research project and posit the use of design fictions as a tool for debating the societal, legal and ethical dimensions of personal health systems. ProtoPolicy was an exploratory pilot research project that ran from June to September 2015[1]. The ProtoPolicy team adopted an inclusive, collaborative and creative approach to engage a range of stakeholders across community groups and Westminster to examine how design fictions could be used to imagine the future implications of political decision-making.

2 Related Work

With an increasing use of personal and pervasive technologies, citizens are becoming data .producers and more knowledgeable about their own health. However, citizen awareness of the level of information sharing and storage garnered in their use of personal health technologies is often low [3]. Several of the new personal health systems available offer self-health management, independent and assisted living and community healthcare benefits. They often rely on personal health data and pervasive monitoring of patients raising many ethical, legal and societal issues, which manifest as both opportunities and challenges [4–7]. The eHealth Action Plan 2012–2020 [8] highlights that patient and public engagement and trust in the ethical, legal and socially considerate use of data is key to leveraging the potential of new technologies. More-over, policy-makers in public health and other sectors are realising the interconnections between decisions in their domains. Increased participation is an ethical and societal opportunity and one increasingly valued in regulatory and legal frameworks [9]. Therefore, there is a need for processes and tools that enable and facilitate the participation of citizens and policy makers in open debate on the social, legal and ethical complexities arising from technological intervention in personal and pervasive health systems, such as smart homes and assisted living environments.

In this paper we propose design fictions as a potential tool for facilitating citizen participation in the social, ethical and legal debates relevant to emergent technologies in healthcare. Speculative design is an approach enabling us to think about the future prospectively and critically [10]. One of its principal assumptions is the negation of the status quo and initiation of a discussion on possible worlds through confrontation with tangible object or process, the so-called design fiction. Speculative design uses design thinking tools and methodologies such as scenarios, brainstorming and rapid proto-typing along with techniques borrowed from art, literature, film, psychology, philos-ophy, anthropology and ecology to create design fictions – provocations or 'narrative elements to envision and explain possible futures for design' [11].

Design fiction is about creative provocation, raising questions, innovation, and exploration [12].' Design fictions go beyond that 'to account for the ways in which cinematic depictions of future technologies demonstrate to large public audiences a technology's need, viability and benevolence' [13]. Therefore one of the key values of design fiction is that is uses a fictional paradigm to catalyse debate about potential

---

[1] See http://imagination.lancs.ac.uk/activities/ProtoPolicy.

futures. As a speculative design practice design fictions do not claim to predict the future; they place potential futures within our imaginative reach for consideration as to their preferability. Fundamentally they act as aids to enable users to act as research participants or debate participants or potentially to explore as real-world policy-makers. Design fictions are concerned with progress, ideas for the better, but they take into account that better means different things to different people [14] and do not focus on implementation, but on discussing 'what-if' scenarios.

3   Research Methodology

A participatory design methodology [15] was used that included three stages, namely problem definition, co-creating design fictions, prototyping and testing.

In stage one, the policy and academic contexts for design negotiating political questions were explored through secondary research and an examination of the government policy documents around the theme of ageing was conducted at the time of the research project (early June 2015). This helped identify a number of related government policy initiatives (such as 'ageing in place', integrated health and social care, ageing well and several others) that could be explored in the second stage with the stakeholders. Extracts of these policies were explored in two co-design [16] workshops in Lancashire (n = 14) and Cornwall (n = 7) with community groups and older citizens. The workshops were conducted in June 2015, with participant ages ranging from 65–95. The first workshop included participants recruited from an Age UK group and lasted half a day, whereas the second workshop included participants at a sheltered accommodation and was run over two days. A range of techniques was used to explore the use of design fictions in negotiating political questions. All speculations, concepts and ideas that emerged from the workshops were captured via audio recording, photography and short video presentations. Stage three focused onto translating the workshop insights and co-designed speculations into design fictions. Analysing and coding the captured data the research team worked with the project collaborator Design Friction to develop a series of concepts for the design fictions. Following this two design fictions were realised and prototyped, namely the SOULAJE, a self-administered euthanasia wearable, and the Smart Object Therapist (SOT), which combines occupational health with experience in pervasive and assisted home technology to ensure that future smart home appliances correspond to user needs. The former design fiction was designed as a response to the workshop co-designers expressed needs for self-control and living with dignity and was aimed at opening further the debate around the ethical and legal aspects of technology-enabled assisted dying. The second design fiction was developed as a response to the government policies of integrated care, ageing in place and assisted living in smart homes and was aimed at extending the debate around the ethical and social aspects of personal health and pervasive technology at home and social inclusion. Given the paper focus and length limitations we will focus on the SOT design fiction in here.

The SOT design fiction[2] comprised of three documents, namely a SOT job application, the SOT intervention report and prescription and a short video breakfast TV style article featuring the SOT and a smart object home user. Set in the year 2020 the SOT interview design fiction sets the speculative scene by presenting the skills a SOT is expected to have in the envisaged integrated health and social care service model, where older people age at home supported by an array of smart appliances. The job of a SOT is not limited to fixing technical faults but is centred around recalibrating human behaviour to facilitate interaction between smart objects and their owners. The SOT intervention report and prescription design fictions present a possible world where the SOT has been called in to intervene between the homeowner and smart home to resolve an issue. The SOT design fiction creates an appropriate and open environment for debate by exploring 'misbehaving' smart home technology, a smart self-refilling fridge that confuses the homeowner for his grandson.

4 Findings and Discussion

Following their development the design fictions and the concepts they encompassed were explored by seeking feedback from policy makers at a policy engagement event in Westminster Palace in London in July 2015 and from citizens at a co-design workshop in Lancaster in September 2015. The event at Westminster and the semi-structured interviews with civil servants and a politician were focused on the barriers and opportunities to using design methods to negotiate political issues with citizens. The co-design workshop, which was run with the same group that initiated the design fictions, was focused on in-depth discussion of the design fictions, the underpinning speculations and the ethical, societal and legal issues they presented. In this short paper, we focus on an analysis of the citizens' discussions in the workshop.

The thematic analysis of discussion that followed the presentation of the SOT design fiction, as well, as the visual material collected during the workshop activities, revealed a number of ethical, legal and societal concerns that participants discussed. In terms of the societal aspects of smart home technology for health systems, workshop participants expressed the need and desire for supporting older people to live independently, especially ones with long-term health conditions.

> 'I have to say although I feel quite hostile to this I have also seen a more primitive version of this work well for somebody living independently with dementia. Their house was set-up with a lot of alarms, so that if she opened the door like at night time and didn't come back straight away then the police would be informed, you know a lot of things like that which meant that she was able live independently for much longer that she would have done otherwise and I suppose this is an extension of the same idea' [Jane]

Some participants used this discussion to also talk about robotics in care but recognised that there is value in health systems that do not diminish independence. In fact reducing independence was a concern that several people raised as a result of living in a home environment over-reliant on technologies. Related to this was a lengthy discussion on

---

[2] See: http://imagination.lancs.ac.uk/outcomes/Smart_Object_Therapist_Design_Fiction.

social isolation being a potential result of peoples' over-reliance on smart home healthcare living environments. Instead of encouraging people to stay more physically active by going out and reinforcing social interactions between people, there was an expression of concern towards encouraging more sedentary and self-isolation behaviours by replacing human contact with 'smart' technology.

> 'An unwanted side effect of that sort of technology is that it would actually keep people in their homes rather than encouraging them out of their home on their day-to-day basis. This would have impact on their health and mental health, it's about interactions, about being stimulated all sort of other things not met by technology' [Maggie]

The SOT design fiction facilitated a discussion around the ethical and legal aspects of similar personal health systems. Trust in the technology to perform as expected and technology replacing humans in terms of healthcare services was a key topic of debate. With regards to the specific SOT design fiction scenario people questioned the training and education background that such a techno-occupational therapist professional would need to have. Questions were raised as to whether such a role would have a person-centred approach and whether the focus will be placed on the human or the smart and personal health technology.

> 'What comes first? Is it an all in one house you move into or does the therapist come first to access your needs?' [Laura]

This led into discussions regarding the financial and legal aspects of personal health systems. A theme, which was extensively discussed, was that of the financial and legal framework of service provision. Questions were raised as to who would pay for the technology installation, home adaptation, technology support, as well as perceived cost and long-term economical value.

> 'This is forwarding thinking of how we are going to carry on with the age of people going to 90s and 100s, how can we stop hospital admissions, how can we save money, even if all this seems fantastical' [Sam]
> 'By the time you paid for all this technology, would it not be cheaper to have somebody pop round for few hours every day' [Claire]

Additional thought was given to accessibility of such future services to the public if a privately funded model is to be selected. A few participants even discussed possible financial models involving big supermarkets (linking it to food restocking), which created discussion around sharing of personal data, habits and personal health records.

> 'You can see how supermarkets the likes of Tesco's would love to something like this. They could restock your [smart] fridge and in the process find out all about your food likes and habits and even your health condition' [Paul]

This led the discussion back to the ethical implications related to agency, personal choice and control between personal health home systems and their users.

> 'This is a clinical solution... you are a diabetic so it's looking at sugar levels in foods, whereas the wheelchair food service does put that on you it's up to you to make the choice, your informed decision' [Sam] 'Thank god for that!' [Jenny]
> 'I tell myself what I want to eat I'm not going to ask any [smart] fridges' [Pam]

5 Conclusion

This paper has argued that research that drives innovation through analysis of ethical, legal and social challenges and opportunities is needed more than ever. Building upon qualitative participatory and speculative design research, it has become clear that, ethics like 'usability' may be usefully based on engagement with directly or indirectly implicated publics and should not be designed into innovation by experts alone.

The design fiction generated a rich discussion on the societal, legal and ethical implications of the presented concept related to personal health systems for independent living. The facilitators used the design fictions as props to initiate discussion and workshop participants used them as prompts to form a debate. Most of the participants employed personal stories and lived experiences to relate to several of the societal and legal aspects of the introduction of smart home technology for healthcare. It was interesting to observe through the recorded data that there was a diversity of views expressed; and that participants who were initially skeptical warmed to the principles underpinning the personal health system concept as a result of working through the socio-ethical issues in debate. Our future work involves testing further the methodologies presented here in different domains, by looking at the ethical and societal aspects around the use of pervasive technology for dementia.

Acknowledgments. The authors would like to thank all workshop participants, Age UK Lancashire, all members of the ProtoPolicy project. The research work was supported by the Arts and Humanities Research Council (Grant no: AH/N003810/1).

References

1. Dishman, E.: Inventing wellness systems for aging in place. Computer **37**, 34–41 (2004)
2. Coughlin, J.F., D'Ambrosio, L.A., Reimer, B., Pratt, M.R.: Older adult perceptions of smart home technologies: implications for research, policy & market innovations in healthcare. In: 29th Annual International Conference of the IEEE EMBS 2007, pp. 1810–1815. IEEE (2007)
3. Batchelor, R., Bobrowicz, A., Mackenzie, R., Milne, A.: Challenges of ethical and legal responsibilities when technologies' uses and users change: social networking sites, decision-making capacity and dementia. Ethics Inf. Technol. **14**, 99–108 (2012)
4. Anthony, D., Henderson, T., Kotz, D.: Privacy in location-aware computing environments. IEEE Pervasive Comput. **6**, 64–72 (2007)
5. Brown, I., Adams, A.A.: The ethical challenges of ubiquitous healthcare. Int. Rev. Inf. Ethics **8**, 53–60 (2007)
6. Dodge, M., Kitchin, R.: 'Outlines of a world coming into existence': pervasive computing and the ethics of forgetting. Environ. Plan. B Plan. Des. **34**, 431–445 (2007)
7. Kim, J., Beresford, A.R., Stajano, F.: Towards a security policy for ubiquitous healthcare systems (position paper). In: Stajano, F., Kim, H.J., Chae, J.-S., Kim, S.-D. (eds.) ICUCT 2006. LNCS, vol. 4412, pp. 263–272. Springer, Heidelberg (2007). doi:10.1007/978-3-540-71789-8_27

8. Digital Single Market: eHealth Action Plan 2012–2020: Innovative healthcare for the 21st century - Digital Single Market - European Commission. https://ec.europa.eu/digital-agenda/en/news/ehealth-action-plan-2012-2020-innovative-healthcare-21st-century

9. Irvin, R.A., Stansbury, J.: Citizen participation in decision making: is it worth the effort? Public Adm. Rev. 64(1), 55–65 (2004)

10. Hales, D.: Design fictions an introduction and provisional taxonomy. Digit. Creativity 24, 1–10 (2013)

11. Tanenbaum, J., Tanenbaum, K., Wakkary, R.: Steampunk as design fiction. In: Proceedings of the SIGCHI Conference on Human Factors in Computing Systems, pp. 1583–1592. ACM (2012)

12. Bleecker, J.: Design fiction. A short essay on design, science, fact and fiction. Near Future Laboratory (2009)

13. Kirby, D.: The future is now: diegetic prototypes and the role of popular films in generating real-world technological development. Soc. Stud. Sci. 40, 41–70 (2009)

14. Dunne, A., Raby, F.: Speculative Everything. Design, Fiction, and Social Dreaming. The MIT Press, Cambridge (2013)

15. Simonsen, J., Robertson, T.: Routledge International Handbook of Participatory Design. Routledge, New York (2013)

16. Sanders, E., Stappers, P.: Co-creation and the new landscapes of design. CoDesign 4, 5–18 (2008)

M3Apps + AALIoT 2016

Engineering IoT Healthcare Applications: Towards a Semantic Data Driven Sustainable Architecture

Rita Zgheib[1]([✉]), Emmanuel Conchon[2], and Rémi Bastide[1]

[1] Laboratoire IRIT, Université de Toulouse, 31062 Toulouse Cedex 9, France
{rita.zgheib,remi.bastide}@irit.fr
[2] Laboratoire XLIM, Université de Limoge, 87060 Limoges Cedex, France
emmanuel.conchon@xlim.fr

Abstract. As the number of developed sensors is growing, new Internet of Things applications are being developed. Healthcare applications offer a perfect domain for Internet of Things since they respond to the challenge of the ageing population while offering safe and quality care in the home. We present in this paper a new Internet Of Things architecture for IoT healthcare applications. The architecture focuses mainly on the principles of weak coupling and of semantic data exchange. We present a software architecture based on a message oriented middleware driven by semantic OWL messages.

Keywords: Home care · Semantic representation · Message oriented middleware (MOM) · Internet-of-things · Health applications

1 Introduction

The world population is rapidly ageing; According to the WHO[1] statistics the number of people aged 65 and over will exceed 15% of the global population by 2050. As the global population ages, the demand for end-of-life care will continue increasing over the years. Elders desire staying in their own homes as long as it is possible and safe. To this end, steps must be taken to provide them with the necessary assistance, ensured by exploiting new technologies.

In the Internet of Things (IoT) [1], intelligent sensors are deployed on a smart space in order to gather real time information. This information can be treated, recorded and correlated to infer new data faster and more accurately, which leads IoT to be an important driver of health care [2]. The combination of assisted living spaces and healthcare applications has been found to provide safe and quality care at home, especially for elders who often incur the risk of many pathologies symptoms and problems.

As the number of sensors is increasing rapidly and encompasses a large number of measurements (temperature, moisture, etc.), many IoT applications have

---

[1] WHO: World Health Organization, http://www.who.int/ageing/en/.

© ICST Institute for Computer Sciences, Social Informatics and Telecommunications Engineering 2017
K. Giokas et al. (Eds.): eHealth 2016, LNICST 181, pp. 407–418, 2017.
DOI: 10.1007/978-3-319-49655-9_49

arisen [3]. The matter of most of these applications focus on data and it does not include the way these data can be gathered or shared. That means data are becoming proprietary for each application. For example, to monitor elders who often incur the risk of many pathologies, a lot of same sensors is required to provide the necessary data to the different applications [4]. For that a semantic and interoperable architecture is needed to inhance information sharing and reusability [5].

In this paper we propose an IoT architecture for healthcare applications providing the following features: 1. the same sensor can potentially be used for several applications reducing the number of connected sensors. And 2. The same information can potentially be provided by different sensors ensuring the redundancy of data in the case of an out of service sensor. For that our architecture is based on semantic representations of sensors and publish/subscribe architecture, ensuring the interoperability between system components.

The remainder of this paper is organized as follow: In Sect. 2 we present the main principles of the proposed architecture, followed by a review of the related work in Sect. 3. We then present our proposal for a semantic middleware architecture for IoT health care application in Sect. 4. Section 5 provides an implementation of the case study which has been used to validate our architecture. We conclude by describing the future directions of this work.

2   Principles of the Proposed Architecture

In the context of home care applications, the aim of our research is long-term monitoring of elders by detecting and monitoring their Activities of Daily Living (ADL) using ambient sensors. In [6] authors show that smart objects and IoT are an essential factor for Ambient Assisted Living (AAL) to support elderly people in their daily routine and to allow an independent and safe lifestyle as long as possible.

In the IoT environment, most applications use a set of dedicated sensors, and each solution has its specific architecture. In order to provide a loosely coupled communication for all IoT system components and to enable information sharing between them, we propose a semantic web of things middleware for healthcare applications. This architecture complies to the principle of "Independent and weakly coupled software components driven by semantic data". It relies on three concepts: semantic interoperability; loose coupling and information pooling; and health requirements.

2.1   Semantic Interoperability

Connected sensors and systems in an IoT environment will have specific technologies and infrastructures. The data sent by any sensor can potentially be used by several different monitoring applications. Likewise, a specific monitoring application should not be concerned about the physical sensors, and should even be able to treat homogeneousremly data sent automatically by sensors and data collected by other means (e.g. by clinical examination and manual entry in a software system). To promote the semantic interoperability between system components, a semantic and homogeneous representation of sensor's data is required. While IoT middleware solutions present a lack of semantic representations [7], ontologies for describing sensor network have been widely used in the literature. Moreover, in [8] authors propose ontologies for knowledge representations and the predominant technique OWL (the Web Ontology Language) for knowledge representation in the web.

For the purpose of representing formally sensors data, we will rely on ontology concept for sensors description. SSN(Semantic Sensor Network ontology) will be used as a base ontology. A location variable the **PatientLocation**(room number and bed) is added to SSN taking into consideration health requirements and the need of tracking a patient at hospital or retirement home. Therefore, the system will be able to exchange localized observations.

2.2   Loosely Coupling and Information Pooling

In IoT solutions presenting a strongly coupled data provider and receiver, each application uses its specific sensors. For example, two monitoring applications that require temperature variable use two temperature sensors for the same patient. And if a sensor breaks, these applications lies with lacks of data accuracy and availability, and they can't handle quickly the arrival of new sensor.

In our work, we are interested in improving sensors sharing between applications, therefore the same sensor can be used by several applications and the same information can be provided by several sensors. For that purpose, a loosely coupled concept between system components is mandated. Likewise, in a multi-pathologies case the pooling of physical devices is required in order to decrease the number of sensors used.

To this end, we propose the use of a middleware, structured as a software communication bus which promotes the interoperability among heterogeneous sensors and allows for the pooling of physical devices.

Publish subscribe architecture: We rely then, on a Message Oriented Middleware (MOM) with a publish/subscribe architecture. In regards to SOA architecture which is often used in IoT solutions, it follows a message-based model. It focuses on the information itself and supports sending and receiving of messages between distributed systems. Among this architecture, data sources (publishers) and destinations (subscribers) are decoupled and anonymous, data objects are filtered and delivered to destinations based on predefined topics expressed as subscriptions. Each subscriber receives over time a personalized set of data related to a specific topic.

The publish/subscribe messaging architecture is therefore a perfect communication and data processing mechanism for IoT environments. It introduces a huge number of heterogeneous devices and applications that are continuously connected to the Internet and able to send and receive real-time data.

2.3 Domain Requirements

Semantic representations are widely used in health applications most of them based on ontology concept for example: Open Biomedical Ontologies (OBO) consortium ontologies, SNOMED [9], etc. Moreover health is an application domain for Internet of things where sensor's value is critical information used by health applications to establish analysis and derive health factors and status. Therefore, it is important to have many **information** sources and then, the application can choose the appropriate one and in a faulty sensor case, another can easily take over. But in a multi-pathologies case, avoiding the accumulation of redundant sensors when several monitoring applications are used simultaneously is necessary to respond to financial concerns, and to the **desire of patients** which prefer to avoid the installation of too many devices in their home.

Time and geographical variables are significant factors for establishing health reports. Time is an important element for an efficient continuous care and follow-up for patients, especially in the context of prevention applications like bedsore risk detection [10]. **Geographic** parameters like latitude and longitude can't be pertinent information, patient's room and bed is more useful information to localize a patient.

By combining the three concepts semantic interoperability, loosely coupling and information pooling and health requirements, we can establish a new semantic MOM architecture principle that introduces an "Independent, weakly coupled software components driven by semantic data" for IoT health care applications.

3 Related Work

This work deals with two main concepts: Semantic representation of sensors data and middleware solutions for IoT applications. These two concepts, the pillar of our proposed architecture, are linked and connected to create a new IoT environment: a semantic middleware for health applications.

3.1 Ontologies for Sensors Description

Ontologies for describing knowledge have been widely used in many IoT applications and artificial intelligence systems. **SSN ontology** (Semantic sensor Network ontology) [11] is a generic and domain-independent ontology introduced by the W3C in 2011. This ontology is compatible and compliant with OASIS (OASIS Group Consortium) standards at the sensors and observations level. It allows the accurate description of sensors and allows the introduction of new domains with the addition of dedicated vocabularies. With SSN, sensors data can be described reflecting the deployment, System, Operating restriction, Platform site, Device, Process, Data and Measuring Capability.

SSN presents some limitations in describing time, space and communication. However it is performed to be compatible with all domains in representing sensors data then, extensions can be added relatively to the needs of areas. According to their domain, many extensions have been created. WSSN in [12] is an extension which addresses the communication limitation. Another SSN extension has been proposed by Roda et al. in [13] for intelligent data analysis, SSN relies on existing extensions to model time and reasoning.

Even if lots of SSN extensions have been provided over the years, there is still no extension that fully meet our requirements. Therefore it has been chosen in this work to propose a SSN extension allowing the description of patient's location to comply with medical location requirements such as in hospitals and retirement homes for instance.

- **OWL representation:** We rely on ontologies in this paper to represent sensors networks, physical aspect and infrastructure. A main advantage of using them is the possibility to generate OWL representations. The Web Ontology Language (OWL) built upon a W3C XML standard can easily be integrated in many programming languages like Java through APIs (Jena or OWL-API).

3.2   Publish/Subscribe Middlewares for Internet of Things

There are many attempts of middleware solution for IoT in the literature. A recent review [7] has analyzed in details several existing solutions according to their architecture type: Event-based, Service-oriented (SOA), Agent-based, database, etc.

Many IoT projects propose publish/subscribe solutions. For instance, CenceMe project [14] aims to automatically infer people's activity (e.g. dancing in the party) based on sensor-enabled smart phone; and to share this activity through social media like Facefook. Another example supporting easy access to sensor data on mobile phones is Pogo [15], a publish/subscribe middleware infrastructure for mobile phone sensing. It uses simple topic-based subscriptions to manage access to sensor data and reports significant energy gains due to topic-based filtering of sensed data on mobile devices.

MQTT (Message Queuing Telemetry Transport) [7] is a lightweight publish-subscribe messaging protocol used in IoT applications. It has been standardized by OASIS since 2014. Several research works have been investigated on publish/subscribe middlewares among which is CUPUS [16]. A comparative study of CUPUS and MQTT have been established by Antonic et al. in [17]. The study shows that MQTT offers basic functionalities of exchanging messages and notifications while CUPUS presents advanced features to manage sensors over the cloud and to process in real-time big data streams.

To summarize, publish/subscribe middleware is used mainly for data acquisition from IoT resources. In our context, MQTT fits our basic requirements since patients will be either at home or in hospital. We are not working in large geographic scope and at the time of writing there is no plan to provide a cloud hosting for patient data.

3.3   Semantic Middlewares

In most of existing IoT solutions, middleware architectures have not been designed with considerations of semantic annotations. Only few attempts address the semantic topic in their proposals. In [18], authors propose a Semantic Middleware for IoT aiming to resolve the interoperability issue between different kinds of protocols (Bluetooth and UPnP). This solution is based on a SOA architecture. SMArc [19] the Smart Middleware Architecture is another SOA-based solution that focus on smart city energy management for smart grid environments.

LinkSmart [20] relies on a semantic model-driven architecture and enables the use of devices as services, the semantic description of devices is based on ontologies using OWL, OWL-s. OM2M [21] is an advanced semantic middleware based on SOA architecture. It is a Machine-to-Machine service based on autonomic computing and semantic annotation to provide an inter-operable system to connect billions of devices.

Another example is the European project OpenIoT [22] that has developed an open-source middleware platform providing a "cloud-of-things". OpenIoT aims to propose on demand access to cloud-based IoT services for internet-connected objects. Trying to use sensing as a service, OpenIoT architecture embeds the CUPUS middleware as a cloud-Based publish/subscribe processing engine and relies on SSN for sensors description. It can be viewed as a federation of several middlewares interconnected with each other targeting applications for smart cities or campus.

As previously mentioned, to provide a loose coupling and information centric solution, SOA-based solutions are not relevant. OpenIoT could have been a good candidate to target IoT health applications but, its complexity due to the variety of middlewares used in its framework can be a major drawback for programmer. Therefore, a new lightweight solution that can provide an effortless programming environment is needed to exchange health related semantic data in a local area network (or even home area network).

4   Semantic Middleware Architecture

The proposed IoT health care architecture, presented in Fig. 1, relies on a message oriented middleware enhanced with a semantic representation of exchanged data. In this architecture, *data sources*, defined as *semantic publisher* send over time personalized data, based on a specific *topic*. These data are delivered to consumers, defined as *semantic subscribers*, based on these specific topics. A *semantic message broker* is responsible of carrying data from a publisher to a subscriber. A semantic representation of all exchanged data is therefore, necessary to promote the interoperability. Therefore, five concepts are defined: **semantic sensor, virtual semantic publisher, semantic subscriber, semantic subscription and semantic message broker.**

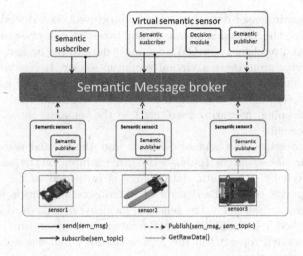

Fig. 1. High-Level semantic Web of Things architecture

```
Bedsore:TemperatureObservation1   rdf:type ssn:Observation;
        ssn:featureOfInterest        Bedsore:waist_skin;
        ssn:observedProperty         Bedsore:Temperature;
        ssn:observationResult
               [rdf:type ssn:SensorOutput;
               DUL:hasDataValue [qudt:numericValue "27"];
               DUL:isClassifiedBy Bedsore:Celsius];
        ssn:observedBy    Bedsore:BD_TemperatureSensor1
               [ssn:OnPlatform [:hasPatientLocation [rdf:type Bedsore:PatientLocation;
                                                      Bedsore:room "2";
                                                      Bedsore:bed "1" ]]];
```

Fig. 2. Semantic localized observation (in room2, bed1) sent by semantic Temperature sensor and received by a semantic subscriber

– **Sensors** represent the data sources. In our design, we distinguish three kinds of sensors: physical sensor, semantic sensor and virtual semantic sensor.

   1. **Physical sensor** is a sensing device capable of detecting stimulus from real world and of sending raw data like "open", "close" in case of contact sensor or "30 C" in case of temperature sensor.
   2. **Semantic sensor** is a software component that converts raw data into semantic data. The semantic sensor requests physical sensors for raw data, represents them using SSN ontology, generates their OWL classes and sends them to the semantic broker.
   3. **Virtual semantic sensor** in [22] authors present the virtual sensor as any entity (device, object or people) capable of observing properties around them. In our architecture, the virtual semantic sensor can be manifested in two roles semantic subscriber and semantic publisher. It is a semantic subscriber since it represents any entity capable of subscribing

for semantic sensor data. Data can be processed via a **decision module** and then, the virtual semantic sensor take the role of **semantic publisher** and publishes new OWL semantic data to the broker. For example an activity monitor is a virtual semantic sensor. It is a semantic subscriber since it receives OWL sensors measurements and analyses their data. It takes then, the semantic publisher role and sends the activity result(sleeping, preparing food, etc.) to the semantic message broker in OWL format.

In our architecture, the semantic sensor and the virtual semantic sensor are semantic data sources (publishers). An example of the semantic message generated by a semantic data source is presented in Fig. 2: this message corresponds to an observation of a temperature sensor identified by "BD_TemperatureSensor1". The sensor is localized in a medical bed situated in room 2 - bed 1 and publishes data related to "temperature" topic which fits the "observedProperty" in the SSN vocabulary and has a data value 27 Celsius at a given time.

- **Semantic subscriber** represents the receiver component connected to the semantic broker. To receive information, the semantic subscriber has to register for the relevant topic. An example of a **semantic subscription** targeting the temperature topic is illustrated in Fig. 3 with the OWL formalism.
- **Semantic Message broker** is the communication relay between all system components. It supplies the monitoring of semantic messages between semantic publishers and subscribers, it managers also semantic subscriptions and notifications.

```
<owl:NamedIndividual rdf:about="&ssn-Bedsore-Detection;Temperature">
    <rdf:type rdf:resource="&ssn-Bedsore-Detection;Property"/>
</owl:NamedIndividual>
```

Fig. 3. Semantic topic represented as an observed property of SSN ontology

5   Bedsore Risk Detection: A Use Case

5.1   Braden Scale

To validate the proposed architecture, a prototype for bedsores risk detection has been designed. Bedsores (also called pressure ulcers) [23] are one of the dangerous diseases that an elder can face. It is a localized injury resulting from prolonged pressure on the skin. It plagues persons who stay in bed or wheelchair for a long period of time. Bedsores are dangerous and can have important consequences, leading to long-term hospitalization.

Bedsore prevention techniques today still rely on human intervention. The caregiver checks regularly (usually every 15 min) the status of the patients and

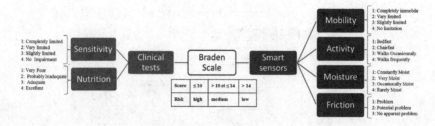

Fig. 4. Braden scale

their changes in body position. In the context of home care for dependent elderly people, the frequent checking are not possible. It is important to have an accurate bedsore detection system based on real time sensors measurements. The Braden scale is the most used method in clinical settings, since it results from a simple calculation based on 6 risk factors as presented in Fig. 4: sensory perception or sensitivity, nutrition, mobility, activity, moisture and friction. For each risk factor a value ranging from 1 to 4 is entered. This value corresponds to the intensity of this factor for the patient. The lower, the lesser risk. A global score is calculated to determine the risk of developing a pressure ulcer.

Based on Braden calculation, we propose to deploy smart sensors in the patients bed or chair as presented in Fig. 4. These sensors can potentially be used to automate the data collection for several factors of the Braden score. For instance, the friction and mobility criteria are monitored by a pressure sensor, activity is monitored by a pedometer and finally the moisture criteria by temperature and humidity sensors. All data is routed to the decision module to calculate the Braden score and potentially to trigger an alarm when the score is worrisome (i.e. $<= 10$). This alarm will then urge the caregiver to change the patients posture.

5.2   Use Case's Software Architectural Design

In accordance with the aforementioned design concepts (semantic interoperability, loosely coupling and information pooling, and health requirements), the bedsore use case has been implemented to validate the proposed architecture. Figure 5 depicts an implementation of our architecture using a UML deployment diagram. This implementation relies on the Mosquitto broker, a lightweight and open source message broker based on MQTT protocol. Mosquito is available in many programming languages like Java and Python for instance. Regards to the bedsore use case, four physical sensors, a humidity a temperature a pressure and a pedometer sensors, are connected to a Raspberry Pi via Grove Pi. The semantic sensor requests the Raspberry Pi for physical sensor observations (temperature, moisture, pressure, friction in a specific room and bed) and then creates a corresponding semantic representation. It then publishes semantic sensors data on the semantic middleware (via the broker) in OWL format.

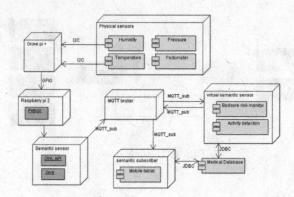

Fig. 5. Deployment diagram of the Web-of-things architecture using Bedsore risk detection use case

Bedsore risk monitor and Activity detection modules are virtual semantic sensors. The Bedsore risk monitor subscribes to the semantic topics related to mobility, activity, moisture and friction. The received semantic data related to topics will be processed withing the Bedsore module to apply Braden scale calculation. A score for the risk of Bedsore is then generated, represented in OWL format and republished on the semantic middleware.

The activity monitor module presented in the diagram is another kind of virtual semantic sensor used to detect person's activity. Even if activity detection is out of the scope of this use case, this module is interesting to highlight the loose coupling and the information centric approach under use. Indeed, this module can subscribe to the same topics as the Bedsore risk monitor module and use the same information provided by the semantic sensors. The Database is used to get medical information about the patient. Indeed, to assess the Braden score, the database is needed to get information that can not be gathered by sensors such as sensitivity and nutrition. The mobile tablet module subscribes to the bedsore-Risk topic via MQTT_sub interface. It will receives in real-time the Braden scale score and in a high risk case, an alarm can be triggered to urge the caregiver.

6   Conclusion

In this paper, we have presented the principles of an IoT software architecture, based on Message Oriented Middleware and on semantic data representation. Our architecture is illustrated by a case study for the detection of bedsore risks. Our ongoing work follows two tracks: On the first hand, we plan to validate our bedsore application through controlled evaluations in a clinical environment, to assess its performance, reliability, safety and usability by the care personnel. On the second hand, we work on developing a reference implementation of our proposed middleware, with the goal of providing a simple software API usable in various application domains, to alleviate the tasks of software developers using the architecture we propose.

Acknowledgments. The work of Rita Zgheib is supported by a grant from Region Midi-Pyrnes and University Champollion.

References

1. Weber, R.H., Weber, R.: Internet of Things: Legal Perspectives, vol. 49. Springer Science & Business Media, Heidelberg (2010)
2. Doukas, C., Maglogiannis, I.: Bringing IoT and cloud computing towards pervasive healthcare. In: 2012 Sixth International Conference on Innovative Mobile and Internet Services in Ubiquitous Computing. Institute of Electrical & Electronics Engineers (IEEE), July 2012
3. Lee, B.M., Ouyang, J.: Intelligent healthcare service by using collaborations between IoT personal health devices. IJBSBT **6**(1), 155–164 (2014)
4. Miorandi, D., Sicari, S., De Pellegrini, F., Chlamtac, I.: Internet of things: vision applications and research challenges. Ad Hoc Netw. **10**(7), 1497–1516 (2012)
5. Atzori, L., Iera, A., Morabito, G.: The Internet of Things: a survey. Comput. Netw. **54**(15), 2787–2805 (2010)
6. Dohr, A., Modre-Opsrian, R., Drobics, M., Hayn, D., Schreier, G.: The Internet of Things for ambient assisted living. In: 2010 Seventh International Conference on Information Technology: New Generations. Institute of Electrical & Electronics Engineers (IEEE) (2010)
7. Razzaque, M., Milojevic-Jevric, M., Palade, A., Clarke, S.: Middleware for Internet of Things: a survey, January 2016
8. Pfisterer, D., Romer, K., Bimschas, D., Kleine, O., Mietz, R., Truong, C., Hasemann, H., Krller, A., Pagel, M., Hauswirth, M., Karnstedt, M., Leggieri, M., Passant, A., Richardson, R.: SPITFIRE: toward a semantic web of things. IEEE Commun. Mag. **49**(11), 40–48 (2011)
9. Rothwell, D.J., Cote, R.A.: Managing information with SNOMED: understanding the model. In: Proceedings of the AMIA Annual Fall Symposium, p. 80. American Medical Informatics Association (1996)
10. Zgheib, R., Bastide, R., Conchon, E.: A semantic web-of-things architecture for monitoring the risk of bedsores (regular paper). In: International Conference on Computational Science and Computational Intelligence (CSCI), Las Vegas, USA, 07/12/15-09/12/15. IEEE, Dcembre 2015. http://www.ieee.org/
11. Compton, M., Barnaghi, P., Bermudez, L., García-Castro, R., Corcho, O., Cox, S., Graybeal, J., Hauswirth, M., Henson, C., Herzog, A., Huang, V., Janowicz, K., Kelsey, W.D., Phuoc, D.L., Lefort, L., Leggieri, M., Neuhaus, H., Nikolov, A., Page, K., Passant, A., Sheth, A., Taylor, K.: The SSN ontology of the W3C semantic sensor network incubator group. Web Semant. Sci. Serv. Agents World Wide Web **17**, 25–32 (2012)
12. Bendadouche, R., Roussey, C., De Sousa, G., Chanet, J.P., Hou, K.M., Hou, K.M.: Extension of the semantic sensor network ontology for wireless sensor networks: the stimulus-WSNnode-communication pattern. In: 5th International Workshop on Semantic Sensor Networks in conjunction with the 11th International Semantic Web Conference (ISWC), November 2012, Boston, United States (2013)
13. Roda, F., Musulin, E.: An ontology-based framework to support intelligent data analysis of sensor measurements. Expert Syst. Appl. **41**(17), 7914–7926 (2014)

14. Miluzzo, E., Lane, N.D., Fodor, K., Peterson, R., Lu, H., Musolesi, M., Eisenman, S.B., Zheng, X., Campbell, A.T.: Sensing meets mobile social networks. In: Proceedings of the 6th ACM Conference on Embedded network sensor systems - SenSys 2008. Association for Computing Machinery (ACM) (2008)
15. Brouwers, N., Langendoen, K.: Pogo, a middleware for mobile phone sensing. In: Narasimhan, P., Triantafillou, P. (eds.) Middleware 2012. LNCS, vol. 7662, pp. 21–40. Springer, Heidelberg (2012). doi:10.1007/978-3-642-35170-9_2
16. Antonic, A., Marjanovic, M., Pripuzic, K., Zarko, I.P.: A mobile crowd sensing ecosystem enabled by CUPUS: cloud-based publish/subscribe middleware for the Internet of Things. Fut. Gener. Comput. Syst. **56**, 607–622 (2015)
17. Antonic, A., Marjanovic, M., Skocir, P., Zarko, I.P.: Comparison of the CUPUS middleware and MQTT protocol for smart city services. In: 2015 13th International Conference on Telecommunications (ConTEL). Institute of Electrical & Electronics Engineers (IEEE), July 2015
18. Song, Z., Cárdenas, A.A., Masuoka, R.: Semantic middleware for the internet of things. In: 2010 Internet of Things, IoT 2010 (2010)
19. Rodríguez-Molina, J., Martínez, J.F., Castillejo, P., De Diego, R.: SMArc: a proposal for a smart, semantic middleware architecture focused on smart city energy management. Int. J. Distrib. Sens. Netw. (2013)
20. Delicato, F.C., Pires, P.F., Batista, T.: Middleware Solutions for the Internet of Things. Springer, London (2013)
21. Alaya, B.M., Banouar, Y., Monteil, T., Chassot, C., Drira, K.: OM2M: extensible ETSI-compliant M2M service platform with self-configuration capability. Procedia Comput. Sci. **32**, 1079–1086 (2014)
22. Kim, J., Lee, J.-W.: OpenIoT: an open service framework for the Internet of Things. In: 2014 IEEE World Forum on Internet of Things (WF-IoT). Institute of Electrical & Electronics Engineers (IEEE), March 2014
23. Webster, J.G.: Prevention of Pressure Sores: Engineering and Clinical Aspects. CRC Press, Boca Raton (1991)

Recognizing Human Behaviour from Temporal Sequential Data with Activity Assignment

Sarah Fallmann[✉] and Johannes Kropf

AIT - Austrian Institute of Technology, Wiener Neustadt, Austria
{sarah.fallman.fl,johannes.kropf}@ait.ac.at

Abstract. A probabilistic system in an ambient assisted living environment is automatically built to detect human behaviour. The focus lies on the early prediction of human activities based on domotic sensor data and on general activity assignment. First recurrent patterns are detected using the Temporal-Pattern (T-Pattern) algorithm and further a probabilistic finite-state automaton is generated out of the patterns. Afterwards the patterns are assigned to specific defined human activities with the help of Fuzzy Logic. The needed rules are learned automatic from an annotated dataset.

Keywords: Behaviour recognition · Fuzzy Logic · T-Pattern algorithm

1 Introduction

The recognition of human behaviour with the usage of non-obtrusive sensors is a challenge, which is of great importance for Ambient Assisted technologies to be accepted by end users [6]. Human behaviour can be very complex, consider, for instance, the preparation of a meal which consists of many sub-activities.

In sensor networks consisting of many sensors, or in environments with multiple persons interacting with the smart home, patterns are very often hidden in data streams and must be discovered with appropriate statistical methods. This in done with the T-Pattern algorithm and a probabilistic suffix tree (PST) [1,7]. Probabilistic suffix trees usually ignore the time between subsequent events and assume no noise in terms of unknown or random events in the data, in marked contrast to merging T-Patterns and probabilistic suffix automata (PSA). Later the probabilistic suffix tree is transformed in an automaton. The assignment of the data is done with an annotated dataset [8] using information as objects, locations, durations and time to construct rules for different activities.

The aim is particularly the detection of human behaviour in regard to time and the automatic assignment of human activities to the detected patterns. The time aspect is important, as data comes from real world settings and different sensors can send at similar timestamps. Moreover, the order and duration of the activities is important, in particular for events which are dependent on past events.

© ICST Institute for Computer Sciences, Social Informatics and Telecommunications Engineering 2017
K. Giokas et al. (Eds.): eHealth 2016, LNICST 181, pp. 419–424, 2017.
DOI: 10.1007/978-3-319-49655-9_50

2   Activity Recognition

Human activity recognition is a fast growing and broad research area. This work focuses on non-obtrusive environmental sensors for activity recognition. Algorithms used in activity recognition can be divided into two major groups. The first one is based on machine learning techniques including supervised and unsupervised learning methods, the second one is based on logical modelling and reasoning [6].

For evaluation, three annotated datasets consisting of several weeks of data are used. This data from conventional home automation sensors in a real-world setting is provided by Kasteren *et al.* [8]. Each dataset belongs to one house which is occupied by one person.

2.1   Algorithm and Concept

The T-Patterns algorithm proposed in [2,3] is used to find recurrent patterns in the sequential data. This data are a set of sensor events, where timestamps represent the beginning and ending time of a specific sensor event. This data in real environments are often sparse during long observational periods and clustered within short periods. The sequential data from the sensors are preprocessed, where false data are deleted. Afterwards the algorithm can be proceeded.

The concept and algorithm behind T-Patterns was first stimulated by research regarding the structure of behaviour and interactions with focus on real-time, probabilistic, and functional aspects, as well as hierarchical and syntactic structure, creativity, routines and planning [2,3]. T-Patterns were chosen, because behaviour patterns are often hidden in a stream of behavioural data and exist at different time scales. The T-Pattern algorithm works with a bottom-up approach. Simple T-Patterns are at the fundamental level just simple pairs of sensor events having a statistical significant interval relationship [3]. The assumption in the T-Pattern approach is a null hypothesis, expecting that each component is independently and randomly distributed over time with its observed average frequency.

The T-Pattern Algorithm is followed by building a PST with the significant T-Patterns. Therefore, each significant T-Pattern stands for one node and the next symbol probabilities are calculated with the Poisson distribution.

The concept how to construct the next symbol probability of states in a PST relies on the idea of maximum duration compare Fig. 1. This means in every pattern-step the longest duration of the patterns in this period is used to calculate the next symbol probability for this transition.

If the maximum duration of pattern-step 11 is interesting, the calculation begins at the pattern @tt. The pattern-step 11 in this example means the transformation of @tt in @ttt, @ttk or @ttx. The duration of every suffix of the pattern @tt{t, k, x} is compared and the maximum duration is chosen to calculate the next symbol probability. All transformation probabilities, which are calculated in the way described before, are put to the correct node, where x describes those cases where nothing significant happens. Therefore, is it ensured

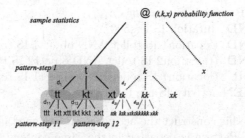

Fig. 1. Concept of next symbol probabilities calculation

that the total cases in one step sums always up to one. This is important, as otherwise no automaton can be constructed out of the PST.

To complete the system, the PST must be transformed in a PSA. In [4] an algorithm can be found for this step. First all leaves are added to the new automaton as recurrent states and a state equal to the root of the PST. The states are connected with each other. In the next step the arcs are built, requiring the next-symbol probabilities of the PST. If there exists a next symbol probability after the given state, the symbol is added, and from the front symbol by symbol is removed until this state can be found in the automaton and an arc is created. The last step is to assign state types. This is done by looking at each node and ascertaining if one of the arcs comes from a recurrent state created in step one, accordingly, this state also becomes a recurrent state. All other nodes are transient states.

3   Activity Assignment

The system described above is able to detect behaviour without annotated data. This is of course important for an automatic system, leading to the problem of which pattern describes which human activities within the system. This is solved during the assignment step, with Fuzzy Logic. The concept of Fuzzy Logic is partial membership in the sense of fuzzy sets and is used also in regard to human activities detection [5].

An annotated dataset for building a system for allocation is necessary and has to be recorded. The activity content consisting of location, objects, time and duration and the detectable activities must be specified before the assignment. Then the general rules for the Fuzzy Logic algorithm can be learned for each person in a specific flat and are for now on used as the basic individual human activity knowledge. This is done with the annotated activity dataset, which is recorded once. Each recorded activity consists of the activity and this information is combined in one rule:

RULE: **IF**   time IS morning
         AND duration IS less500
         AND (location1 IS toilet AND object1 IS toiletdoor)
         AND ((location2 IS toilet AND object2 IS toiletflush)
          OR   (location1 IS toilet AND object1 IS toiletflush))
         THEN activity IS use toilet

On the basis of this construct the activities are assigned using Fuzzy Logic. This means each T-Pattern is departed in the same content with the information 'timestamp begin', 'timestamp end' and the included 'sensors'. Later each pattern is compared with each rule, where the fulfilled rules are combined to one specific activity from the knowledge basis. This activity is assigned to the pattern, finally.

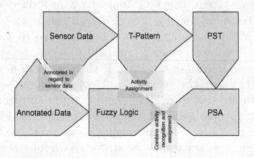

Fig. 2. Construct of behavior recognition model

To get an overview of the concept, Fig. 2 shows the relation and combination of the different parts within the system of behavior recognition. Meaning the assignment and the activity recognition part are merged together and the chain of recognition can be seen.

4   Results

In this section the results of the methods are discussed. The data from Kasteren *et al.* [8] are used to evaluate the T-Pattern algorithm. First the results of the T-Pattern algorithm is shown. The last part focuses on the results from the algorithm constructing a PSA.

4.1   T-Pattern Analysis

The T-Patterns are evaluated with the annotated dataset. In this analysis the significance test for the T-Patterns is done by the Binomial distribution. In the first evaluation the T-Pattern algorithm finds too many T-Patterns. This is the reason why a fine tuning of the recognized T-Patterns has been done to get more appropriate patterns. Especially those patterns which do not intersect with an activity or only intersect with at most 10% are a problem for further evaluation. In consequence, the first step is to leave out the T-Patterns which consist of only one sensor event, leading to a huge improvement. This fine tuning is expanded by blurring the activities 10% each side, ignoring specific patterns, useless patterns and bad pattern, leading finally to an appropriate result.

The significance analysis indicate that 0.005 or 0.001 levels seems to be most appropriate. The significance level is lowered with the consequence of less patterns being recognized. These patterns are those which match an annotated activity with higher percentage.

4.2 Probabilistic Suffix Tree and Probabilistic Suffix Automata

In Fig. 3 a result of the used system can be seen. In this case the sensors 7 and 8 are considered to build a PST. The probabilities are described in percentage, where the state 8_0 means 'toilet flush usage ended', 8_1 'toilet flush usage started', 7_0 'toilet door contact opened' and 7_1 means 'toilet door contact closed'. The results show that the probabilities are reasonable, as in each step the probabilities get smaller. This is of course true, because the occurrence of event A is at least as probable as the occurrence of pattern AB.

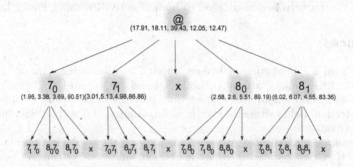

Fig. 3. PST based on sensor 7 and 8 with pattern length 2

In Fig. 4 the PST is transformed into a PSA with the already mentioned method. The result is an automaton, because for each state exists a subsequent state. If the activity, for instance 'using the toilet', is finished, the activity concludes with the state x, describing all events excluding the important ones 7 and 8. The two probabilities in Fig. 4 assigned to arrows pointing in both directions describe the probability to the left node, indicated by the number above, and to the right node, indicated by the number below.

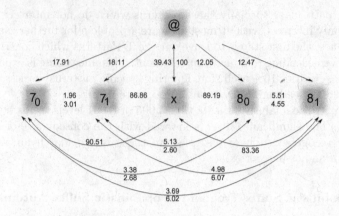

Fig. 4. PSA transformed from PST in Fig. 3

5 Conclusion and Outlook

This work gives an overview of a behavior system which is able to deal with sequential data from domotic sensors. This sensor data are used to detect patterns and transform this patterns into knowledge. This is done with the transformation of the T-Pattern sample statistic to a PST and later to a PSA. Furthermore, the pattern are associated to human activities using Fuzzy Logic.

References

1. Li, K., Yun, F.: Prediction of human activity by discovering temporal sequence patterns. IEEE Trans. Pattern Anal. Mach. Intell. **36**(8), 1644–1657 (2014)
2. Magnusson, M.S.: Discovering hidden time patterns in behavior: T-Patterns and their detection. Behav. Res. Methods Instrum. Comput. J. Psychon. Soc. Inc. **32**(1), 93–110 (2000)
3. Magnusson, M.S.: Repeated patterns in behavior, other biological phenomena. In: Oller, D.K., Griebel, U. (eds.) Evolution of Communication Systems: A Comparative Approach, pp. 111–128. MIT Press, Cambridge (2004)
4. Mazeroff, G., De, V., Jens, C., Michael, G., Thomason, G.: Probabilistic trees and automata for application behavior modeling. In: 41st ACM Southeast Regional Conference Proceedings, pp. 435–440, January 2003
5. Medjahed, H., Istrate, D., Boudy, J., Dorizzi, B.: Human activities of daily living recognition using fuzzy logic for elderly home monitoring. In: IEEE International Conference on Fuzzy Systems, 2009. FUZZ-IEEE 2009, pp. 2001–2006, August 2009
6. Nugent, C.N., Biswas, J., Hoey, J.: Activity Recognition in Pervasive Intelligent Environments (Google eBook). Springer, New York (2011)
7. Ron, D., Singer, Y., Tishby, N.: The power of amnesia: learning probabilistic automata with variable memory length. Mach. Learn. **25**(2), 117–149 (1996)
8. Kasteren, T.L., Englebienne, G., Kröse, B.J.A.: Human activity recognition from wireless sensor network data: benchmark and software. In: Chen, L., Nugent, C.D., Biswas, J., Hoey, J. (eds.) Atlantis Ambient and Pervasive Intelligence, vol. 4, pp. 165–186. Atlantis Press, Amsterdam (2011)

Emotion Recognition in the Wild: Results and Limitations from Active and Healthy Ageing Cases in a Living Lab

Evdokimos I. Konstantinidis, Antonis Billis, Theodore Savvidis,
Stefanos Xefteris, and Panagiotis D. Bamidis$^{(\boxtimes)}$

Lab of Medical Physics, Assistive Technologies and Silver-Science Group,
Medical School, Aristotle University of Thessaloniki, Thessaloniki, Greece
evdokimosk@gmail.com, {ampillis,bamidis}@med.auth.gr,
teosavv@yahoo.gr, sxefteris@auth.gr

Abstract. The work presented in this paper relies on the recognition of emotions during pilot trials with elderly people in an ecologically valid living lab. The emotion recognition is processed by cloud based service and the photos for processing are captured from Kinect based on the skeleton presence and information. The Kinect publishes its information to a channel where the clients subscribe efficiently either to the skeleton or the RGM images channel.

Keywords: Emotion · Living lab · AAL · Elderly · IoT

1 Introduction

In the research field of Ambient Assisted living, a shift towards monitoring elderly people status remotely, providing the physicians with information not only on physical, but also the psychological health [1, 2] has been identified. The emerging trends are behavioral profiling and activity monitoring in the wild as parts of decision support implementations in AAL context [3, 4]. Face [5], body language and vocal cues [6, 7] are the dominant modalities for emotion recognition.

So far, in the unobtrusive emotion recognition domain, efforts are mostly made in "in-vitro" ideal set-ups while the real challenge is multimodal emotion recognition in the wild, in ecologically valid environments. Although a lot of facial expression recognition systems have emerged with good accuracy [8], emotion recognition in the wild remains a challenging problem due to diversity in scenes in the form of head pose, illumination, occlusion and background noise [9].

2 Materials and Methods

The work presented in this paper relies on the recognition of emotions during pilot trials with elderly people in an ecologically valid living lab. The emotion recognition is processed by cloud based service and the photos for processing are captured from Kinect based on the skeleton presence and information.

© ICST Institute for Computer Sciences, Social Informatics and Telecommunications Engineering 2017
K. Giokas et al. (Eds.): eHealth 2016, LNICST 181, pp. 425–428, 2017.
DOI: 10.1007/978-3-319-49655-9_51

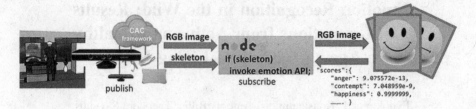

Fig. 1. Architecture of the emotion recognition approach exploiting the IoT infrastructure in Active and Healthy Ageing related pilots in living labs.

2.1 Architecture

The Controller Application Communication framework (CAC-framework) [10], based on the publish/subscribe messaging pattern in line with the IoT paradigm, is a cross device/application framework built on top of the Webockets. Design to support high throughput for real time streaming of information published from gaming controller, such as Kinect, Wii and Emotiv [11], JSON messages are exchanged among the devices and applications in the same session [12].

In the work presented in this paper (cf. Fig. 1), a NodeJs client subscribes to the skeleton information of the Kinect. Every time a skeleton is detected, the NodeJs client subscribes to the RGB image channel of the Kinect, gets the first streamed image and unsubscribes from this channel to avoid wasting bandwidth. Thereafter, the image is sent to the Emotion API of the Project Oxford[1] [13] and the emotion information is returned back. This information is then enriched with information pertaining to the skeleton position and rotation (from the body shoulders). The NodeJs application does not capture images more frequently than 5 s.

2.2 Experiment

Lab pilots ran in Thessaloniki, in the Active & Healthy Aging Living Lab (http://aha-livinglabs.com). There, a living room environment and a kitchen environment were set up in the same room and equipped unobtrusively with the necessary recording infrastructure, including the Kinect sensor. Each participant visiting the Living Lab was going through some daily activities [14], interaction with smart devices and exergaming play [15] for approximately 60–90 min (cf. Fig. 2). This study presents results of 6 sessions for 2 seniors. The CAC Playback Manager [16] was utilized to reproduce the experiment by playing back the recorded datasets.

---

[1] https://www.projectoxford.ai/demo/emotion#detection.

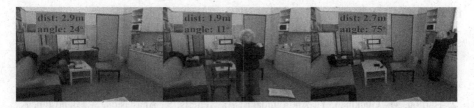

Fig. 2. The senior in the AHALL along with the skeleton detected information.

3 Results

In Table 1 emotions detected represents the number of images where at least one face emotion has been detected (along with the average value of three emotions) while the images analyzed is the total number of images sent to the Emotion API for processing. The max distance and body angle (shoulders rotation) are the maximum corresponding values of the skeleton when an emotion is detected.

Table 1. Emotions detected along with the seniors position and rotation

Actor#	Day#	Duration (mins)	Emotions detected	Images analyzed	Max distance (m)	Max body angle	Anger	Happy	Sad
1	1	87	334	667	2.42	41	0.005	0.008	0.017
1	2	88	252	665	2.5	68	0.004	0.024	0.003
1	3	124	350	1191	2.48	78	0.004	0.033	0.005
2	1	103	210	1035	2.44	39	0.009	0.100	0.051
2	2	135	347	1738	2.43	41	0.021	0.048	0.069
2	3	98	147	1305	2.54	42	0.012	0.070	0.033

4 Discussion

This work presents a first approach towards identifying the limitations of emotion recognition in the wild. Since the existing methodologies are far from perfect, a contextual approach to application should be considered. For example, since our findings indicate that existing algorithms perform better when the subject is less than 2.5 m away and with facing angle up to 70°, it follows that context aware emotion recognition could be more accurate in the IoT domain. On the other hand, the purpose of this work is to underline existing limitations and provide points on which we could focus our research for improving existing methodologies.

Acknowledgments. This work was supported in part by the UNCAP Horizon 2020 project (grant number 643555), as well as, the business exploitation scheme of the ICT-PSP funded project LLM, namely, LLM Care which is a self-funded initiative at the Aristotle University of Thessaloniki (www.llmcare.gr).

References

1. Xefteris, S., Baboshin, A., Tserpes, K., Androulidakis, A., Glickman, Y., Varvarigou, T., Haritou, M., D'Andria, F.: Enabling risk assessment and analysis by event detection in dementia patients using a reconfigurable rule set. In: Proceedings of the 4th International Conference on PErvasive Technologies Related to Assistive Environments, p. 47 (2011)
2. Haritou, M., Glickman, Y., Androulidakis, A., Xefteris, S., Anastasiou, A., Baboshin, A., Cuno, S., Koutsouris, D.: A technology platform for a novel home care delivery service to patients with dementia. J. Med. Imaging Heal. Inform. **2**, 49–55 (2012)
3. Xefteris, S., Andronikou, V., Tserpes, K., Varvarigou, T.: Case-based approach using behavioural biometrics aimed at assisted living. J. Ambient Intell. Humaniz. Comput. **2**, 73–80 (2010)
4. Billis, A.S., Papageorgiou, E.I., Frantzidis, C.A., Tsatali, M.S., Tsolaki, A.C., Bamidis, P.D.: A decision-support framework for promoting independent living and ageing well. IEEE J. Biomed. Health Inform. **19**, 199–209 (2015)
5. Ekman, P., Friesen, W.V., Ellsworth, P.: Emotion in the human face. In: Guidelines for Research and an Integration of Findings (2013)
6. Singh, S., Sharma, V., Jain, K., Bhall, R.: EDBL-algorithm for detection and analysis of emotion using body language. In: 2015 1st International Conference on Next Generation Computing Technologies (NGCT), pp. 820–823 (2015)
7. Martinez, L., Falvello, V.B., Aviezer, H., Todorov, A.: Contributions of facial expressions and body language to the rapid perception of dynamic emotions. Cogn. Emot., 1–14 (2015)
8. Song, K.-T., Lin, C.-Y.: Robust facial emotion recognition using a temporal-reinforced approach. In: 2014 14th International Conference on Control, Automation and Systems (ICCAS), pp. 804–807 (2014)
9. Dhall, A., Ramana Murthy, O.V., Goecke, R., Joshi, J., Gedeon, T.: Video and image based emotion recognition challenges in the wild: EmotiW 2015, pp. 423–426 (2015)
10. Konstantinidis, E.I., Antoniou, P.E., Bamparopoulos, G., Bamidis, P.D.: A lightweight framework for transparent cross platform communication of controller data in ambient assisted living environments. Inform Sci. **300**, 124–139 (2014)
11. Konstantinidis, E., Conci, N., Bamparopoulos, G., Sidiropoulos, E., De Natale, F., Bamidis, P.: Introducing Neuroberry, a platform for pervasive EEG signaling in the IoT domain. In: Proceedings of the 5th EAI International Conference on Wireless Mobile Communication and Healthcare - "Transforming Healthcare Through Innovations in Mobile and Wireless Technologies." ICST (2015)
12. Konstantinidis, E.I., Antoniou, P.E., Billis, A., Bamparopoulos, G., Pappas, C., Bamidis, P. D.: leveraging web technologies to expose multiple contemporary controller input in smart TV rich internet applications utilized in elderly assisted living environments. In: Stephanidis, C., Antona, M. (eds.) UAHCI 2014. LNCS, vol. 8515, pp. 118–128. Springer, Switzerland (2014). doi:10.1007/978-3-319-07446-7_12
13. Microsoft Project Oxford seconds that emotion: Biometric Technol. Today **2016**, 2 (2016)
14. Billis, A.S., Katzouris, N., Artikis, A., Bamidis, P.D.: Clinical decision support for active and healthy ageing: an intelligent monitoring approach of daily living activities. In: Pereira, F., Machado, P., Costa, E., Cardoso, A. (eds.) EPIA 2015. LNCS (LNAI), vol. 9273, pp. 128–133. Springer, Switzerland (2015). doi:10.1007/978-3-319-23485-4_14
15. Konstantinidis, E.I., Bamparopoulos, G., Bamidis, P.D.: Moving real exergaming engines on the web: The webFitForAll case study in an active and healthy ageing living lab environment. IEEE J. Biomed. Health Inform. (2016). Accepted
16. Konstantinidis, E.I., Billis, A.S., Bratsas, C., Bamidis, P.D.: Active and healthy ageing big dataset streaming on demand. In: HCI International 2016 (2016)

Smart Adaptable System for Older Adults' Daily Life Activities Management

Kostas Giokas[1]([✉]), Athanasios Anastasiou[1],
and Dimitrios Koutsouris[2]

[1] Applied Informatics in m-Health (AiM) Research Team,
Biomedical Engineering Laboratory,
National Technical University of Athens, Athens, Greece
{kgiokas,aanastasiou}@biomed.ntua.gr
[2] Biomedical Engineering Laboratory, National Technical University of Athens,
Athens, Greece
dkoutsou@biomed.ntua.gr

Abstract. In this paper we propose a system that will act as the main platform for a number of low-cost, mature technologies that will be integrated in order to create a dynamically adaptive Daily Life Activities Management environment in order to facilitate the everyday life of senior (but not exclusively) citizens at home. While the main target group of platform's users is the ageing population its use can be extended to all people that are vulnerable or atypical in body, intellect or emotions and are categorized by society as disabled. The classes of assistive products that are well defined in the international standard, ISO9999 such as assistive products for personal medical treatment, personal care and protection, communication, information and reaction and for personal mobility, will be easily incorporated in our proposed platform. Furthermore, our platform could integrate and implement the above classes under several service models that will be analyzed further.

Keywords: Mobility · Safety · Assistance · Smart Home

1 Introduction

The field of home computerization is extending quickly as electronic innovations merge. The home system envelops interchanges, stimulation, security, comfort, and data frameworks. Our platform advancement addresses the change of the living-at-home nature of elderly people. Maturing is a worldwide pattern that will proceed for future eras. Currently, 19 of the world's 20 "eldest" countries - those with the largest percentage of elderly people (65 or older) - are in Europe. In Italy, the world's most seasoned nation by these measures, more than 19 percent of the populace is elderly. This figure is required to achieve 28 percent by 2030. In Germany, future is required to achieve 90 by 2050. Encompassing helped living and the change of the living-at-home quality for the elderly populace is a European as well as a worldwide issue. This issue however pinpoints the limit for a European wide effect of our proposed platform. Through the proposed platform, we mean to convey a framework that

© ICST Institute for Computer Sciences, Social Informatics and Telecommunications Engineering 2017
K. Giokas et al. (Eds.): eHealth 2016, LNICST 181, pp. 429–437, 2017.
DOI: 10.1007/978-3-319-49655-9_52

can drag out the stay of elderly natives at their own home. This will be accomplished by coordinating existing advances into a shrewd home environment, for example, seniors can appreciate computerized consideration and help at their own premises. Our proposed solution will give "flat" administrations at a container European level. The horizontality of the arrangement will give the capacity of simple adjustment in order to meet diverse societal and social needs and in addition monetary limitations that may contrast crosswise over Europe.

2   The Platform

2.1   Researched Service Models

ABLE through Localisation Assistance at Home, will permit enhancement of the client's development inside the home. By utilizing the neighborhood data administration benefit the client will make the minimum conceivable developments required to finish a particular undertaking. The accompanying innovations will be actualized:

1. Real time localization services with Wi-Fi tags. Tags are placed on ordinarily misplaced things like mobile, glasses, automobile and residential keys. Location of those things are displayed on the central information monitor overlaid on a plan of the house
2. An inconspicuous transferrable electronic device as is described below.
   In like manner, the Local data administration, will ensure that the client knows about every conceivable "state" of the innovations as well as administrations that are coordinated in the platform. The accompanying innovations are imagined:

   • A focal data screen - this screen will serve as the primary data purpose of our platform. It will be arranged near the passage of the home so that the client will have simple and significant access. This can be a dynamic reflect or brilliant surface. This screen will caution the client in all cases furthermore introduce him/her with significant data.
   • Call focus reconciliation - a devoted call focus will get ready information and will have the capacity to make calls to the client's home in the event of crisis.
   • General Memory Aids can either be a piece of the wellbeing booth or fall under the general correspondence entryway of the house (this can be the client's PC). An electronic coordinator for regular data administration, PC applications particularly intended for clients with psychological impedances will be utilized for preparing.

3. Also, under the Telemedical Assistance at Home administration, a Health Kiosk will assemble, store and transmit wellbeing data utilizing advanced innovations. This wellbeing booth - this will be the primary wellbeing estimation station of our incorporated framework. It will comprise of the accompanying:

   • Drug update System: in spite of the fact that went for clients with memory weakness a solution update framework like the MD2 can expand adherence, kill drug abuse and treatment disappointment.

4. Late advances in ICT for maturing admirably (and dynamic maturing) have concentrated on the improvement and approval of innovations, instruments, methods and general answers for the successful administration of falls. Through the Safety@Home administration the accompanying innovations will be incorporated:

- Floor sensors in the lavatory and kitchen floors (where most deadly falls happen) for flaw identification. The framework will have the capacity to raise prompt alarms if a fall happens in either room.
- PtZ cameras: all rooms will be fitted with idle cameras that have a point-to-zoom office. A camera will be enacted once it gets the ready call from the fall identification sensors and the sensor on the convenient gadget.
- An unpretentious convenient electronic gadget (the measure of an advanced camera) fitted with fall discovery accelerometers and a frenzy catch. This gadget will have the capacity to convey through Wi-Fi with the home's focal data center furthermore incorporate a sensor that will draw in the PtZ cameras upon fall discovery.
- Sleep Management Hypnogram administration: The platform will contain a rest engineering observing framework keeping in mind the end goal to help the client keep up his circadian cadence. The SAMS will have the capacity to distinguish Seasonal Affective Disorder and/or Delayed Sleep Phase Syndrome and caution the call focus as needs be. It will likewise incorporate a rest apnea observing framework.

5. Shrewd Engine Everything gets keen. This is a typical origination in the examination field of Pervasive Computing. The Smart Engine administration which is proposed in our platform will recognize any unusual conduct as right on time as could be allowed keeping in mind the end goal to trigger a caution or initiate another fitting procedure as fast as would be prudent. A brilliant home is a private setting outfitted with an arrangement of cutting edge hardware, sensors and computerized gadgets particularly intended for consideration conveyance, remote checking, early location of issues or crisis cases and advancement of private security and personal satisfaction.

It expects to target elderly clients that don't have a casual carer living close-by. It plans to augment these clients' autonomy with the goal that they are supportable while living alone. These clients might have an assigned formal carer however our platform will help them more dynamic and upbeat in their homes. It will be generally welcomed by the "old" and "old-old" gatherings.

It is effectively comprehended that the plenty of sensors fitted all through the home does not constitute an incorporated arrangement until the data got is prepared and gone through a guidelines motor that produces important yields and a general mix arrangement has been executed.

At long last, our platform goes for expanding the acknowledgment level of assistive innovation from Reluctant to Grateful or shockingly better Internal [1].

2.2 An Example Scenario

Olivia is forty-four years recent and had an automobile accident some years ago. She lives alone and so as to complete her daily tasks reception needs help since her quality is restrained. The projected application can permit her to confirm her freedom within the house by optimizing her movement as so much because the location of many objects within the house as involved. it'll be ready to prompt her drug treatment, keep track of her daily activity and organize her tasks or maybe alert her to things like "oven continues to be on". Likewise, the embedded floor sensors, can permit hindrance of any fall, minimizing the chance for any injuries. Last however not least this sensible system are ready to adapt its services although customization, to Olivia's wants, resulting in an easier life.

3 Platform's Architecture

The Aimed Service Models can permit optimization of the user's movement inside the house through quality help reception service. By persecution the native info management service the user can build the less potential movements needed to accomplish a particular task. the most innovation of this service is that the reduction of physical effort to the minimum from the top user. The technology behind it's out there these days (at least in terms of hardware, sensors, etc.) and therefore the demand is that the coaching of the system inside a particular house (user's home) by modelling the resident's activity supported their past movements (LeZi formula [2], Hidden Markoff Models). so as to assemble more information on movements within the house, IR sensors area unit put in on top of every area entrance and at foot level within the room and passageway. 2 RFID systems area unit wont to establish the residents, one active and therefore the different passive. the previous uses 315 MHz waves, whereas the latter operates within the pair of .45 GHz band. Active scanners area unit settled on top of the ceiling of every area, and sight RFID tags whenever a theme enters. Passive system antennas area unit embedded within the walls around every area entrance, and browse out information on the tag once someone passes through [3].

Moreover, the Local data administration will ensure that the client knows about every conceivable "state" of the advancements as well as administrations that take an interest in our platform. All significant data will be shown in the principle screen near the home way out [4, 5]. For instance, there will be a notice when the client moves towards the exit having overlooked his telephone at home. The detecting modules of the room record the conditions of the floor, bed, table and switches. The mix of these information is characterized as the "room state". A calculation named "outline" was additionally created, which sections the aggregated sensor information at focuses where the yields change definitely. The sections are coordinated with and appointed to "room states". The calculation additionally tries to dispose of repetitive states that have changed just somewhat. The framework incorporates switch sensors on various apparatuses, notwithstanding the table, seat and bed [6]. These sensors are adequate to distinguish whether a human is standing or dozing, to identify the position of their hands on the table, and to recognize the positions of items on the table. The cooler, icebox, microwave, toaster, windows, and bureau are all furnished with switch sensors to identify whether their entryways are open or shut [7]. A useful adjusted to the particular client bunch, User Interface is accessible introducing key data to client.

The Health Kiosk will assemble, store and transmit wellbeing data utilizing advanced innovations through the Telemedical help at home administration model. It will utilize the accessible sensors (circulatory strain, temperature, amplifier, and so forth.) that catch/record imperative signs (beat, breath, development) and investigations it through Fuzzy rationale. In the event that cautions are raised (in light of the Smart Engine) the Safety@Home Service (through the Alert Management highlight) will empower the intercession of the call focus and triage operations will be started.

The Safety@Home administration model will incorporate Fall counteractive action, Alert Management and Intrusion Detection Recent advances in ICT for maturing great (and dynamic maturing) have concentrated on the improvement and approval of advances, devices, systems and general answers for the compelling administration of falls. The separate arrangements incorporate sensors for the auspicious location of falls, inescapable applications for activating alerts, actuators for enhancing the encompassing environment (e.g., lighting conditions. Interruption Detection frameworks (cost/esteem proportion considering) will be coordinated in the platform.

The Smart Engine will apply decides that will make a comprehensive systemic way to deal with home wellbeing. Everything gets shrewd is a typical origination in the examination field of Pervasive Computing. A great deal of items and gadgets that we use in day by day life are as of now keen. Similarly, our living spaces get to be more quick witted step by step. Keen homes and situations are these days no more sci-fi. One point of Smart Environments and Product is to upgrade the solace of the tenant and the client separately. All these solace can be a key advantage for individuals with inabilities or elderly people. Such prepared situations can repay a few incapacities of the tenant. It can improve their day by day lives and decrease the reliance on different people. They can utilize all the gave usefulness of the earth themselves, fortify their autonomy and individual opportunity and can thusly stay longer in their standard environment. Along these lines Ambient and Assisted Living is one vital field of use for Smart Homes taking into consideration custom fitted intercessions. These frameworks can possibly bolster maturing and enhance personal satisfaction and basic leadership for individuals in need, debilitated and maturing individuals. The prosperity Domain incorporates a scope of components like wellbeing, wellness, depressive side effects and subjective working. The proposed structure will watch exercises and practices, which are identified with these variables, and it will progressively create controls and activate forms keeping in mind the end goal to weaken, standardize or invigorate the different prosperity aspects [8, 9].

Keeping in mind the end goal to make an agreeable domain for the client, home mechanizations with respect to the ecological control will be put in the home and coordinated to the platform making the Home Environment Controls. To wrap things up, some fundamental Home Entertainment incorporation will be offered (principle based TV control, and so on.) (Fig. 1).

The prevalence of the many pilots across totally different EU countries can facilitate the moral adjustment of the platform so as to make sure that legal and social problems area unit addressed. Initial of all, any legal, elementary and moral diversifications for

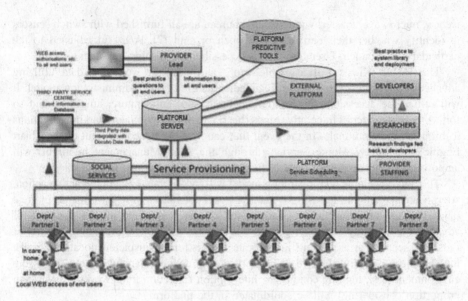

Fig. 1. Platform's architecture

every land concerned are going to be assessed throughout the pilot part and any obligatory amendment to the merchandise are going to be incorporated. Additionally, as a result of the unfold of the pilots at totally different European countries the ability and cultural adaptation (language, bioengineering etc.) are going to be addressed like the planned system can be wide used across Europe [10]. At now, we should always additionally underline that the platform is going to be adjustable supported the wants and value limitations of the patron. though a good vary of services are going to be obtainable through the platform, the user can have the prospect to accommodate less services (if desired) within the platform supported his wants. This practicality, can enable voters with totally different wants or economical restrictions to afford the merchandise. Finally, we should always underline that each one parts of the planned system do take under consideration from their early style part, the actual fact that the EU market is targeted with all its disparities and cultural no uniformity. Even so, the measurability and generic and standards-based approach permits to ideate all necessary adaptation different national or local's implementation necessities. Exploitation are going to be potential to evolve in parallel with the technical work and it'll become a lot of intense whereas approaching the mop up of the merchandise. During this approach the ultimate product are going to be thought of from a spread of various views. We'll be able to perceive in additional detail what we've to supply and reveal the business price of such service within the context of many countries. Once the exploitation part is running, factors like maturity, current trends and users' expectations are going to be addressed across the platform's life time. The user organizations piloting the service can function feedback suppliers on the practicableness of the technical approach still on give input regarding the marketability of the merchandise in every country. Through such organizations we have a tendency to additionally expect to spot potential

European-wide actors that may give a transparent plan concerning the market conditions during which the planned platform are going to be commercial such they may be taken into thought. additionally, merchandise and ideas to be enclosed are going to be addressed against cultural protocols and aim to include them [11]. Any ability and standardisation problems that would contribute to the creation of a generic and ascendable product to be adjustable within the wants of every totally different user are going to be evaluated.

4 Platform's Benefits

The computerized observing and reacting of telecare frameworks gives true serenity to families that a check is being continued their adored one, and if any of various unsafe events emerges then this will be distinguished and will be given. The client additionally has the consolation of realizing that they will be aided if such events emerge. Assessments of this innovation have demonstrated that it gives great backing to its clients [12] and in reality in more than one case had been a key element in counteracting significant damage. The significant effect has been through utilizing the more direct sensors, for example, entryway sensors and development sensors. Sensors intended to recognize more unpredictable practices such disregarding running showers and flooding bathrooms, and abuse of cookers, were observed to be less successful. It has ended up being very hard to identify complex human conduct from the utilization of basic sensors, and a few applications, for example, distinguishing abuse of shower taps obviously requires faster reactions than can be given through the convoluted reaction course by means of call focuses to somebody going to give assistance. The general population being upheld by telecare establishments are for the most part delicate elderly individuals in their own particular homes, yet work has additionally been completed to investigate the use of the innovation to all the more extremely crippled gatherings. There are potential cost funds for wellbeing and social consideration suppliers utilizing telecare on the grounds that there is not the same requirement for consistent checks by domiciliary staff, and helping somebody to stay autonomous in their own home as opposed to going into consideration could spare expansive entireties without a doubt. Additionally, the identification of some behavioral circumstances, for example, going outside amidst the night, could decrease human services costs as the more serious results of such activities would be diminished. A reasonable confinement of telecare establishments is the need to include call focuses in the reaction circle. The call focus staff can give some remote verbal backing however in the event that assistance is required then they need to contact individuals on their rundowns to visit and resolve whatever issue had emerged, with an inescapable deferral while this happens. All the more inconspicuously for the client these frameworks are fundamentally simply observing their conduct. They can send help on the off chance that it is judged important yet can't empower the clients themselves to manage issues, and in that sense they are not exceptionally engaging.

5 Conclusions

Interest for astute assistive innovation for more established grown-ups is becoming quickly. The utilization of shrewd homes to bolster powerless individuals is still in its earliest platforms however is as of now demonstrating that it can give an abnormal state of backing. The essential sensors and bolster gear innovation is very basic, and the way to its prosperity is standing out the shrewd home establishment is designed utilizing these advancements to suit the requirements of the client. Proof is developing that these advancements are going to give numerous a huge number of individuals with enhanced autonomy and control of their lives, and ought to wind up very standard in the years ahead.

Keeping up utilitarian autonomy is a high need for some more established grown-ups. Quiet information observing is a key issue for wellbeing and ailment administration [13]. Often, staying in their own particular homes is critical to such autonomy. Progresses in data interchanges innovation and related computational force are giving a wide exhibit of frameworks and related administrations that shape the premise of keen home advancements to bolster the wellbeing, security and freedom of more seasoned grown-ups. While these innovations offer critical advantages to more established individuals and their families, they are additionally changing more established grown-ups into lead adopters of another every minute of every day way of life of being observed, overseen, and, on occasion, persuaded, to keep up their wellbeing and health. PC innovation can possibly help with this objective by supporting the regular undertakings of more established people, and in addition by helping parental figures and relatives. Our platform will investigate how computational capacities can upgrade everyday exercises under Daily Life Activities Management environment. Shrewd home situations normally are furnished with various types of sensors and GPS beacons for setting mindful administration provisioning. While from one viewpoint, individuals need to exploit the solace and included estimation of customized connection mindful administrations, protection and traceability turns into a genuine worry then again he PC is not an apparatus to be grabbed, utilized, and after that put aside [14]. It ought to be a steady accomplice in day by day exercises. The test is to plan interfaces that reflect and backing progressing exercises of everyday life yet not be improperly meddling. Our platform will be intended to meet day by day mindfulness needs of grown-up youngsters worried about the prosperity of a senior guardian, and another that can give surrogate memory helps to family unit assignments. It will show the many-sided quality of the issues required in outlining the computationally competent SMART home without bounds and give heading to future innovative work endeavors.

References

1. The Engineering Handbook of Smart Technology, Abdelsalam Helal, Mounir Mokhtari
2. Bhattacharya, A., Das, S.K.: LeZi-Update: an information-theoretic approach to track mobile users in PCS networks. In: Proceedings of the 5th Annual ACM/IEEE International Conference on Mobile Computing and Networking (MobiCom 1999), Seattle, USA, August 17–19 (1999)

3. Schmitt, L., Falck, T., Wartena, F., Simons, D.: Novel ISO/IEEE 73 Standards for Personal Telehealth Systems Interoperability
4. Yao, J., Warren, S.: Applying the ISO/IEEE 11073 Standards to Wearable Home Health Monitoring Systems
5. http://www.continuaalliance.org/about-the-alhance.html. Accessed 7 Dec 2013
6. Parkka, J., et al.: Activity Classification Using Realistic Data From Wearable Sensors (2006)
7. Home Care Technologies for Ambient Assisted Living Ratko Magjarevic
8. http://en.wikipedia.org/wiki/KNX_(standard)
9. http://www.eetimes.com/design/embedded/4025721/Catching-the-Z-Wave
10. Al-Ali, A.R., Al-Rousan, M., Ozkul, T.: Implementation of experimental communication protocol. Comput. Stand. Interfaces **28**, 523–530 (2006)
11. Liang, L.L., Huang, L.F., Jiang, X.Y., Yao, V.: Design and implementation of wireless smart-home sensor network based on ZigBee protocol. In: International Conference on Communications
12. Waddington, P., Downs, B.: The sandwell telecare project. J. Integr. Care **13**, 40–48 (2005)
13. Monton, E., Hernandez, J.F., Blasco, J.M., Herve, T., Micallef, J., Grech, I., Brincat, A., Traver, V.: Body area network for wireless patient monitoring. IET Commun. **2**, 215–222 (2008)
14. Technologies.   http://users.freenet.am/~file/DownDB/CISCO_PDF/SecurityTechnologies_ CISCO.pdf

An Ambient Assisted Living Technology Platform for Informal Carers of the Elderly

Ahmad Lotfi[1]([⊠]), Caroline Langensiepen[1], Pedro A. Moreno[2],
Enrique J. Gómez[2], and Saisakul Chernbumroong[1]

[1] School of Science and Technology, Nottingham Trent University, Clifton Lane,
Nottingham NG11 8NS, UK
ahmad.lotfi@ntu.ac.uk
[2] Bioengineering and Telemedicine Group, ETSI Telecommunication,
Technical University of Madrid, 28040 Madrid, Spain

Abstract. Family care is the most accepted and preferred care setting for both long-term care patients and their relatives. However, many of these caregivers are elderly people themselves, and often reach the point where they also need support. Care poses a substantial burden, so often it is not the health of the patient but the overload of stress for the caregiver that results in the need for much more expensive professional care and even residential care. An ambient assisted living technology platform is developed to support both older adults and their carers to overcome the challenges of the care. The platform offers informal carers support by means of monitoring Activities of Daily Care as well as their psychological state, and will provide orientation to help them improve the care given. Monitored information will be registered by means of home-installed and personal sensor technologies based on Internet of Things (IoT), which will be as unobtrusive as possible for the house inhabitants.

Keywords: Health care · Ambient Assisted Living · Ambient Intelligence · Elderly · Dementia · Assistive technology · Sensors · Internet of Things

1 Introduction

The world population is currently suffering progressive ageing which can have dramatic effects on health systems due to increasing costs and a higher demand of socio-healthcare services to maintain the elderly's independence and quality of life. The four major themes that are important for older adults to age in their own homes and community are [5]; safety and independence, social interaction, use of technology, and the desire for support. In addition, many older adults prefer to age in their own home rather than in an assisted living facility, even though they require long-term care due to diseases associated with ageing and assistance in their Activities of Daily Living (ADLs) [3]. Therefore, a significant increase in care responsibilities, which is typically performed by family and friends, appears

© ICST Institute for Computer Sciences, Social Informatics and Telecommunications Engineering 2017
K. Giokas et al. (Eds.): eHealth 2016, LNICST 181, pp. 438–442, 2017.
DOI: 10.1007/978-3-319-49655-9_53

and implies a need for innovative support approaches for family members and their carers.

This demographic change will lead to significant and interrelated modifications in the health care sector and technologies promoting independence for the elderly. Therefore, an enormous interest is growing in the use of technological solutions and specifically Information and Communication Technologies (ICT) to support elderly people to live independently for longer period in their homes and connect the older adults to geographically dispersed family and friends. In order to deal with this issue, the Ambient Assisted Living (AAL) initiative [4] promotes the creation of products, systems and solutions based on ICT for the support of the elderly's life independence. AAL services can be enclosed in the Ambient Intelligence (AmI) concept which implies a seamless environment of computing, advanced networking technology and specific interfaces providing users with context-aware, personalized, adaptive, ubiquitous and interoperable systems [1]. Additionally, AAL might need to support or collaborate with informal carers, such as relatives and friends, who play important roles in the lives and care of older adults [2].

2   Technological Needs

In order to initially establish the needs and concerns of the elderly and their carers, domain analysis was carried out. In a business context, a system would generally be based purely on pcs and servers, and the end users would probably be the primary stakeholders. They would be interviewed and user stories solicited. However for AAL systems, the sensors and AmI are as necessary as the servers, and the end users include formal care organisations, informal carers and the elderly. It is thus difficult to apply the usual open interview techniques since they may have no ideas of what they want from such systems. To provide an initial perspective on the problems and concerns of the stakeholders, without rejudging what is important to them, an automated method of finding contextual information was applied. Lexical analysis of over 34000 words from different Alzheimers Carers' forum threads has indicated some of the key concerns of the carers and issues for the elderly. Although the terms 'mum', 'mother', 'dad' and 'care' obviously dominate, the terms 'social', 'health', 'friends', 'services', 'people' were used surprisingly frequently, whereas specific care issues were not so dominant. These appeared to indicate that the carers were more concerned about the general well-being of the older adult.

The intelligent care guidance and learning services platform for informal carers of the elderly (iCarer) project has made an attempt to develop a personalized and adaptive platform to offer informal carers support by means of monitoring Activities of Daily Care (ADC) as well as their psychological state, and will provide orientation to help them improve the care given. Monitored information will be registered by means of home-installed and personal sensor technologies based on Internet of Things (IoT), which will be as unobtrusive as possible for the house inhabitants. Registered data will be analysed and fed into the platform

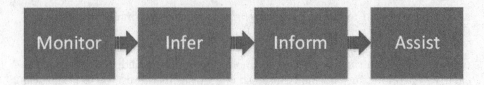

Fig. 1. Stages of iCarer platform.

in order to model the ADC based on behavioural patterns. With this information, and if the informal caregiver is absent at the time, the platform will act as a 'virtual carer', giving support to the older adult and providing information to the carer in case a daily activity is done incorrectly. Additionally, iCarer will provide e-Learning services and an informal carers' learning network. As a result, caregivers will be able to expand their knowledge, supported by the experience provided by expert counsellors and fellow carers. The coordination between formal and informal carers will be improved, offering the informal carers flexibility to organize and combine their assistance and social activities.

3   iCarer Platform

Considering the contextual situation of the elderly and their carers, the iCarer project proposes a personalized and adaptive platform to offer informal carers support by monitoring their ADC and psychological state, as well as providing an orientation to help them and improve the care provided. Monitored information will be registered by means of home-installed and personal sensors. Registered data will be analysed and fed into the platform in order to model the ADC based on behavioural patterns. With this information the platform can infer possible problems in the informal carer's activities or status. Thus, the platform will act as a "virtual carer" providing to the carer with recommendations to solve the issue. If the informal carer is absent at the time from the older adult's home, the platform will give support to the older adult in case a daily activity is done incorrectly. Additionally, iCarer will provide e-Learning services and an informal carers' learning network. As a result, carers will be able to expand their knowledge. The coordination between formal and informal carers will be improved, offering the informal carers flexibility to organize and combine their assistance and social activities. The platform is aimed at informal carers living with elderly adults (co-residents, commonly another elderly adult) who suffer cognitive impairment at any stage (from mild to severe).

The platform comprises four stages of: monitoring, inferring, informing and ultimately assisting the carer of an older adult as shown in Fig. 1. Unobtrusive sensors around the house are used to monitor activities of older adults and send data to the Cloud for analysis. To infer activities from the data, Computational Intelligence techniques are used to determine the activities and whether these are as expected. If the activities change from the usual pattern, fuzzy models are

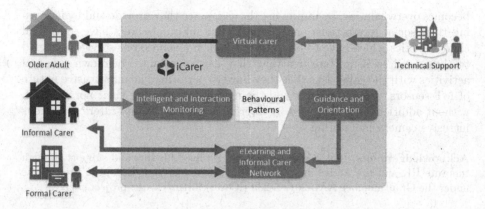

Fig. 2. The iCarer platform architecture.

used to deduce potential problems e.g. with sleep behaviour. Once a problem is identified, the carer is warned about the problem, and offered strategies to solve it, and hence reduce their stress.

In order to achieve the previous goals defined, the iCarer platform will be composed of a suite of modules, which provide the different services to support the informal carer, as shown in Fig. 2 and described briefly below.

– Intelligent and Interaction Monitoring - The iCarer platform provides a monitoring environment where the assistance tasks (ADCs) are monitored to detect early symptoms of carers' burden and stress.
– Guidance and Orientation - After analysing the data monitored, behavioural patterns of both informal carers and older adult will be inferred in this module. In the case of the informal carer, once the behavioural patterns have been inferred, this module is also responsible to determine if a problem is occurred in assistance tasks.
– Virtual Carer - The iCarer platform through this module proposes a service to support the care process reducing the carer's burden. Once the informal carer's problem or mistake is detected in ADC or ADL performance, the "Virtual Carer" will provide them with suitable guidance to improve the care activity or reduce the burden level of the informal carer.
– eLearning and Informal Carer Network - By employing a content management system (CMS) this module will offer to the carer a personalised selection of video based e-Learning contents in order to reduce their workload and improve the effectiveness of the provided care.

4   Conclusions

Informal carers feel thrown into the caring role without receiving enough assistance, lacking education and training for their role as carers. Informal carer's quality of life will be improved by detecting their burden and stress before it becomes overwhelming, by improving the assistance they provide and by increasing their social interactions and support. The informal carers have individual characteristics which have to be considered when a solution or service is offered to them, and so iCarer ensures that they can coordinate their own personal activities with the care tasks that they have to perform. The unobtrusive nature of IoT sensors allows the carer and the elderly to carry out their normal ADL without additional stress caused by interference from external carers or obvious intrusive camera monitoring.

Acknowledgements. The iCarer project has received funding and support through Innovate UK and the Active and Assisted Living (AAL) joint European programme under the Grant number AAL-2012-5-239 (iCarer) [http://icarer-project.eu/].

References

1. Aarts, E., de Ruyter, B.: New research perspectives on ambient intelligence. J. Ambient Intell. Smart Environ. **1**(1), 5–14 (2009)
2. Bamidis, P.D., Antoniou, P., Sidiropoulos, E.: Others: using simulations and experiential learning approaches to train careers of seniors. In: 2014 IEEE 27th International Symposium on Computer-Based Medical Systems (CBMS), pp. 119–124. IEEE (2014)
3. Hossain, M.A., Ahmed, D.T.: Virtual caregiver: an ambient-aware elderly monitoring system. IEEE Trans. Inf. Technol. in Biomed. **16**(6), 1024–1031 (2012)
4. Kubitschke, K., Cullen, K., Müller, S.: ICT and ageing: European study on users. Markets and Technologies, Final report (2010)
5. Van Hoof, J., Kort, H.S.M., Rutten, P.G.S., Duijnstee, M.S.H.: Ageing-in-place with the use of ambient intelligence technology: perspectives of older users. Int. J. Med. Inform. **80**(5), 310–331 (2011)

Volume Visualization Tools for Medical Applications in Ubiquitous Platforms

Ander Arbelaiz[1]([✉]), Aitor Moreno[1], Luis Kabongo[1],
and Alejandro García-Alonso[2]

[1] Vicomtech-IK4, Paseo Mikeletegi, 57, 20009 Donostia/San Sebastián, Spain
{aarbelaiz,amoreno,lkabongo}@vicomtech.org
[2] University of the Basque Country,
Paseo Manuel de Lardizabal 1, 20018 Donostia/San Sebastián, Spain
alex.galonso@ehu.es

Abstract. This paper presents three required functionality when volume datasets are aimed to be visualized in ubiquitous platforms: *(i)* support of segmented volume datasets, *(ii)* navigation inside the volume and *(iii)* direct visualization of DICOM datasets. DICOM is the de-facto standard in the medical imaging field. The results shows that these functionalities can be achieved using the Volume Rendering component implemented in X3DOM in several web browsers in different platforms (from desktop computer to tablets and mobile phones).

Keywords: Volume rendering · Medical imaging · DICOM · Visualization · X3DOM · Ubiquitous platforms

1 Introduction

In the medical field, the volumetric datasets are key in several phases of the medical procedures. The CT or MRI scans produce a large amount of information of a patient, normally as a set of 2D slices. These slices can be visualized and analyzed one by one, but they provide more information if they are considered as a whole volumetric dataset. The introduction of volume rendering techniques in desktop platforms was a milestone in the medical field. New methodologies and algorithms were implemented to take into account the 3D information embedded in the set of 2D slices that compose the scans.

In the last years, the new mobile paradigm has changed the landscape of the information sharing and the visualization schemes. The graphical power of the mobile devices has made possible to render interactive 3D content (commercial games, etc.). It was a matter of time to get open standards to deal with the 3D content generation and visualization without worrying about the underlying platform (hardware or software). The X3D standard aim to accomplish this challenge and X3DOM provides a WebGL implementation of the standard.

The volume rendering nodes in X3D are specified, but they do not materialize the precise functionality that the users require to interact with the volumetric datasets.

© ICST Institute for Computer Sciences, Social Informatics and Telecommunications Engineering 2017
K. Giokas et al. (Eds.): eHealth 2016, LNICST 181, pp. 443–450, 2017.
DOI: 10.1007/978-3-319-49655-9_54

This work presents three functionalities that have been detected as missing in the web-based volume rendering toolkits, including X3DOM. A solution has been devised for all the three functionalities and the results show that the new functionality works in different platforms.

The next section provides a summary of the bibliography and the related work. Section 3 presents the three functionalities to include in the volumetric visualization toolkits and how we have provided a solution for them. This paper concludes with the conclusions and future work.

2   Related Work

This section is divided in two parts: the first one describes previous work and the second one describes the volume ray-casting algorithm implemented in WebGL.

2.1   Previous Work

Volumetric visualization has been extensively studied over the years. Nowadays it is currently used on a variety of fields, but especially in medicine. Different volume visualization techniques can be found in the literature; our work focuses in ray-casting. Originally introduced by Kajiya and Herzen [5], ray-casting method was later translated to the GPU by Kruger and Westermann [6].

The growth of mobile devices and their rapid adoption on every days work has made them a target platform for computationally expensive applications like medical visualization. Rodríguez et al. [9] analyzed different volume rendering algorithms on mobile devices. More recently, Schiewe et al. [10] reviewed the status of volume rendering with the latest graphics APIs available on iOS devices.

WebGL-based rendering positions as the only choice to achieve a ubiquitous volumetric visualization. The first WebGL-based ray-casting method was introduced by Congote et al. [2]. In this direction, improvements have been published by Mobeen et al. [7]. Also, the volume size constraints of this approach have been addressed by Noguera and Jiménez [8]. The web browser is a common denominator in current devices; this has promoted initiatives to create web based medical oriented visualization tools. Between the current available scientific frameworks we should mention XTK [4], VJS [11], and X3DOM [1].

2.2   WebGL Volume Ray-Casting

Our work is integrated in the X3DOM framework under the volume rendering component. Volumetric rendering is performed with a single-pass ray-casting algorithm. In the scene a cube is rendered and it will be used to place the actual volume data during the ray-casting. Using the programmable pipeline provided by the WebGL API, a single pair of vertices and fragment shaders is used. In the vertex shader, each vertex position of the cube is multiplied by the Volume `ModelView` matrix and the `Projection` matrix, transforming the vertices into clip space.

In the fragment shader, the ray traversal is actually computed. When the triangles of the cube are rasterized into fragments, the interpolated vertices of the unitary cube represent 3D texture coordinates. From the inverse `ModelView` matrix the camera position can be obtained. After, by subtracting the interpolated vertex position with the camera position the ray direction can be determined. Taking both the interpolated position as the ray origin and the ray direction, using a fixed length loop statement in the fragment shader the ray traversal is created. For an in depth description of the single-pass approach, we refer the reader to Mobeen et al. [7].

The ray traversal is discretized into a series of steps. At each step the position of the ray is used as a 3D texture coordinates to fetch the volume data. However, WebGL does not support 3D textures, as first stated by Congote et al. [2] this can be overcome using a texture atlas (*ImageTextureAtlas*): the cross sectional slices that compose the volume are tiled into a matrix configuration to compose a single 2D texture.

3   Medical Visualization

Volumetric data is often used in the medical field in a large variety of situations: from research and diagnosis to educational purposes. In terms of visualization interactivity and usability, mobile platforms should provide the same tools as their desktop counterpart.

In pursuit of a ubiquitous medical volumetric visualization, we have detected three features that we consider that a ubiquitous volume visualization toolkit must provide: *(i)* the visualization of segmented data, *(ii)* camera navigation inside the 3D volume and *(iii)* the support of DICOM file format, a widely used medical data exchange format.

3.1   Segemented Medical Data

Volume visualization must be extended to provide the tools that the medical use cases require. Trained specialists in medical imaging segment regions of interest from the cross-sectional slices that compose a volume. The segmentation of the volume is important to focus the attention or to limit further work at the region of interest. Thus, any medical visualization tool must be capable of helping the user to discern the region of interest from the whole volume.

We have extended the initial ray-casting algorithm presented at Sect. 2.2 to support segmented visualization. In the ray-casting loop the ray traverses the volume accumulating color and opacity. The segmented data acts as an identifier on each voxel to allow the selection of an alternative accumulation algorithm at the region of interest. Using a distinctive color and opacity in sections where the ray traverses, allows standing out a region by visually enhancing the segmented area from the whole volume. The algorithm at Fig. 1 describes how the segmented data must be implemented inside the ray-casting loop.

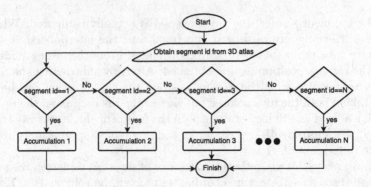

Fig. 1. Flowchart describing the segmentation algorithm in the ray traversal

As Fig. 1 shows, the segment data fetching is actually translated into a switch or selection statement that is performed in the ray-casting loop at a per step basis. From a performance point of view, this must be carefully considered as branching is not well supported in mobile devices. The type of variation in the accumulation process (see Fig. 1) will change depending of the use case, e.g., mapping colors with a transfer function (TF), modifying the opacity given the camera view and discarding the data. Figure 2 shows two renders of datasets with segmented regions. Each one has been generated with different accumulation processes to make them distinguishable from the volume.

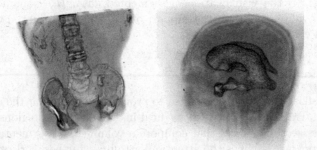

Fig. 2. Segmented data renderings of the aorta ($512 \times 512 \times 97$) and the *Head MRI* [12] ($256 \times 256 \times 124$) datasets. On the left, the edges of the segmented bones have been enhanced with color. On the right, the segmented ventricles had been colored with blue tones (Color figure online)

We have seen that it is advisable to specify a user-defined argument to explicitly know the maximum number of segments beforehand. The maximum number of segments limits the branching statements and they are dynamically added at the fragment shader creation time. Otherwise, the number of branching statements will be unbounded and a big amount of unnecessary comparison operations will be performed with a potential impact on the GPU performance.

In our implementation, the segmented data is tiled into a matrix configuration with the same procedure that must be performed with the volume data (see Sect. 2.2). To gain performance the segmented data could be stored in the alpha channel of the original volume data texture atlas, however, it is better and easier to create a separate texture. In first place, communication between server and client should be considered. The segmentation can be processed automatically or manually in an off-line tool and be loaded when required.

In second place, the texture atlas resolution should be considered. Due to memory restrictions in GPU mobile devices compared to desktop computers, the segmented texture atlas can be stored with a smaller texture size than the original texture atlas, and the same position coordinates would be valid to fetch the data from both textures. This technique will imply a precision loss of the segmented region.

3.2 Inside Exploration of Volume Data

Another visualization requirement in the medical environment is related to the interaction and immersive experience that volumetric data can provide. This can be conceptualized as the ability to explore the data from within the volume. An inside exploration allows the user to easily discern the internal composition of the volume rather than looking at the cross-sectional 2D images. In our implementation we have allowed the exploration of the volume by dynamically changing the initial position of the ray origin. Figure 3 describes the algorithm used. In this case, the cube is of unitary size.

First the camera position is obtained from the inverse ModelView matrix. Then using the maximum and minimum boundaries of the cube, it can be determined whether or not the camera is inside the volume. If the camera is outside the cube, the ray origin is assigned as the interpolated vertex position from the output of the vertex shader (varying vertex position), if not, the ray origin is the camera position. Figure 4 shows an external and internal rendering of the *Head MRI* dataset [12]. Without changing the ray origin, the camera face

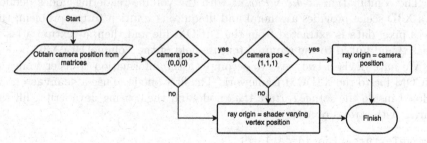

Fig. 3. Flowchart describing the ray origin computation in the single-pass ray-casting algorithm

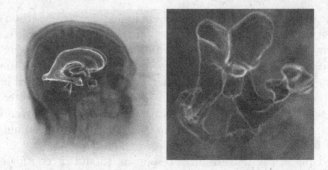

Fig. 4. Rendering of the *Head MRI* dataset (256×256×124) [12] enhancing a segmented area. On the left, the camera is outside the volume. On the right, the camera is inside the volume

of the cube will be clipped, making not possible an examination of the inside. Thus, back face culling must be disabled when internal exploration is required. When the camera is moved into the cube, the ray-casting direction for each ray is obtained by subtracting the interpolated back face vertex position with the camera position.

3.3 DICOM Visualization

Medical imaging devices do not only produce the actual 2D set of slices. They are linked with a large amount of metadata with related information about the patient and other medical procedures. DICOM is the medical image standard to store and transfer all this information from and between imaging devices and medical image storage repositories. The wide utilization of DICOM by all manufacturers had a major impact on usability of the file format. Resulting sometimes in a variable set of tags to be read, interpreted and combined in order to achieve coherent restitution of the images for the final user.

Cornerstone JavaScript library [3] provides a set of functions to read and interact with the 2D set of slices stored in DICOM files and it relies on *dicomParser* to load DICOM tags, including pixel data.

The combination of *dicomParser* with the volume rendering nodes defined in a X3D scene provides a general and ubiquitous solution to the problem: the slices pixel data is extracted from the DICOM file and then, a texture atlas is created and linked to the required texture field of the VolumeData X3D node.

We have devised two ways to accomplish the information transfer from the DICOM file to the X3DOM framework. The first one is to use a `<canvas>` node defined inside the *ImageTextureAtlas* node and then, using JavaScript, fill the canvas with a texture atlas.

```
<ImageTextureAtlas id="atlas">
    <canvas id="voxelCanvas"></canvas>
</ImageTextureAtlas>
```

The second integration method is to use the same auxiliary <canvas> node but defined out of the *ImageTextureAtlas* node. The *VolumeData* node uses an empty *ImageTextureAtlas* (no real URL is given). The JavaScript loader draws the atlas texture in this canvas as before, and then, the correct URL is provided as a *DataURL*, which means that the whole volumetric information is encoded and passed in the URL.

```
<ImageTextureAtlas id="atlas" url="data:"></ImageTextureAtlas>
document.getElementById("atlas").setAttribute(
        'url',
        document.getElementById("voxelCanvas").toDataURL()
);
```

4   Conclusions

This work has introduced three functionalities required by the users in the visualization and inspection of volumetric datasets, especially in the medical field. The utilization of segmented datasets has been made possible via the *Segmented-VolumeData* node of the X3D in combination with the X3DOM framework. The ability to visualize the volumetric information from inside the dataset enables novel capabilities like vessel navigation. Finally, DICOM files have been read and parsed in the web and different methods to pass the volumetric information to the interactive volume rendering X3D nodes have been explored. All these functionalities are currently available in the developer version of the X3DOM framework and they will be part of the next stable release.

The Fig. 5 shows how the presented functionality in this work can be used in the web browser in desktop and mobile platforms. Next steps will be oriented toward the further integration of DICOM in the web environment, as right now

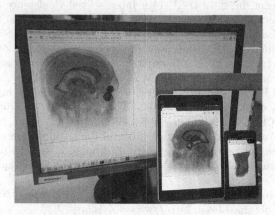

Fig. 5. Ubiquitous volume rendering with WebGL in multiple platforms using segmented medical datasets

only the scanned images are used in the visualization. More fields and metadata could be used to generate better immersive experiences in the volumetric data.

The utilization of modern VR devices like Oculus Rift, HTC Vive or Microsoft Hololens will increase the immersiveness in the information, but novel user interfaces should be provided. WebVR [13] proposes a preliminary solution to integrate VR devices into the Web and currently, there are sample demos of X3D scenes rendered in such devices. A responsive web application could provide a specific immersive visualization of volumetric datasets for VR devices or a mobile oriented visualization if a smartphone is detected.

References

1. Behr, J., Eschler, P., Jung, Y., Zöllner, M.: X3DOM: a DOM-based HTML5/X3D integration model. In: Proceedings of the 14th International Conference on 3D Web Technology, pp. 127–135. ACM, June 2009
2. Congote, J., Segura, A., Kabongo, L., Moreno, A., Posada, J., Ruiz, O.: Interactive Visualization of volumetric data with WebGL in real-time. In: Proceedings of the 16th International Conference on 3D Web Technology, Web3D 2011, pp 137–146. ACM, New York(2011)
3. Cornestone JavaScript library to display interactive medical images including but not limited to DICOM. https://github.com/chafey/cornerstone
4. Hähn, D., Rannou, N., Ahtam, B., Grant, P.E., Pienaar, R.: Neuroimaging in the browser using the X toolkit. Front. Neuroinform. (2014). Conference Abstract: 5th INCF Congress of Neuroinformatics
5. Kajiya, J.T., Von Herzen, B.P.: Ray tracing volume densities. In: Christiansen, H. (ed.) Proceedings of the 11th Annual Conference on Computer Graphics and Interactive Techniques (SIGGRAPH 1984), pp. 165–174. ACM, New York (1984)
6. Kruger, J., Westermann, R.: Acceleration techniques for GPU-based volume rendering. In: Visualization, VIS 2003, pp. 287–292. IEEE, 24 October 2003
7. Mobeen, M., Feng, L.: High-performance volume rendering on the ubiquitous WebGL platform. In: 2012 IEEE 14th International Conference on High Performance Computing and Communication, 2012 IEEE 9th International Conference on Embedded Software and Systems (HPCC-ICESS), pp. 381–388 (2012)
8. Noguera, J., Jimenez, J.: Visualization of very large 3D volumes on mobile devices and WebGL. In: 20th WSCG International Conference on Computer Graphics, Visualization and Computer Vision, WSCG 2012, June 2012
9. Rodríguez, M.B., Alcocer, P.P.V.: Practical volume rendering in mobile devices. In: Bebis, G., et al. (eds.) ISVC 2012. LNCS, vol. 7431, pp. 708–718. Springer, Heidelberg (2012). doi:10.1007/978-3-642-33179-4_67
10. Schiewe, A., Anstoots, M., Krüger, J.: State of the art in mobile volume rendering on iOS devices. In: Bertini, E., Kennedy, J., Puppo, E. (eds.) Eurographics Conference on Visualization (EuroVis) - Short Papers. The Eurographics Association (2015)
11. VJS Medical Imaging Sugar for ThreeJS. https://github.com/FNNDSC/vjs
12. Volume Data obtained from, http://www.volvis.org
13. WebVR Bringing virtual reality to the web. http://webvr.info/

Analysis of Mobility Management Solutions for Mobile Medical Multimedia Transmission in HetNet Environments

Norbert Varga[✉] and László Bokor

Department of Networked Systems and Services,
Multimedia Networks and Services Laboratory (MediaNets),
Budapest University of Technology and Economics, Budapest, Hungary
{vnorbert,bokorl}@hit.bme.hu

Abstract. By 2020 the number of mobile-connected devices will reach 11.6 billion, including smartphones, tablets, wearable devices, sensors among others, which will exceed the world's projected population at that time. Wirelessly connected devices by their nature imply that users are able to be part of a network, giving space for new-generation, novel fields such as mobile healthcare applications. Such pervasive and ubiquitous services rely advanced network architectures designed to provide reliable communication and high quality data transmission in any mobility scenario. Increasingly growing heterogeneous network (HetNet) technologies hold the potential to address longstanding challenges in healthcare domain, to ensure advanced communication solutions for critical mHealth services and to support patient-centric, 'care anywhere' concept. The focus of this article is to present and evaluate the effects of an optimized HetNet-aware mobility management proposal on mHealth applications with intense multimedia transmission.

Keywords: Mobile healthcare (mHealth) · Mobility management · Heterogeneous networks (HetNet) · Mobile medical multimedia · Quality assessment · Performance evaluation

1 Introduction

Ever growing penetration of connected-devices, data-hungry, real-time and pervasive applications like social media, M2M (machine-to-machine), mobile healthcare services create serious challenges for the traditional network infrastructures, which cannot offer reliable connection with an acceptable quality for both emergent traffic growth and ubiquitous applications. To enable the highest quality experience for demanding mobile device users, HetNet technologies have been recognized as a key-important solution [1,2]. HetNet covers the combination of several wireless technologies such as cellular architectures (2G/3G/4G), WLANs, pico- and femtocells to provide efficient network resource usage and enhance the user experience of real-time, pervasive applications, furthermore improves the

© ICST Institute for Computer Sciences, Social Informatics and Telecommunications Engineering 2017
K. Giokas et al. (Eds.): eHealth 2016, LNICST 181, pp. 451–458, 2017.
DOI: 10.1007/978-3-319-49655-9_55

coverage of access networks and increases the network capacity. A large part of mobile Health (mHealth) use-cases requires advanced and reliable mobile communication solutions to provide efficient multimedia transmission with strict medical level Quality of Service (QoS) and Quality of Experience (QoE) provision [3,4]. HetNet can be a promising technique to fulfill the requirements of such mHealth services [5,6]. Critical mHealth applications, on which a life may depend, are going to require the 'always available,' high capacity capabilities of HetNet systems.

Aiming to solve the above challenges of real-time mHealth service provision in our previous works [7–9] we designed and implemented a Mobile IPv6-based, cross-layer optimized flow mobility framework. The goal of this article is to analyse our scheme in the light of existing mobility management standards and to present the evaluation of medical multimedia transmission quality in various mobility scenarios.

The rest of the paper is organized as follows. In Sect. 2 we present the related work on advanced mobility management schemes already applied for real-time mHealth services. Section 3 recaps our advanced flow mobility architecture, the signalling framework, and the integrated multi-criteria decision engine. Section 4 presents the comparison of our proposal with standard mobility management schemes performed in scenarios focusing on simultaneous transmission of multiple medical multimedia streams over HetNet. In Sect. 5 we conclude the paper and describe our future work.

2   Backgorund and Related Work

The deployment of HetNet covers the aggregation of various wireless access schemes, hereby integrates traditional mobile solutions such as 3G/4G cell with WLAN technologies for pervasive, and seamless communication techniques in any mobility event without connection drops and access network failures. Benefits of such heterogeneous environments can only be exploited if mobility between the different wireless accesses is efficiently handled. The Mobile IPv6 protocol (MIPv6) family aims to provide reliable communication and solves the session continuity for mobile nodes on the move. MIPv6 [10] allows that each mobile node always can be identified by its home address, regardless of its current point of attachment to the Internet (e.g., in case of moving between different Wi-Fi access points). A mobile node is also associated with a care-of address (CoA) provided by the foreign network. IPv6 packets addressed to a mobile node's home address are transparently routed to its CoA thanks to the Home Agent (HA) entity of the MIPv6 concept. The protocol enables IPv6 nodes for mobile nodes to create bindings between the home address and the CoA, thus any packets destined for the mobile node can directly sent to its CoA. Recently mobile devices are equipped more network interfaces like Wi-Fi, 3G/4G, Bluetooth among others. For matters of cost, bandwidth, delay it is useful for the mobile node to get Internet access through multiple accesses simultaneously, in which case the mobile node would be configured with multiple active IPv6 CoA. However MIPv6 cannot be applied in multi-access environments, since it enables only one care-of address binding at a time with its home address, so mobile nodes cannot use multiple interfaces to send and receive packets while taking advantage of session continuity provided by MIPv6. In order to exploit the advantages of such heterogeneous solutions Multiple-care of Address extension of MIPv6 [11] (MCoA) was designed in the IPv6 domain. MCoA enables a mobile node to register multiple CoAs for a home address and create multiple binding cache entries. If HA receives Binding Update (BU) message, creates a separate bindings. MCoA exploits the network resources provided by heterogeneous networks. A possible MCoA handover mechanism was introduced in [12]. The solution relies on overlapping radio access networks (RANs), and in case of an appearing new access network on an unused interface, moves every traffic to this new RAN by activating symmetric policy rules for all the MR transmissions (e.g., between LTE and Wi-Fi). Due to the limitations of MCoA, further optimization is required with the help of Flow Bindings extension of MIPv6 [13] (FB). FB enables to bind a particular flow to a particular CoA directly with correspondent nodes/mobility agents (i.e., home agents and mobility anchor points), such creates a fine grained mobility management and offloading tool for HetNets. However, neither MCoA nor FB handover execution schemes are able to work efficiently without proper handover decision and control, which requires a complex mobility architecture to implement for real life mHealth use-cases [8].

3 A Review of Our Proposed Mobility Architecture

In this section we briefly introduce our mobile device driven, flow-aware mobility architecture designed for real-time mobile medical multimedia transmission. Only a high-level overview of the main components are discussed in this section, while a detailed description can be found in our previous works [7,8]. In our proposed framework a highly customized Android-based mobile device plays the role of the central entity responsible for the client-based flow-aware mobility management and provide reliable communication in various mobility event in heterogeneous access environment. Our solution relies on MIP6D-NG [14], which is a novel Mobile IPv6 [10] implementation extended with multi-access, flow mobility, and advanced cross-layer communication support among others. A key part of the architecture is the network discovery and selection module, which collects static and dynamic information (e.g., throughput in the uplink/downlink, rate of erroneously received and discarded packets, number of discarded packets and number of users) of Wi-Fi APs or cellular. We consider both built-in Android APIs (e.g., WiFiManager, Telephony, NeighboringCellInfo etc.), external tools running on the router (e.g., OpenWrt Bandwidth Monitoring tool[1] and network-assistance mechanisms [15,16] for the comprehensive network discovery process. The network selection module relies on a widely-used multi-criteria decision technique, namely Analytical Hierarchy Process [17]. Our proposed AHP-based decision engine decides about the optimal network(s) for the selected med-

---

[1] OpenWrt bmon tool: https://wiki.openwrt.org/doc/howto/bwmon.

ical multimedia flow(s) based on the collected information and directs the network management module to connect the mobile to the selected network(s). The proposed solution adaptively follows the changes in the network environment and dynamically modifies assignments of flows and networks/interfaces. Another important part of our architecture from the healthcare point of view is the Sensor Data Aggregator module collecting data from connected diagnostic devices and medical sensors, device-integrated sensors, etc., and sends the multimedia data towards a correspondent node, which is typically a hospital or an emergency centre.

4   Testbed and Measurement Results

4.1   Testbed Environment

A multi-flow mHealth streaming application was used to test and compare different mobility management techniques and mobility scenarios in a heterogeneous testbed environment depicted in Fig. 1.

The measurement story-line focuses on a real-time, continuous medical multimedia transmission from a diagnostic clinic's ultrasound and ECG device to a medical specialist on the move. Our IPv6-based HetNet environment combines traditional 3G/4G mobile network and Wi-Fi access points located in the campus of Budapest University of Technology and Economics (BME). In the presented setup these networks are covered by two Wi-Fi access points belonged to the campus of BME and by a commercial 3G/LTE mobile network. Wi-Fi APs ensure native IPv6, contrarily Android devices do not support native IPv6 through 3G/4G interface. To enable IPv6 communication on the cellular interface we applied a TAP-based OpenVPN tunnel. The detailed description of our testbed setups is presented in our previous work [7,9].

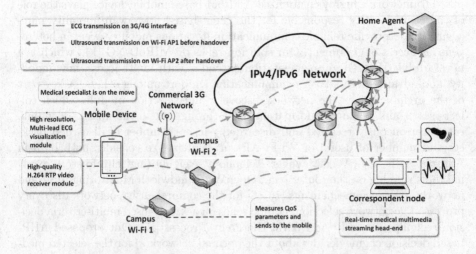

Fig. 1. HetNet testbed for multi-flow mobile medical multimedia transmission

4.2   Measurement Results

For the analysis we transferred two different medical multimedia flows (an ECG flow and an ultrasound video stream) from the correspondent node (playing the role of the mobile medical multimedia streaming head-end) to a medical experts' smartphone device. The used ECG flow is pre-recorded data provided by PhysioNet [18]. The chosen signal records contain 12 standard leads records from patients undergoing tests for coronary artery disease with 257 Hz sampling rate [19]. These digital ECG signals were transmitted and received using a custom packetizer with a simple UDP socket-based implementation at 950 kbps. The transmitted video was a colour ultrasound stream of a fetal heart with HD resolution (720 × 1280 pixel), 30 fps frame rate and 880 kbps UDP/RTP encoded with H.264 and provided by the Mátyásföldi Klinika diagnostic clinic. For the real-time ultrasound transmission and objective evaluation we used the software components of the Evalvid framework [20]. We have also initiated TCP background traffic (BT) generated with iperf3[2] toolset. In this section ten different mobility scenarios are described as Table 1 shows.

Table 1. The defined mobility scenarios

ID	Available network(s)	Used network(s)	BT (Mbit/s)	Applied MM technologies
#1	3G	3G	no	None
#2	3G	3G	5	None
#3	LTE	LTE	no	None
#4	LTE	LTE	5	None
#5	Wi-Fi	Wi-Fi	no	None
#6	Wi-Fi	Wi-Fi	5	None
#7	Multiple WiFi APs, 3G	Multiple WiFi APs	5 (WiFi)	MIPv6
#8	WiFi, 3G	WiFi, 3G	5 (WiFi)	MIPv6+MCoA
#9	Wi-Fi, 3G	Wi-Fi, 3G	5 (WiFi)	MIPv6+MCoA+FlowB
#10	Wi-Fi, LTE	Wi-Fi, LTE	5 (WiFi)	MIPv6+MCoA+FlowB

To perform the analysis by evaluating the quality of the transmitted medical multimedia flows we applied the cumulative distribution and probability density functions (CDF and PDF) of end-to-end delay for the ultrasound video, and the packet loss rates for both the ultrasound and the ECG streams. The measurement scenarios have been categorized based on the available/used network interfaces and IPv6 protocol family extensions applied to the mobility management mechanism (MM).

In scenario 1–6 only one interface was used for transmission of both medical flows and the additional background traffic without any mobility mechanisms. In these scenarios both medical flows suffer significant packet loss due to the

---

[2] iperf3 tool: https://iperf.fr/.

limited throughput capacity of 3G, LTE or even of Wi-Fi, which cannot guarantee the suitable bandwidth for both ultrasound and ECG flows in case of higher
background traffic volumes.

Scenario 7–10 depict a mobility event, where the mobile device is moving and
changing its Internet point of attachment through accesses belonging to different
IP domains, thus IP level handover is required. In scenario 7 the mobile device
executes a handover between two Wi-Fi APs using MIPv6 causing extra packet
loss in the transmitted data. Scenario 8 shows a condition, where two Wi-Fi
APs, and a 3G network are available, however, due to the lack of flow mobility,
the device cannot separate medical flows between the available interfaces, thus
both medical flows are moved from 3G to Wi-Fi using a simple MCoA handover.

Thanks to our solution integrated with multi-access and flow binding support,
we can provide flow-aware decision and proper handover execution in scenarios
9 and 10. It means that the mobile device transfers mobile medical multimedia
flows bound to appropriate interfaces based on fine grained coupling of applications and available access networks. Scenario 9 still includes small degradation
on both flows due to the limited capability of 3G, however the proposed solution
provide optimal mobility management in LTE and Wi-Fi environments as shown
in scenario 10. Our multi-access, flow-level architecture and decision intelligence
eventuate medical quality simultaneous ECG and ultrasound transmission even
in mobile environments and other active background TCP sessions. As an important performance indicator, Fig. 2 summarizes the above and shows the packet
loss rate of both ECG and ultrasound flows in before-described mobility conditions.

The application policies of the incoming ECG flow prefer the 3G/4G interface
of the mobile device in order to benefit from the enhanced QoS provisioning and
security capabilities of a 3GPP operator. Policies of the ultrasound transmission
favour Wi-Fi for more bandwidth and lower delays, as well as of any TCP-based
(background) traffic.

As another important performance indicator we examined end-to-end delay
of transmitted ultrasound video.

Figure 3 shows the empirical cumulative distribution and estimated probability density function of end-to-end delay of video frames. We can observe that
3G cause significant end-to-end delay on the multimedia video, approximately

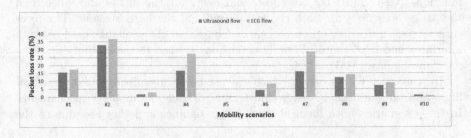

Fig. 2. Packet loss rate of ECG and ultrasound flows in different mobility scenarios

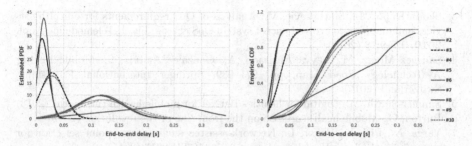

Fig. 3. Estimated PDF (left) and empirical CDF (right) of ultrasound video's end-to-end delay in different mobility scenarios

around 120 ms, while the transmission over LTE implies in average 25 ms. Using our intelligent flow-based Wi-Fi offloading for the ultrasound transmission the average end-to-end delay of the real-time stream closes the pure Wi-Fi case which is under 10 ms.

5   Conclusion

Increasingly spreading heterogeneous network (HetNet) concepts offer the possibility to provide reliable, advanced and pervasive communication solutions for critical mHealth services and to support patient-centric scenarios. The goal of this article is to analyse our cross-layer optimized, multi-access, flow mobility framework designed and developed in our previous works in the light of existing mobility management standards and to present the evaluation of medical multimedia transmission quality in various mobility scenarios. Results of the introduced evaluation show that our framework gives an efficient and fine-grained mobility solution for quality-sensitive real-time and pervasive mHealth services.

As a part of our future work we are planning to provide a comprehensive mapping between QoS (e.g., Packet Loss), objective QoE (e.g., PSNR), and subjective QoE (i.e., diagnostically relevant quality) metrics for different mobile medical multimedia applications with the help of medical experts.

Acknowledgement. The work leading to these results has been partly funded by the National Research, Development and Innovation Office's Hungarian-Montenegrin Bilateral Research Project (TET-15-1-2016-0039) and also by the ÚNKP-16-4-I. New National Excellence Program of the Ministry of Human Capacities of Hungary.

References

1. Moura, J., Edwards, C.: Future trends and challenges for mobile and convergent networks. CoRR, abs/1601.06202 (2016)
2. Nokia Solutions and Networks. Heterogeneous networks (HetNet) - deliver a high quality mobile broadband service using a hybrid network with unified control and optimization (2015)

3. Skorin-Kapov, L., Matijasevic, M.: Analysis of QoS requirements for e-health services and mapping to evolved packet system QoS classes. Int. J. Telemedicine Appl. **2010**, 9:1–9:18 (2010)

4. Sanchez Meraz, M., Leyva Alvarado, A., Gonzalez Ambriz, S.: Mobile Health: A Technology Road Map, pp. 971–989. Springer International Publishing, Switzerland (2015)

5. Sumner-Smith, M.: Digital for health - HetNet for mobile health (mHealth) (2013)

6. Burton, C.: Mobile healthcare: Be on the front line of the revolution (2015)

7. Varga, N., Piri, E., Bokor, L.: Network-assisted smart access point selection for pervasive real-time mHealth applications. In: ICTH 2015 (2015)

8. Varga, N., Bokor, L., Takacs, A.: Context-aware IPv6 flow mobility for multi-sensor based mobile patient monitoring and tele-consultation. In: Concerto 2014, September 2014

9. Varga, N., Bokor, L., Piri, E.: A network-assisted flow mobility architecture for optimized mobile medical multimedia transmission. Ann. Telecommun. **71**, 1–14 (2016)

10. Perkins, C., Johnson, D., Arkko, J.: Mobility support in IPv6. Number 6275 in Request for Comments. IETF, Published: RFC 6275, July 2007

11. Wakikawa, R., Devarapalli, V., Tsirtsis, G., Ernst, T., Nagami, K.: Multiple care-of addresses registration. Number 5648 in RCF. IETF, October 2009

12. Bokor, L., Jeney, G., Kovács, J.: A study on the performance of an advanced framework for prediction-based NEMO handovers in multihomed scenarios. Infocommun. J. **VI**, 16–27 (2014)

13. Tsirtsis, G., Soliman, H., Montavont, N., Giaretta, G., Kuladinithi, K.: Flow Bindings in Mobile IPv6 and Network Mobility (NEMO) Basic Support. Number 6089 in RFC. IETF, Published: RFC 6089, January 2011

14. Takács, A., Bokor, L.: A distributed dynamic mobility architecture with integral cross-layered and context-aware interface for reliable provision of high bitrate mhealth services. In: Godara, B., Nikita, K.S. (eds.) MobiHealth 2012. LNICS, vol. 61, pp. 369–379. Springer, Heidelberg (2013). doi:10.1007/978-3-642-37893-5_41

15. 3GPP TS 24.312. Access Network Discovery and Selection Function (ANDSF) Management Object (MO), Rel. 11, April 2013

16. IEEE Standard for Local and metropolitan area networks- Part 21: Media Independent Handover. IEEE, January 2009

17. Saaty, T.L., Ozdemir, M.S.: Why the magic number seven plus or minus two. Math. Comput. Modell. **38**, 233–244 (2003)

18. Goldberger, A.L., Amaral, L.A., Glass, L., Hausdor, J.M., Ivanov, P.C., Mark, R.G., Mietus, J.E., Moody, G.B., Peng, C.K., Stanley, H.E.: PhysioBank, PhysioToolkit, and PhysioNet: components of a new research resource for complex physiologic signals. Circulation **101**, 215–220 (2000)

19. Bousseljot, R., Kreiseler, D., Schnabel, A.: Nutzung der EKG-ignaldatenbank CARDIODAT der PTB ber das internet. Biomedizinische Technik **40**, 317–318 (1995)

20. Klaue, J., Rathke, B., Wolisz, A.: EvalVid – a framework for video transmission and quality evaluation. In: Kemper, P., Sanders, W.H. (eds.) TOOLS 2003. LNCS, vol. 2794, pp. 255–272. Springer, Heidelberg (2003). doi:10.1007/978-3-540-45232-4_16

On the Extraction of Anthropometric Parameters by Visual and Non-visual Means

Ondrej Kainz[(⊠)], Ján Forgáč, Miroslav Michalko,
and František Jakab

Department of Computers and Informatics,
Faculty of Electrical Engineering and Informatics,
Technical University of Košice, Letná 9, 042 00 Košice, Slovak Republic
{ondrej.kainz,jan.forgac,miroslav.michalko,
frantisek.jakab}@tuke.com

Abstract. In this paper the system for collection of anthropometric data is presented, along with the novel techniques for extraction of such data. System is built on selected open-source platform having developed various plugins as a part of the project. Means for extraction follow two approaches: visual and non-visual. The first presumes the acquiring of data from static 2D image, the latter gets data through the direct measurement. Visual approach utilizes several principles following the image processing and related face recognition algorithms. Moreover known anthropometric relations are utilized to estimate other proportions. The output in the form of data of individual user may serve as for statistical comparison with other users. Further such data is to be used for correlation studies with several diseases and changes of overall health condition.

Keywords: Anthropometer · Computer vision · Image processing · Skeleton model · Static image · Structural anthropometry · Human body

1 Introduction

Measurement of specific parts of human body has been carried out way before the advent of computer machines, this part of the medical science is referred to as anthropometry - specifically structural anthropometry, where the human body movement is not the concern of measurement. Knowledge of these measurements may be helpful in diagnosis of growth disorders or uncover correlation to other forms of health problems. Other uses of this data is in the field of ergonomics, where the data is used to help designers to predict and correctly adjust the products. The principal focus in this research is the extraction of human body dimensional parameters. Traditional form of such estimation utilized specific devices directly designed for this purpose, e.g. GPM anthropometer. Advance in computer science and related technologies allowed partial replacement of these devices. The following sections present novel visual techniques that enable estimation of several human body dimensions. To check correctness of estimation, the developed hardware anthropometric device for data collection is utilized.

© ICST Institute for Computer Sciences, Social Informatics and Telecommunications Engineering 2017
K. Giokas et al. (Eds.): eHealth 2016, LNICST 181, pp. 459–467, 2017.
DOI: 10.1007/978-3-319-49655-9_56

2 Human Face Anthropometry and Its Detection

In the following section the anthropometry of human face is introduced and further we will focus on the face and its segmentation and detection processes.

2.1 Anthropometry of Face

One of the common human body features is the structure of a human face, i.e. set of two eyes and ears, one mouth and nose. All of these are set symmetrically in a bilateral symmetry. Similarities in this structure allow its utilization in the field of anthropometry.

Anthropometry, as defined by [1], is the "science of measurement and the art of application that establishes the physical geometry, mass properties, and strength capabilities of the human body". There are many uses of anthropometry, e.g. the same authors note: posture evaluation, clearances definition, separation of person from hazards etc. Authors in [2] use this field of science to estimate the length of the prosthetic hand. [3] define face anthropometry as a branch of research dealing with measurement and analysis of absolute quantities and proportion related to human head and face. Further authors note that these measurements are to be done by medical personnel using tools for measurement (ruler, tape etc.). Landmarks, help to find the relations in proportions and may be used for statistical purposes, e.g. age progression.

More information on the face and its parameterization and morphing is in [4]. Same authors also point out that the anthropometry may be used as a solution for artifacts presence or occlusion using laser scanning or stereo images. In [5] authors used anthropometry to reconstruct face model. Worth of mentioning is also FACS, short for Facial Action Coding System, term originally comes from 1978 as defined by [6] to describe facial activity, e.g. used in recognition systems [7].

One of the relations present in the nature and which also may be found at human being is the golden ratio or π. This ratio is useful in the face detection, authors in [8] used it to estimate the position of eyes, also research by [9] utilized the golden ratio for the face location. Another form of implementing ratio onto a human face is its division to thirds.

2.2 Face Segmentation and Detection

Techniques used in image processing for allocation of groups in digital image based on specified criteria are called segmentation. On the other hand, the detection of objects in the image is generally a complex process, which requires implementation of various techniques. In [10] the detection is defined as a tool for identifying the location of object such as face. One of the requirements set within this paper is also research in the field of face detection. Definition of term detection represents for us only localization of face in the image. Recognition in this case is not being taken into account, i.e. categorization of object into categories or subcategories.

Authors in [11] categorize detection of faces into four categories:

Skin color model-based technique - color of human face is used as a feature for human face detection, advantage is its invariance towards rotation, however lightning conditions are crucial. Research on skin color technique was carried out by [12] and [13], the latter declares HSV color model to have the best performance, yet no specific data on efficiency of the solution is provided. Skin color detection together with AdaBoost algorithm was used by [14] with detection rate of 92.86%. Another research by [15] used mixed color model of YCbCr and RGB in their framework, detection rate was over 99%.

Template matching-based approach - predefine template is used to locate the face in the image, in this case the template is not invariant to rotation and also scaling. In [16] the authors used image pyramids to achieve scale invariance. This technique was used in the framework described by [17] for the identification of person.

Feature-based approach - selected features of face are used for its detection, e.g. eyes, ears etc. Research in [18] used combination of skin color model and feature model, allowing enhanced generalization for the detection. As the facial features were selected eyes, mouth, authors do not provide information about efficiency of proposed solution. Similar approach was taken by [19], in this care authors estimated the location of eyes, accuracy of the testing proved to be slightly over 90%. The last research we present is [20], which also uses skin color model and feature-based model, which is being employed after skin segmentation. Lip color model and search for eyes based on geometry textures proves solution to have accuracy over 98%.

Statistical model-based approach - statistical methods are employed to achieve the face detection. Such approach together with skin color model was utilized by [21], authors created face and non-face model as a product of multidimensional histograms. Aim of the project was to achieve detection and subsequent tracking of face, authors achieved detection rate of 90.5%, very similar research [22] deals also with face detection in video. More recent research is presented by [23] developed probabilistic method for face detection from multiple views. In [24] authors developed statistical model for face detection based on extracted multi-resolution image features. In model the illumination, pose and face variations are resolved. Authors claim approach to be significantly better compared to other approaches.

The broad review on human face detection and slightly different approach to division of approaches is presented in [25]. From the above described we can conclude that the most often employed technique is the skin color model approach used together with some other approach.

3   Face Detection in Parameters Estimation

The crucial part of the whole process is the face detection, which is being carried out as the first processing step. Input image may be acquired in two ways. In the first, only the face, is being used only to enhance the future calculations. In the second, the image of the person standing is the input to the system. In both cases, the system presumes persons in the input images to be facing the camera directly.

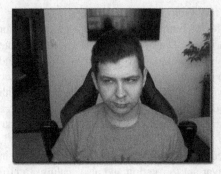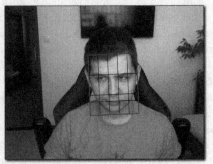

Fig. 1. Face and eyes detection with masking.

The first case, presumes only image of a face to be provided to a system. Further the face and eyes are being detected using the Haar-like features. Onto this image is applied the mask which divides the face into the 5 equal parts in vertical and three equal parts in horizontal direction. Note that this mask is only for future purposes and is being stored in database. In the future research these images are to be used to validate the presumption of dividing the face to thirds/fifths.

Once the eyes are detected the constant of 65 mm is applied as a reference value, marking the distance between the eyes. This value was estimated based on several tests on a larger number of tests subjects. Value is then used to acquire the length and width of the head, i.e. limits that delimit the head itself. Same process may be applied of the second image, however using close-up proved to be more accurate. Detected face with the mask is show in the Fig. 1.

Analogous process is carried out for the second image, providing the first image is not available. If the image is available, the height and the width of head is not calculated but extracted from a prior image.

4   Skeleton Model Mapping and Parameters Extraction

Human model mapping is following the concept of a skeleton model consisted of edges and vertices. Vertices are primarily of synovial joints type and edges are connection between vertices, mostly representing real bone structures. In our research another step of parameters extraction is mapping of this model onto an image of a full body. Such mapping is possible due to constant and symmetrical properties of human body and the fact that human body may be located in the one vertical plane, i.e. no special poses are being taken into account in this phase of a project. This presumption allows mapping of several vertices, in total were selected twelve. Automatic detection of border nodes is fairly easy; however, six joints require semiautomatic approach. Once the skeleton model is mapped the extracted information of distance between the eyes is compensated to a second image, together with the information about the head height and width. Compensated distances are then used to extract the individual information of the edges length. To measure the person's height, the marginal points (upper and lower extremes)

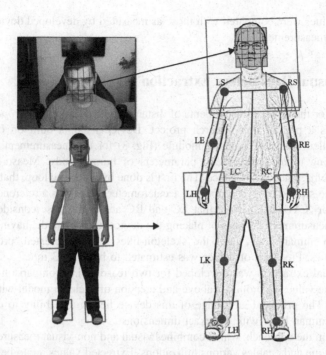

Fig. 2. Skeleton model mapping (first *L* is for *left*, vice versa *R* for *right*, *LH – hand*, *LE – elbow*, *LS – shoulder*, *LC – hip* or *coxa*, *LK – knee*, *LH – heel book*).

are being used, however for case of lower extreme the node of heel bone is being taken into account. This measurement also utilizes the information about person's head height and width with relation to human eyes. In the Fig. 2 is depicted the mapping of vertices being connected be the edges, each vertex is numbered and considered as sole node that may be connected only with particular node. Hands (carpal bones), shoulders (humeral head) and heel bones are detected automatically and adjusted manually if required, the rest is using the semiautomatic detection, i.e. elbows, hip joints and knees (patella). When taking the image as a whole body certain presumptions have to be met considering the angle and camera height. Tests were carried out in the laboratory environment, however pose reconstruction and compensation is to allow omit these using the developed mobile application.

Testing of approach on several testing subjects (20 in total) proved to be success in the measurement of height, with total deviation of 20 mm. The precision of skeleton model parameters is rather inferior, with the average deviation of 50 mm, having the worst results for distance between hip joints and heel bones. Principal cause may be in the nature of skeleton model and reference value. Overall mapping of 2D skeleton model onto 3D scene is possible and provides promising results, however optionally 3D complex model might provide superior outputs. In the future research we plan to utilize such model and implement composite reference values in combination with the ratios existing in the human body. This will enable the pose to be in various position.

Extracted values were compared with those as measured by developed device for body proportions measurement.

5 Non-visual Parameters Extraction

The device for the direct measurements of distance units so called *anthropometer* was developed as a part of this research project. Device itself is built on open-source hardware called Arduino. Separate module (Fig. 3) for the measurement was developed, allowing to measure several parameters of human body. Measured are two aspects, circumference and distance. The first is done by hardware loop, that serves as a meter and the second by gyroscope and accelerometer, having as a reference point the LH (0,0,0 for X,Y,Z axis). Note that LC and RC are in this case considered as one node. The measurement consists of placing the device node by node, having the direct contact with human body, until the skeleton-like model is created, providing the required values. Precision of device was estimated to be up to 3 mm.

Non-visual extraction was developed for two reasons, i.e. comparison and evaluation with the values as proposed above and creation of skeleton model with the exact dimensions. The principal advantage of this device lies in the ability to create a 3D model of a human body with the exact dimensions.

Novelty in the approach, which combines visual and non-visual measurements is in this field unique and enables various utilizations. Extracted values are to be used in the future medical-based projects and also for recognition enhancement.

Table 1 compares selected extraction results as acquired by visual and non-visual approach. Comparison of parameters is also enabled via created web interface, separate for every user, e.g. height to total average of the heights for specific gender and age. Skeleton model parameters may be put into a ratio with a group of other parameters and their tracking over specific duration of time is possible.

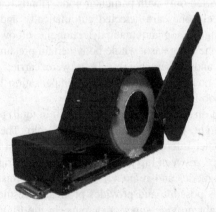

Fig. 3. Anthropometer for manual parameter extraction.

Table 1. Selected parameters: extraction technique (IET) vs. anthropometer (ANT). Testing subject: male, 25 years old.

Parameter	Measured IET	Measured ANT	Total mean ANT (20 subjects)
Height	190 cm	188 cm	185.5 cm
LH-LK	53 cm	57 cm	54.2 cm
LK-LC	46 cm	50 cm	45.4 cm
LS-RS	55 cm	51 cm	51.0 cm
LS-LE	30 cm	32 cm	29.1 cm
LE-LH	27 cm	30 cm	26.4 cm

6 Conclusion

In this research we introduced two techniques for extraction of human body parameters. The first was visual computer-based extraction that utilized image processing algorithms and enabled extraction of dimensional parameters from the static 2D image containing human body in one plane. The latter technique is based on direct measurement of body parameters via created device, so called anthropometer. This device, as well as visual approach allows to develop skeleton model of a human body with the exact dimensional units. Visual approach proved success rate in estimation to be over 85%, while utilizing reference distance between the eyes and semi-automatic skeleton model mapping. Non-visual approach has success rate of 100%, proving the proper conditions for measurement are met. Values acquired were used as a reference for the further comparison. Another analysis was between the set of total extracted values to single user. Due to nature of testing set only male subjects of the age from 20 to 30 were considered. This set is to be expanded in the future research, moreover multiple reference values or ratios will be used in the visual technique to enhance the overall output.

Acknowledgments. We support research activities in Slovakia/This project is being co-financed by the European Union. Paper is the result of the Project implementation: University Science Park TECHNICOM for Innovation Applications Supported by Knowledge Technology, supported by the Research & Development Operational Programme funded by the ERDF.

References

1. Prado-Lu, J.L.D.: Anthropometric measurement of Filipino manufacturing workers. Int. J. Ind. Ergon. **37**(6), 497–503 (2007)
2. Razak, N.A.A., Osman, N.A.A., Gholizadeh, H., Ali, S.: Development and performance of a new prosthesis system using ultrasonic sensor for wrist movements: a preliminary study. BioMed. Eng. OnLine **13**(1), 23 (2014)
3. Lin, A.J., Lai, S., Cheng, F.: Growth simulation of facial/head model from childhood to adulthood. Comput. Aided Des. Appl. **7**(5), 1–10 (2010)

4. Deng, Z., Noh, J.: Computer Facial Animation: A Survey. Springer, London (2008)
5. Decarlo, D., Metasas D., Stone, M.: An anthropometric face model using variational technique. In: Proceeding SIGGRAPH 1998, Proceedings of the 25th Annual Conference on Computer Graphics and Interactive Techniques, pp. 67–74 (1998)
6. Ekman, P., Friesen, W.V.: Facial action coding system. Consulting Psychologist Press, Palo Alto (1978)
7. Gavrilescu M.: Proposed architecture of a fully integrated modular neural network-based automatic facial emotion recognition system based on Facial Action Coding System. In: 10th International Conference on Communications (COMM), pp. 1–6 (2014)
8. See, Y.CH., Noor, N.M., Rijal, O.M.: Hybrid method of iris detection based on face localization. In: IEEE Region 10 Conference TENCON, pp. 1–5 (2014)
9. Yun, J.-U., Lee, H.-J., Paul, A.K., Baek, J.-H.: Robust face detection for video summary using illumination-compensation and morphological processing. In: Third International Conference on Natural Computation, vol. 2, pp. 710–714 (2007)
10. Amit, Y.: 2D Object Detection and Recognition: Models, Algorithms, and Networks. MIT Press, Cambridge (2002)
11. Ajmera, R., Saxena, N.: Face detection in digital images using color spaces and edge detection techniques. Int. J. Adv. Res. Comput. Sci. Softw. Eng. 3(6), 718–725 (2013)
12. Ghmire, D., Lee, J.: A robust face detection method based on skin color and edges. J. Inf. Process. Syst. 9(1), 141–156 (2013)
13. Sandeep, K., Rajagopalan, A.N.: Biometric Facial Recognition Database Systems. http://www.inf.pucrs.br/~pinho/CG/Trabalhos/DetectaPele/Artigos/Human%20Face%20Detection%20in%20Cluttered%20Color%20Images%20Using%20Skin%20Color.pdf
14. Li, Z., Xue, L., Tan, F.: Face detection in complex background based on skin color features and improved AdaBoost algorithms. In: IEEE International Conference on Progress in Informatics and Computing (PIC), vol. 2, pp. 723–727 (2010)
15. Wang, X., Xu, H., Wang, H., Li, H.: Robust real-time face detection with skin color detection and the modified census transform. In: International Conference on Information and Automation, pp. 590–595 (2008)
16. Tang, L., Huang, T.S.: Automatic construction of 3D human face models based on 2D images. In: International Conference on Image Processing, vol. 3, pp. 467–470 (1997)
17. Junior, J.C.S.J., Moreira, J.L., Braun, A., Musse, S.R.: A template matching based method to perform iris detection in real-time using synthetic templates. In: 11th IEEE International Symposium on Multimedia, pp. 142–147 (2009)
18. Widjojo, W., Yow, K.CH.: A color and feature-based approach to human face detection. In: 7th International Conference on Control, Automation, Robotics and Vision, vol. 1, pp. 508–513 (2002)
19. Chan, Y.H., Abu-Bakar, S.A.R.: Face detection system based on feature-based chrominance colour information. In: International Conference on Computer Graphics, Imaging and Visualization, pp. 153–158 (2004)
20. Wang, Y., Xia, L.: Skin color and feature-based face detection in complicated backgrounds. In: International Conference on Image Analysis and Signal Processing (IASP), pp. 78–83 (2011)
21. Wu, H., Zelek, J.S.: The extension of statistical face detection to face tracking. In: First Canadian Conference on Computer and Robot Vision, pp. 10–17 (2004)
22. Tariq, U., Jamal, H., Shahid, M.J.S., Malik, M.U.: Face detection in color images, a robust and fast statistical approach. In: 8th International Multitopic Conference, pp. 73–78 (2004)
23. Anvar, S.M.H., Yau, W.-Y., Teoh, E.K.: Fast face detection and localization from multi-views using statistical approach. In: 8th International Conference on Information, Communications and Signal Processing (ICICS), pp. 1–5 (2011)

24. Ying Z., Castanon, D.: Statistical model for human face detection using multi-resolution features. In: International Conference on Information Intelligence and Systems, pp. 560–563 (1999)

25. Sharifara, A., Rahim, M.S.M., Anisi, Y.: A general review of human face detection including a study of neural networks and haar feature-based cascade classifier in face detection. In: International Symposium on Biometrics and Security Technologies (ISBAST), pp. 73–78 (2014)

m-Skin Doctor: A Mobile Enabled System for Early Melanoma Skin Cancer Detection Using Support Vector Machine

Muhammad Aleem Taufiq[1], Nazia Hameed[2(✉)], Adeel Anjum[1], and Fozia Hameed[3]

[1] COMSATS Institute of Information Technology, Islamabad, Pakistan
{aleem.taufiq,adeel.anjum}@comsats.edu.pk
[2] Anglia Ruskin University, Chelmsford, UK
nazia.hameed@pgr.anglia.ac.uk
[3] King Khalid University, Abha, Saudi Arabia
fhameed@kku.edu.sa

Abstract. Early detection of skin cancer is very important as it is one of the dangerous form of cancer spreading vigorously among humans. With the advancement of mobile technology; mobile enabled skin cancer detection systems are really demanding but currently very few real time skin cancer detection systems are available for general public and mostly available are the paid. In this paper authors proposed a real time mobile enabled health care system for the detection of skin melanoma for general users. Proposed system is developed using computer vision and image processing techniques. Noise is removed by applying the Gaussian filter. For segmentation Grab Cut algorithm is used. Support Vector Machine (SVM) is applied as a classification technique on the texture features like area, perimeter, eccentricity etc. The sensitivity and specificity rate achieved by the m-Skin Doctor is 80% and 75% respectively. The average time consumed by the application for classifying one image is 14938 ms.

Keywords: Skin cancer · Melanoma · Computer aided systems · Mobile application · Health care systems · Machine learning

1 Introduction

Human skin consists of different layers with unique, distinct functions and optical properties. Epidermis being an outermost layer protects the human from harmful sunlight and ultraviolet (UV) radiations. It largely composes of the connecting tissues and also contains melanin producing cells, melanocytes and melanin; product of melanocytes and its producing cells as shown in Fig. 1. Melanin is the pigment which absorbs the light in the ultra violet spectrum and protects the deeper layers of the skin. Then come the dermis layer; which is made up of collagen fibers and it contains sensors, receptors, nerve ends and the blood vessels [1].

Skin cancer is the abnormal growth of tissues in the skin. At present the skin abnormal tissues are mainly classified in two types: benign and malignant. Benign

© ICST Institute for Computer Sciences, Social Informatics and Telecommunications Engineering 2017
K. Giokas et al. (Eds.): eHealth 2016, LNICST 181, pp. 468–475, 2017.
DOI: 10.1007/978-3-319-49655-9_57

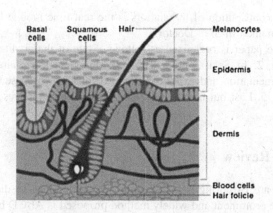

Fig. 1. Skin layers and their components [1]

tissues are not cancerous whereas the malignant skin tissues are dangerous and can invade their neighbouring tissues. In benign lesions, melanin is normally present in the epidermis layer and is not life threatening. When this melanin penetrates into the dermis layer, it becomes life threatening [2, 3].

In United States, approximately 73,870 new malignant skin cancer cases were estimated in year 2015. Out of these 73,870 cases, 9,940 death cases were found [4]. Therefore its early detection is very much important. The most and the frequent method used for the skin cancer detection are the ABCD rule of dermoscopy [5, 6], the 7-point checklist [7], image processing and pattern analysis and the Menzies method [8, 9].

Currently mostly skin cancer detection systems are based on combination of image processing and machine learning techniques [1]. These systems are not the replacement of the dermatologists but really helpful to dermatologists in diagnosing the skin cancer. Most of the world population lives in the backward and rural areas and they don't have an easy access to the skin specialists. To the best of our knowledge currently there are very few smartphone application for skin cancer. There are some short coming in these existing applications. Firstly, majority of applications are IOS based [10] and people living in the backward areas don't have easy access to IOS devices because IOS devices are costly then android [11]. Secondly majority of applications only provide the news and skin cancer information [12, 13]. Other applications asks for a skin lesion image and then send the image to any dermatologists for expert opinion. Patient has to wait for a long time for the results [14–16] and because of these delays, strength of the disease may increase. These types of systems are not very effective for the people living in remote areas. Only few applications are available for real time skin analysis and mostly are the paid. Nowadays a wide variety of android based smart phone applications with high processing speed and advanced operating systems are available in the market and everybody has an easy access to smartphones; therefore there should be some automated healthcare diagnostic systems for these areas. Healthcare applications should be provided to the general public living in the rural as well as urban areas. Therefore smartphone based skin cancer detection applications are required for general public. The main contribution of the authors is the real time mobile base skin cancer detection system named m-Skin Doctor.

The rest of the paper is organized as follows. State of the art literature review is described in Sect. 2. In Sect. 3 proposed methodologies is explained in detail. In Sect. 4 the implementation and experimentation details are discussed and results are discussed in Sect. 5. Last but not the least conclusion and future research is summarized in Sect. 6.

2   Literature Review

Different authors are exploring and inventing new techniques to diagnose the skin cancer. One of the prominent and widely method proposed is ABCD by Nachbar et al. Asymmetry, Border irregularity, colour and diameter are the key features used in ABCD rule. In [17] Jain et al. have used image processing techniques to find the melanoma. Karargyris et al. [18] propose an iOS application for the detection of the skin cancer. The proposed technique starts with the identification of the ROI. In the pre-processing step the original RGB color is transferred into the HSV color space. Afterwards the image is binarized by setting the H-V threshold values followed by applying SVM on extracted features.

Classification algorithm proposed by Abuzaghleh et al. [19] has been divided into two main parts. In the first part authors have introduced a novel equation to compute the time for skin burn and developed a real-time alert system. Second component is an automated image analysis module which classify the skin cancer. Abderrahim et al. have described an innovative mobile based health care system for detecting the skin cancer. Multilayer perceptron is used for the detection purpose [20]. A mobile application has been developed by Doukas et al. that can acquire, identify and classify the moles into benign, nevus and melanoma. The proposed system also includes a cloud infrastructure for better storage and computation [21]. An Android application has been developed by Kiran et al. for early melanoma detection [22]. In the proposed algorithm the skin image is converted to the monochrome image. Main purpose of this conversion is the outline contour detection. Shape and color features were extracted. KNN is used as the classifying algorithm.

Setiawan et al. proposed an automated algorithm for early detection of melanoma with an accuracy rate of 83% [23]. Proposed system was divided into three stages. In segmentation, several color spaces can be selected by the user followed by learning algorithms. Noise is removed by applying morphological filters in filtering steps. In the localization step, connected component labelling and K-means technique are used for objects classification.

3   Proposed Methodology

In this papers authors have proposed an efficient real time skin cancer detection technique for smartphone applications. Proposed methodology is divided into three main steps i.e. pre-processing, segmentation, feature extraction and classification (Fig. 2).

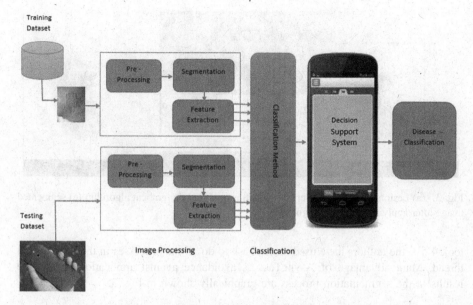

Fig. 2. Proposed Methodology for m-skin Doctor

Dermoscopic images of skin lesion from Klinik und Poliklinik für Dermatologie und Allergologie, Technische Universitat Munchen, Germany is used for training and testing purpose.

3.1 Pre-processing Step

The first stage of the proposed methodology aims to enhance the image quality. All the images are in RGB format. All images should be of same dimension and noise free before segmentation so that better segmentation results should be achieved and so as the main task of our technique pre-processing step. All images are resized first to 640×480 dimensions and then Gaussian filter with window size 3 has been applied on the resized images to remove the noise.

3.2 Segmentation

For efficient training the suspected skin image should be segmented from the healthy skin portion. For segmentation of images Grab Cut algorithm is used. Grab cut algorithm is an interactive segmentation technique for images [24] and divide the image in the image into four portions, i.e. Exactly Background, Probably Background, Exactly Foreground and Probably Foreground. The main reason of selecting the grabcut algorithm is that it provide good segmentation results in real time. While keeping the easiness of user's, authors provide the facility to select the cancerous area. User can draw the rectangle around the lesion part. The segmentation process is a bit long and

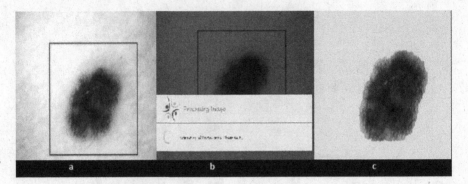

Fig. 3. (a) Lesion selection by user (b) m-Skin is applying the grabcut algorithm (c) segmented image after applying Grab Cut algorithm

took 4-5 s, the authors have used AsyncTask to do all the processes in the background thread. Main advantage of AsyncTask is avoidance against application crash. The results of the segmentation process are graphically shown in Fig. 3.

3.3   Feature Extraction and Classification

After extracting the region of extract (ROI) from segmentation process, meaningful features have been extracted. While proposing the melanoma detection algorithm for mobile applications, memory consumption and processing time are most important factors to consider. There are many features that can be extracted from the segmented image but the main challenge was to select the features while considering the processing time. While considering the mobile limitations authors have selected minimal features so that processing speed will not be affected. Mainly histogram and ABCD features have been used. Authors have extracted area of lesion, perimeter of lesion, eccentricity, mean, standard deviation, L1 norm, L2 norm angle of lesion, major and minor axis of lesion from the segmented image. We randomly split the dataset images into training and testing images. The system was trained using the SVM classifier. Main reason for selecting SVM is that is empirically proved that SVM outperforms among different machine learning techniques for skin cancer segmentation.

4   Implementations Details

Android is an operating system developed by Google and offers a wide selection of functions to the developers. For our application we have also used some of the build in libraries. For image processing authors have used open source computer vision library (OpenCV). OpenCV offers impressive computer vision and machine learning capabilities [25]. OpenCV provides a common infrastructure for computer vision and it was first developed by Intel Inc. Initially OpenCV was developed for the personal computers but later on its libraries were ported for mobile phones thus making mobile phones a powerful device and yet the replacement for the personal computers. Minimum version to run the m-Skin Doctor is Android 4.0. Authors have used Extensible Mark-up Language (XML) to create the layouts and have used java for all the business logics. For capturing the skin images by default android camera application has been used.

5 Results and Discussion

Dataset from Klinik und Poliklinik für Dermatologie und Allergologie, Technische Universitat Munchen, Germany is used for training and testing purpose. All images are without any distracting elements like jewellery, clothes and any background. For each image the region of interest was manually selected that contains both normal and malignant skin pigments. We randomly split the dataset into two parts i.e. training and testing part with ratio 70%|30%. Support vector machine is used for classification purpose. 84 images consisting both melanoma and non-melanoma images with same proportion are used for the training purpose of the support vector machine and other 36 images with same proportion of melanoma and non-melanoma images are used for testing. Through testing 80% images predicted correctly as melanoma and 75% non-melanoma images correctly identified by our application. All the images were pre-processed in advance. The overview of the obtained accuracy is shown in Table 1 below. The average time consumed by the application for classifying one image is 14938 ms. Average time classifier consumed for training is 30405 ms.

Table 1. Accuracy results achived by m-Skin Doctor

	Melanoma	Non-melanoma
Melanoma	80%	20%
Non-melanoma	25%	75%

6 Conclusion and Future Research

In this paper author's have developed real time application for skin cancer detection. In the pre-processing step the images are resized and the noise has been removed from the skin images. Grab cut algorithm is used for the segmentation purpose. Reason of choosing the grab cut algorithm is that it provides good segmentation in real time. Area, perimeter, eccentricity, mean, standard deviation, L1 norm, L2 norm angle of lesion, major and minor axis of lesion are the main features that have been extracted in the feature extraction phase. For classification purpose Support Vector Machine has been used. Reason of choosing the support vector machine is that it provides good classification results in real time on smart phone. The smartphone application has been tested on the dataset provided by the Munchen University Germany.

Still there are a lot of research issues that need to be addressed on the smart phone based skin health care systems. Mostly work has been done on the skin melanoma. Proposed application can be extended by including other skin diseases like psoriasis,

474   M.A. Taufiq et al.

eczema, skin rashes, skin burns etc. Mobile based health care systems should consume less power and deliver efficient results in real time. Optimal feature selection for smartphone based systems is another open area of research for researchers.

Acknowledgements. We want to say special thanks to Klinik und Poliklinik für Dermatologie und Allergologie, Technische Universitat Munchen, Germany for providing the classified dataset. We would also like to thanks Dr. Asad Ali Safi and Dr. Alamgir Hossain for his continuous support and guidance.

References

1. Maglogiannis, I., Doukas, C.N.: Overview of advanced computer vision systems for skin lesions characterization. IEEE Trans. Inf. Technol. Biomed. **13**(5), 721–733 (2009)
2. Abuzaghleh, O., Barkana, B.D., Faezipour, M.: Noninvasive real-time automated skin lesion analysis system for melanoma early detection and prevention. IEEE J. Transl. Eng. Health Med. **3**, 1–12 (2015)
3. Melanoma Skin Cancer. http://www.skincancer.org/skin-cancer-information/melanoma. Accessed 4 Feb 2016
4. American cancer society. Cancer facts & figures 2015. Atlanta: American cancer society. Technical report, American Cancer Society (2015)
5. Nachbar, F., Stolz, W., Merkle, T., Cognetta, A.B., Vogt, T., Landthaler, M., Bilek, P., Braun-Falco, O., Plewig, G.: The ABCD rule of dermatoscopy. High prospective value in the diagnosis of doubtful melanocytic skin lesions. J. Am. Acad. Dermatol. **30**, 551–559 (1994)
6. Binu Sathiya, S., Kumar, S., Prabin, A.: A survey on recent computer-aided diagnosis of melanoma. In: 2014 International Conference on Control, Instrumentation, Communication and Computational Technologies, pp. 1387–1392 (2014)
7. Argenziano, G., Fabbrocini, G., Carli, P., De Giorgi, V., Sammarco, E., Delfino, M.: Epiluminescence microscopy for the diagnosis of doubtful melanocytic skin lesions. Comparison of the ABCD rule of dermatoscopy and a new 7-point checklist based on pattern analysis. Arch. Dermatol. **134**, 1563–1570 (1998)
8. Argenziano, G., Soyer, H.P., Chimenti, S., Talamini, R., Corona, R., Sera, F., Binder, M., Cerroni, L., et al.: Dermoscopy of pigmented skin lesions: results of a consensus meeting via the Internet. J. Am. Acad. Dermatol. **48**(5), 679–693 (2003). http://www.sciencedirect.com/science/article/pii/S0190962203003530
9. Peter Braun, R., Rabinovitz, H.S., Oliviero, M., Kopf, A.W., Saurat, J.-H.: Dermoscopy of pigmented skin lesions. J. Am. Acad. Dermatol. **52**, 109–121 (2005)
10. Kassianos, A.P., Emery, J.D., Murchie, P., Walter, F.M.: Smartphone applications for melanoma detection by community patient and generalist clinician users: a review. Br. J. Dermatol., 1507–1518
11. Android phones are getting cheaper. http://uk.businessinsider.com/android-iphone-price-disparity-increase-2015-2. Accessed 28 Feb 2016
12. Dermatology Planet by Edizioni Scripta Manent. https://itunes.apple.com/us/app/dermatology-planet/id499547735?mt=8. Accessed 4 Feb 2016
13. Melanoma Watch, IOS application by Stroika. https://itunes.apple.com/gb/app/melanoma-watch/id381272252?mt=8. Accessed 4 Feb 2016

14. Dermlink.md, IOS application by Dermlink.Inc. https://itunes.apple.com/us/app/dermlink.md/id548549220?ls=1&mt=8. Accessed 4 Feb

15. iDoc24 - Ask the dermatologist today!, IOS application by iDoc24 Inc. https://itunes.apple.com/gb/app/idoc24-ask-dermatologist-today!/id481226133?mt=8. Accessed 5 Feb 2016

16. OnlineDermClinic, IOS application by OnlineDermClinic.com LLC. https://itunes.apple.com/us/app/onlinedermclinic/id573545197?mt=8. Accessed 5 Feb 2016

17. Jain, S., Jagtap, V., Pise, N.: Computer aided melanoma skin cancer detection using image processing. In: International Conference on Computer, Communication and Convergence, vol. 48, pp. 735–740 (2015)

18. Karargyris, A., Karargyris, O., Pantelopoulos, A.: DERMA/care: an advanced image-processing mobile application for monitoring skin cancer. In: 2012 IEEE 24th International Conference on Tools with Artificial Intelligence, vol. 2, pp. 1–7 (2012)

19. Abuzaghleh, O., Faezipour, M., Barkana, B.D.: Skincure: an innovative smartphone-based application to assist in melanoma early detection and prevention. Sig. Image Process. Int. J. 5 (6), 1–15 (2014)

20. Bourouis, A., Zerdazi, A., Feham, M., Bouchachia, A.: M-Health: skin disease analysis system using smartphone's camera. In: The 8th International Symposium on Intelligent Systems Techniques for Ad hoc and Wireless Sensor Networks (IST-AWSN), pp. 116–1120 (2013)

21. Doukas, C., Stagkopoulos, P., Kiranoudis, C.T., Maglogiannis, I.: Automated skin lesion assessment using mobile technologies and cloud platforms. In: 34th Annual International Conference of the IEEE EMBS, pp. 2444–2447 (2012)

22. Ramlakhan, K., Shang, Y.: A mobile automated skin lesion classification system. In: 23rd IEEE International Conference on Tools with Artificial Intelligence, pp. 138–141 (2011)

23. Hadi, S., Tumbelaka, B., Irawan, B., Rosadi, R.: Implementing DEWA framework for early diagnosis of melanoma. In: International Conference on Computer Science and Computational Intelligence, Procedia Computer Science, vol. 59, pp. 410–418 (2015)

24. Rother, C., Kolmogorov, V., Blake, A.: "GrabCut" — Interactive Foreground Extraction using Iterated Graph Cuts. Microsoft Research Cambridge

25. OpenCV. http://opencv.org/about.html. Accessed 19 Jan 2016

Perceptual Quality of Reconstructed Medical Images on Projection-Based Light Field Displays

Peter A. Kara[1,4(✉)], Peter T. Kovacs[2,3], Suren Vagharshakyan[3], Maria G. Martini[1], Sandor Imre[4], Attila Barsi[2], Kristof Lackner[2], and Tibor Balogh[2]

[1] Wireless Multimedia and Networking Research Group, Kingston University, London, UK
{p.kara,m.martini}@kingston.ac.uk
[2] Holografika, Budapest, Hungary
{p.kovacs,a.barsi,k.lackner,t.balogh}@holografika.com
[3] Department of Signal Processing, Tampere University of Technology, Tampere, Finland
{peter.t.kovacs,suren.vagharshakyan}@tut.fi
[4] Department of Networked Systems and Services,
Budapest University of Technology and Economics, Budapest, Hungary
{kara,imre}@hit.bme.hu

Abstract. With the appearance of light field displays, users may enjoy a much more natural sensation of 3D experience compared to prior technologies. This type of autostereoscopic, glasses-free visualization allows medical applications to improve both in usability and efficiency. The high angular resolution of medical images is resource-consuming, but can only be reduced while maintaining a sufficient level of overall quality through continuous parallax. A dense image set can also be achieved by applying the synthesis of intermediate views. In this paper we provide the analysis of the effect of reduced angular resolution and image synthesis on Quality of Experience in medical applications. Two separate series of subjective quality assessment measurements were conducted with 20 participants each, one focusing on angular resolution reduction and another one comparing the effect of such reductions with the quality of reconstructed images.

Keywords: Quality of experience · Perceived quality · Medical QoE · Light field display · Angular resolution · Light field reconstruction · View synthesis · Image-based rendering

1 Introduction

Autostereoscopic displays enable 3D experience without any special head gear (e.g., 3D glasses). Unlike stereoscopic display technologies, where the number of views is exactly 2, glasses-free systems do not define such a value. Although it needs to be at least 2, no theoretical upper limit exists; the number of views is only bounded by device capabilities.

Using more views to display a specific content requires more resources but, on the other hand, an insufficient number of views may result in serious degradation of the perceived quality [1] and can completely ruin usability. Immersive visual applications –

© ICST Institute for Computer Sciences, Social Informatics and Telecommunications Engineering 2017
K. Giokas et al. (Eds.): eHealth 2016, LNICST 181, pp. 476–483, 2017.
DOI: 10.1007/978-3-319-49655-9_58

such as those with medical content – necessitate high quality at the user side [2] in order to prevent certain incidents, i.e. flawed diagnosis.

In certain cases, it might not be possible to acquire enough visual inputs to support a display with sufficient image density. In case of light field displays, the reconstruction of intermediate views – also known as light field reconstruction – enables continuous motion parallax [3, 4], so that no discrete borders may appear between views.

In this paper we wish to address two research questions. The first one focuses on the relationship between angular resolution and the perceived quality of medical images, and the second one compares the effect of angular resolution reduction with light field reconstruction. While image synthesis directly affects the quality of the image, a lower number of views alters the way the image is displayed, diminishes continuous parallax and thus disturbs perception. Both may degrade the experience and impair usability, but the question is which one of these two makes a higher impact on the Quality of Experience.

The paper is structured as follows: Sect. 2 introduces the research setup of the series of measurements carried out, Sect. 3 presents the obtained results and Sect. 4 concludes our findings.

2   Research Configuration

Although the research was performed in two parts, both series of measurements used the same light field display and the test stimuli were based on the same reference stimulus (see Fig. 1). The display was a HoloVizio C80 [5, 6], a LED-based 3D projection unit with a 40° field of view. The core stimulus was the 3D still image series of a rendered human heart in 1024 × 576 resolution. During the experiment, the test participant had to make at least a slight movement to the left and the right in order to properly observe the stimuli and to witness issues with continuous motion parallax during test cases with lower angular resolutions.

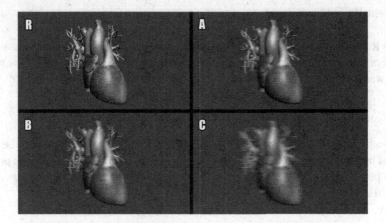

Fig. 1. Test stimuli of the research measurements. Stimulus R is there reference quality, stimulus A, B and C are the reconstructed images.

2.1 Research 1 – Angular Resolution

The first part of the research was the evaluation of angular resolution. For this, we selected 10 views, running from view number 15 to 150 with intervals of 15 (15, 30, 45 etc.). Assessment was performed on a quantitative 10-point Absolute Category Rating (ACR) [7], running from 1 to 10, where 1 was the lowest possible score and 10 was the reference quality. The subjective assessment of quality always began by showing the reference test case – which is just to be observed and not to be rated – followed by a randomized sequence of test cases. The reference test case had 150 views, thus it was identical to one of the test cases, making a hidden reference in the test measurement.

2.2 Research 2 – Light Field Reconstruction

In the second part of the research, there were six test cases in total. Three of them were identical to the ones in the previous experiment, namely those with 30, 60 and 90 number of views. The other three (see Fig. 1) were created with light field reconstruction using shearlet transform [8, 9], based on the reference image. Stimulus A was decimated by a factor of 2 (meaning that every 2nd row was retained while the others were zeroed) and this value was 3 for stimulus B. In case of stimulus C, in order to generate an input with significantly inferior quality, representing a poorly designed reconstruction solution, the setup was tuned so that the maximum disparity between two images was too high for the algorithm, resulting in a high level of blur and distortion.

The algorithm used for reconstruction generated 1024 views, from which every 4th (256 views) was used for the research measurement. Similarly to Research 1, the assessment was performed on a 10-point ACR scale, but the test participant had to simultaneously take into consideration the changing image quality and the number of views. Also, the measurement started with the reference quality, followed by the 6 test cases in random order.

3 Results

In both Research 1 and 2, a total of 20 test participants provided scores for the test cases. 8 of them were medical experts and 12 were non-experts. The average age of the participants was 26.

3.1 Research 1

The results of Research 1 (see Fig. 2) show the breakpoint of excellence to be at 75 views. The three lowest number of views (15, 30 and 45) cannot be considered to provide an acceptable level of quality for medical purposes. Sufficient angular resolution can be obtained at 60 views and above.

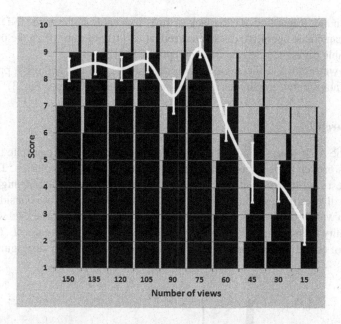

Fig. 2. Results of measurement series Research 1. The black columns provide the actual scores of the test cases, while the points with vertical bars in the white curve represent the Mean Opinion Score with confidence interval.

In case of 45 views, the upmost score extremes can be witnessed, since one particular test subject could not distinguish it from the reference quality, while another deemed it to be absolutely unacceptable. Such outliers can of course distort the mean results, not to mention other types of cognitive bias, like the avoidance of extreme values.

The reason of the sudden high scores of 75 could be the contrast effect if test cases had not been random; while for most people test case 60 provided certain perceptual artefacts, such as ghost image parts or perceivable discrete borders between images, 75

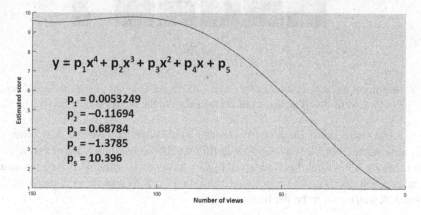

Fig. 3. Estimated Mean Opinion Score model for number of views.

had nearly none. Regarding 90, the lack of Just Noticeable Difference (JND) between 75 and 90 can create cognitive dissonance reduction [10], during which the preconception of notable differences overwrites perception [11, 12].

In case we remove outliers and inconsistent scores, we can acquire a preliminary model that maps between number of views and estimated MOS (see Fig. 3).

3.2   Research 2

Based on the ACR scores obtained for Research 2 (see Fig. 4), we can state that image quality was proven to be a more important aspect than angular resolution. The reason why most test cases of different view numbers (30 and 60) received notably higher scores than identical ones in Research 1 is that image quality was taken into consideration as well, which was the same as the reference quality. Test case 90 was assessed with a very similar quality rating compared to the top 4 number of views in Research 1. This is due to the lack of cognitive bias, because these test cases were evidently distinguishable for most.

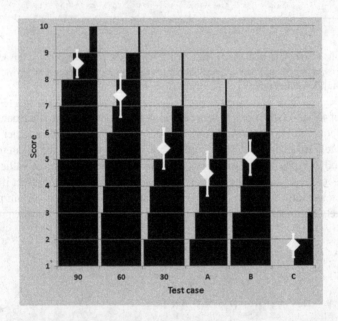

Fig. 4. Results of measurement series Research 2. The black columns provide the actual scores of the test cases, while the white diamonds are the values of the Mean Opinion Score.

As it can also be seen, the properly reconstructed images received slightly lower yet quite alike scores than test case 30, suggesting similar acceptability. However, what is rather curious is that stimulus B received higher scores than stimulus A. As a reminder, stimulus A was decimated by a factor of 2 and stimulus B by a factor of 3, meaning that stimulus A was meant to be the better one.

If we observe the score distribution of test case 30, A and B (see Fig. 5), we can see great diversity among the results. 8 test participants declared test case 30 to have a better quality than the reconstructed light fields, 5 evaluated in the opposite direction, 3 could not distinguish the overall quality of these test cases and 4 provided mixed results. With respect to test case A and B, B received higher scores 9 times, A and B were given the same scores also 9 times, and A was evaluated to be better 2 times. These differences are usually just 1 or 2, but can be even 7, on a scale from 1 to 10.

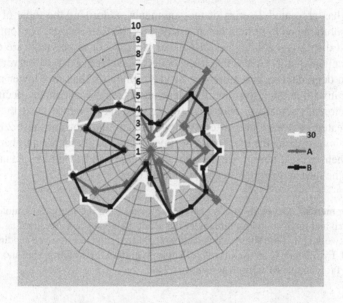

Fig. 5. Score distribution of test case 30, A and B.

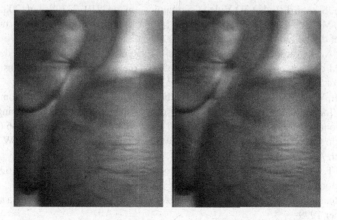

Fig. 6. Comparison of detail of stimulus A (left) and B (right).

The assessments of Research 2 favored test case B, because even though decimation by a factor of 3 provides lesser quality, some points of the stimulus actually appeared to be sharper, less blurry, due to some overlapping visual artefacts, creating higher contrast (see Fig. 6).

4   Conclusions

The paper has presented 2 series of measurements, addressing the topic of sufficient angular resolution and light field reconstruction for medical images. We found that for a light field display for 40 degrees of field of view, 75 or more views are enough to provide excellent quality. According to the collected subjective data, observers are more sensitive to degradations in texture due to view synthesis than to a lower number of views. The investigation also shows that depending on medical content, decimation by a higher factor may actually provide better overall visual experience due to the increased contrast created by overlapping artefacts. Possible continuations of these 2 researches are closely investigating the breakpoint in experienced quality for the number of views, compare them with different view synthesis methods and to utilize actual medical footage in the measurements instead of rendered ones.

Acknowledgments. The work in this paper was funded from the European Union's Horizon 2020 research and innovation program under the Marie Sklodowska-Curie grant agreement No 643072, Network QoE-Net. The research leading to these results has received funding from the PROLIGHT-IAPP Marie Curie Action of the People programme of the European Union's Seventh Framework Programme, REA grant agreement 32449.

References

1. Ijsselsteijn, W., Seuntiens, P., Meesters, L.: Human factors of 3D displays. In: Scheer, O., Kauff, P., Sikora, T. (eds.) 3D Video Communication, pp. 219–233. Wiley (2005)
2. Butt, A., Mahoney, M., Savage, N.W.: The impact of computer display performance on the quality of digital radiographs: a review. Aust. Dent. J. **57**, 16–23 (2012)
3. Ouazan, A., Kovacs, P.T., Balogh, T., Barsi, A.: Rendering multi-view plus depth data on light-field displays. In: 3DTV Conference: The True Vision – Capture, Transmission and Display of 3D Video (3DTV-CON), Antalya, pp. 1–4 (2011)
4. Farre, M., Wang, O., Lang, M., Stefanoski, N., Hornung, A., Smolic, A.: Automatic content creation for multiview autostereoscopic displays using image domain warping. In: IEEE International Conference on Multimedia and Expo (ICME), Barcelona, pp. 1–6 (2011)
5. HoloVizio C80 3D cinema system. http://www.holografika.com/Products/NEW-HoloVizio-C80.html. Accessed February 2016
6. Balogh, T.: The HoloVizio system. In: Proceedings of SPIE, Stereoscopic Displays and Applications XIII, vol. 6055 (2006)
7. ITU-T Rec. P.910: Subjective video quality assessment methods for multimedia applications, September 1999
8. Vagharshakyan, S., Bregovic, R., Gotchev, A.: Image based rendering technique via sparse representation in shearlet domain. In: IEEE International Conference on Image Processing (ICIP), Quebec City, pp. 1379–1383 (2015)

9. Vagharshakyan, S., Bregovic, R., Gotchev, A.: Light field reconstruction using shearlet Transform. CoRR, (2015)
10. Festinger, L.: A Theory of Cognitive Dissonance. Stanford University Press, Stanford (1957)
11. Kara, P.A., Sackl, A., Mourão, M., Bokor, L.: What your phone makes you see: investigation of the effect of end-user devices on the assessment of perceived multimedia quality. In: 7th International Workshop on Quality of Multimedia Experience (QoMEX), Costa Navarino, Messinia, Greece, pp. 1–6 (2015)
12. Sackl, A., Zwickl, P., Egger, S., Reichl, P.: The role of cognitive dissonance for QoE evaluation of multimedia services. In: IEEE Globecom Workshops (GC Wkshps), pp. 1352–1356 (2012)

A Survey on Multimedia Quality of Experience Assessment Approaches in Mobile Healthcare Scenarios

Tamás Péteri[⊠], Norbert Varga, and László Bokor

Department of Networked Systems and Services,
Multimedia Networks and Services Laboratory (MediaNets),
Budapest University of Technology and Economics,
Műegyetem rakpart 3-9., Budapest 1111, Hungary
peteritom@gmail.com, {vnorbert,bokorl}@hit.bme.hu

Abstract. The digital revolution in healthcare presents day after day new solutions to us. As one of the major roles in healthcare is the prevention of being diseased by the popularization of healthier living and doing sports, a vast majority of digital applications aims at self-monitoring and activity tracking via new wearable gadgets and smartphone apps. Also there are solutions for making the work of physicians and medical specialists easier and change their attitude for digital resolutions. This article gives an overview of mobile healthcare status respect to general and multimedia-related solutions and highlights the importance of the respect of Quality of Experience in these applications.

Keywords: Quality of experience (QoE) · mobile healthcare (mHealth) · electronic healthcare (eHealth) · Mobile medical multimedia · Quality assessment

1 Introduction

The term eHealth[1] exists from 1999 [1]. It describes the use of electronic communication and information technology in healthcare. eHealth also includes the transmission and storage of digital data for clinical, educational scenarios and their administration [2]. A research from 2005 found out that under the term eHealth specialists mean a large spectrum of themes but there was not a solid definition about what is eHealth [3]. Therefore eHealth involves several topics such as telemedicine, homecare and clinical information systems [4,5].

A new idea in eHealth should be well mature and prepared towards to a solution that is suitable for the medical practice and accepted by physicians and patients as well. However, another important aspect when discussing about eHealth services is the patient - health professional relationship. In several cases patients are more involved in the case of eHealth services than in the case of regular healthcare services, in short eHealth brings closer the patient to the doctor [6].

---

[1] electronic healthcare.

© ICST Institute for Computer Sciences, Social Informatics and Telecommunications Engineering 2017
K. Giokas et al. (Eds.): eHealth 2016, LNICST 181, pp. 484–491, 2017.
DOI: 10.1007/978-3-319-49655-9_59

As the mobile world has started its exponential evolution from the early 2000s, a new term has appeared stem from eHealth: the mHealth[2]. Under this theme, there are increasingly popular solutions that use the possibilities of ever-changing telecommunication networks and mobile devices in medical practice and supporting for the everyday user's health-related intentions (self-"patient monitoring") as well [7]. An example for patient-monitoring application is Laborom, a free to use iOS and Android app which brings the medical data (e.g., diabetes records) about the patient to their pockets and they can send them in a report format to their doctors [8].

The wireless networks that deliver the mHealth services to users need well-defined QoS[3] parameters (e.g., bandwidth and delay) that grant the reliable transmission. These QoS parameters are often unknown so they need to be predicted, like it is presented in [9]. However, a mHealth application itself could set extra QoS requirements that should be taken into consideration in addition to network's demands. For example in a real-time scenario, an ECG[4] signal should be transmitted without noticeable delay [10].

The increase of available gadgets that communicate to the smartphones in wired or wireless way causes a raise in the world of mHealth applications. This is the case with a smartphone dongle which can make a laboratory-quality diagnosis of infectious diseases, such as HIV and syphilis within 15 min. It simplifies the diagnosis procedure with reducing the laboratory costs and waiting time for the results [11].

A large group of these applications deals with the transmission, visualization and storage of multimedia content in mobile equipments, created by medical devices [12]. In this scenario a product made by Philips, called Lumify implements a simple portable ultrasound solution. Lumify includes a handheld ultrasound device and its smartphone/tablet application which enables the user to watch and store lively the ultrasound recording [13].

The available bandwidth and other parameters should be considered when transmitting multimedia signals in various wireless telecommunication systems. Therefore the image and video content should be compressed to satisfy the bandwidth requirements [14]. The level of quality degradation caused by compression and transmission could be measured by evaluating the quality perceived by specialists and outsiders. The respect of QoE[5] when designing an eHealth or mHealth services is a cardinal issue since it is the most important factor of the implementation. The goal of this paper is to provide a survey on topics of Quality of Experience assessment in medical multimedia applications and mHealth services.

This article has the following structure: it begins with an explanation of the role of QoE in eHealth and mHealth services, after that a review of various QoE-based service improvement approaches in mHealth is presented. Finally, in Sect. 4 we conclude the paper.

---

[2] mobile healthcare.
[3] Quality of Service.
[4] Electrocardiography.
[5] Quality of Experience.

2 The Role of QoE in Electronic and Mobile Healthcare Services

To realize a mHealth (or an eHealth) application is a challenge. A wide range of aspects should be concerned, such as: the human demands (both non-specialists and medical specialists), technology limits, economical considerations and legal issues. A statistic from article [15] points out that the most important factor for an eHealth service implementation is the user acceptance.

The importance of adequate QoE in eHealth is obvious. For example: data loss could cause false judgments in diagnosis and latency or delay has effect e.g. to the remote surgeon's performance. It is essential to realize the characteristics of eHealth services and define the role of QoE in acceptance of these services. It is supposed that eHealth in general should follow the same standards of quality and safety as that in the traditional healthcare. Therefore eHealth services could have several quality requirements depending on the "application purpose", which could be for example: professional, clinical interest or non-clinical interest (i.e. educational). It is noticeable that clinical applications have the most strict requirements. Other subjective sights of a service could affect the quality requirements and the user perception as well, i.e., content type (video, audio, image) and user context (emergency, hospital or primary care). The quality requirements of an eHealth application also depend on the context of use: real-time and non real-time solutions have different quality demands [16]. Based on the above mentioned remarks it is obvious that the user acceptance should be in the centre of an eHealth system and every stakeholders of this system should operate to subserve the user acceptance of the system [15,17]. In the acceptance process of. an electronic or mobile healthcare solution the users are both the patients and healthcare specialists [18].

When planning a mobile or electronic healthcare application that will be used in a medical establishment, QoE has an undealt conception: the diagnostic relevance. This means that medical specialists should be involved in the right segment of the implementation. Only they could validate an IT innovation in medical practice. Some researches (e.g., [19–22]) investigate in lossy compression methods in the case of medical videos in order to reduce the need to huge bandwidth and high compression ratios. However, impairing a medical video could cause quality degradation regarding to the diagnostical relevance too. To examine this lessened diagnostical quality in medical recordings a quality evaluation method could be used. The article [23] classifies and specifies the different medical image and viceo quality assessment approaches in eHealth services.

Nedia Nouri et al. in [19] used the DSCQS[6] measurement method recommended by the ITU[7] [24]. Seven expert surgeons were involved in the subjective test. Reference and impaired videos were shown to the attendants and they had to evaluate the sequences regarding to the diagnostical relevance based on their medical experience. The outcome of the analysis is that a compression ratio

---

[6] Double-stimulus continuous quality-scale.

[7] International Telecommunication Union.

of around 90:1 can be achieved with MPEG-2[8] compression in robotic-assisted surgery videos. A more complex task in telesurgery is the implementation of 3D video which is a complex multimedia signal regarding to the human perception. 3D video uses higher bandwidth and storage capacity compared to other 2D medical video thus it is necessary to use the compression method with a setup which results degradation under the surgeons' perception [20].

The research [21] used the DSCQS evaluation method for similar purpose. M. Razaak et al. reviewed the usage of HEVC[9] compression coding in the case of ultrasound videos. The huge result of this measurement is that diagnostic quality videos can be obtained at the compression ratio range of 140:1 to 420:1 by HEVC compression.

The H.264 coding standard for ultrasound and CT[10] recordings was examined in article [22]. In this case the DSCQS method was used to verify the efficiency of a new rate control scheme in H.264 standard proposed by Hongtao Yu et al. The result is that the proposed model can achieve better perceptual quality than the existing method implemented in H.264.

In this section the importance of QoE and diagnostical relevant quality assessment in electronic and mobile healthcare services was presented with some examples. The next section introduces several service improvement approaches based on having respect for QoE in mHealth services.

3   QoE-Based Service Improvement Approaches in mHealth

Mobile healthcare services as eHealth, bring together the IT sector's innovations and the demands of the healthcare services. mHealth takes advantage of mobile networks, mobile computing and medical sensors [25] and produces new wireless solutions in e.g. telemedicine and telemonitoring with using wearables in body area networks. With worn and/or implanted sensors several physiological parameters could be monitored, such as blood pressure, body temperature and ECG signals [26]. ECG signals are measured in project [28] which realizes telemonitoring system's mobile adaption for patients with cardiovascular diseases in Georgia with using 3-channel ECG Loop Recorder communicating with smartphones via Bluetooth. ECG and other patient vital signal types are one of the influence factors in QoE of remote monitoring services. Other QoE factors and their details are discussed in [29,30]. In [27] in order to satisfy the medical level QoE/QoS requirements in multi-sensor based mobile patient monitoring services a proper Wi-Fi network selection method is presented which is using a multi-criteria decision engine.

It is necessary to run the mHealth service on a robust wireless broadband network that can grant a connection for the desirable bandwidth. The bandwidth requirement is crucial in the case of mHealth applications that realize solutions

---

[8] Moving Picture Experts Group 2 standard.
[9] High Efficiency Video Coding (H.265).
[10] Computed tomography.

in e.g., wireless diagnostic system for patients living in a distance, hospital consultation with streaming medical video content and emergency scenarios where data transfer between the scene and the hospital [31]. To optimize the service that uses the wireless network, the QoS requirements of the mHealth application should be defined. A comprehensive overview of QoS demands (e.g., delay and loss) of different types of eHealth and 4G mHealth applications could be found in [32,33]. A possible optimization could obtain by using cross-layer designed network (e.g., 3G and 4G systems) concept that allows the medical video streaming [39]. The priorization of the traffic of eHealth services with different QoS requirements can be done based on QoE management [40].

In an ubiquitous health monitoring service with heterogeneous networks, the medical images should be perfect in regarding to pixel loss that might influence the diagnostic process. The article [34] summarizes the objective, subjective and quasi-subjective metrics in medical-image quality evaluation. Objective quality metrics are serving instant information about quality thus they are suitable in real-time scenarios [35]. Objective metrics mentioned in [34] are suitable to reflect to the quality percieved by medical experts [36,37]. The article [38] analyses the quality with subjective and objective metrics in the case of mobile robotic tele-ultrasound system that sends ultrasound images through 3G network.

More than 165,000 health-related apps exist in the online smartphone application stores for general purposes for everyday users, e.g.: fitness, workout assistant, bodyweight tracker, sleep monitoring applications. Only few of these applications have reasonable quality reviews. The problem is that there is no standardized quality evaluation method for smartphone apps [41,42]. In [43] several health-related app evaluation and selection methods are proposed to healthcare service providers to make the app recommendation to their patients easier. The tool [44] measures the QoE in the case of mHealth apps. The measurement is based on a survey which contains 21 questions about several quality factors of a health-related application, e.g., content quality, security, use, availability, performance and accuracy. The similar MARS mHealth app quality rating tool [45] relies on quality indicators, such as: subjective quality, engagement, functionality, aesthetics and information quality, that were extracted from previous mHealth literature and researches.

4   Conclusion

This paper reviews a few solutions from the area of eHealth and mHealth services and features the term of Quality of Experience. It discusses several mHealth service improvements based on increasing the QoE by the help of quality assessment methods. This article grounds for further works that takes account of Quality of Experience in the field of mobile healthcare.

Acknowledgement. The work leading to these results has been partly funded by the National Research, Development and Innovation Office's Hungarian-Montenegrin Bilateral Research Project (TET-15-1-2016-0039) and also by the ÚNKP-16-4-I. New National Excellence Program of the Ministry of Human Capacities of Hungary.

References

1. Mitchell, J.: From Telehealth to e-health: The Unstoppable Rise of e-health. Commonwealth Department of Communications, Information Technology and the Arts, Australia (1999)
2. Della Mea, V.: What is e-Health (2): the death of telemedicine? J. Med. Internet Res. **3**(2), e22 (2001)
3. Oh, H., et al.: What Is eHealth (3): a systematic review of published definitions. J. Med. Internet Res. **7**(1), e1 (2005)
4. eHealth Industries Innovation Centre: What is eHealth? a new definition for eHealth. http://www.ehi2.swan.ac.uk/en/what-is-ehealth.htm
5. Svensson, P.-G.: eHealth applications in health care management. eHealth Int. **1**, 5 (2002)
6. European Patients Forum - User acceptance of eHealth: hype, hope or reality? (2012). http://www.eu-patient.eu/News/News-Archive/User-acceptance-of-eHealth-hype-hope-or-reality-/
7. World Health Organization (WHO): mHealth - new horizons for health through mobile technologies: based on the findings of the second global survey on eHealth. Global Observatory for eHealth series, vol. 3 (2011)
8. Laborom. http://www.laborom.org/
9. Wac, K.: Towards quality of service-awareness of mobile healthcare services. In: Jordanova, M., Lievens, F. (eds.) Electronic Proceedings of the International eHealth, Telemedicine and Health ICT Forum for Educational, Networking and Business - Med-e-Tel, pp. 288–292 (2009)
10. Sanchez Meraz, M., et al.: Quality of service in wireless technologies for mhealth service providing. In: Adibi, S. (ed.) Mobile Health. Springer Series in Bio-/Neuroinformatics, vol. 5, pp. 971–989. Springer, Heidelberg (2015)
11. Laksanasopin, T., et al.: A smartphone dongle for diagnosis of infectious diseases at the point of care. Sci. Transl. Med. **7**(273), 273re1 (2015)
12. Razaak, M., et al.: A study on quality assessment for medical ultrasound video compressed via HEVC. IEEE J. Biomed. Health Inf. **18**, 2168–2194 (2014)
13. Philips - Lumify (2015). https://www.lumify.philips.com/web/
14. Axis Communications: An explanation of video compression techniques. White paper (2008)
15. Rojas-Mendizabal, V.A., et al.: Toward a model for quality of experience and quality of service in e-health ecosystems. Procedia Technol. **9**, 968–974 (2013)
16. Ullah, M., et al.: On the ambiguity of quality of service and quality of experience requirements for eHealth services. In: Medical Information and Communication Technology (ISMICT) (2012)
17. Da, X., et al.: Improving quality of experience in M-health monitoring system. In: 35th Annual International Conference of the IEEE EMBS, pp. 2271–2274 (2013)
18. Rehman, I.U., Philip, N.Y.: M-QoE driven context, content and network aware medical video streaming based on fuzzy logic system over 4G and beyond small cells. In: International Conference on Computer as a Tool, EUROCON 2015. IEEE (2015)
19. Nouri, N., et al.: Subjective MPEG2 compressed video quality assessment: application to tele-surgery. In: IEEE International Symposium on Biomedical Imaging: From Nano to Macro, pp. 764–767 (2010)
20. Hewage, C.T.E.R., et al.: Quality evaluation of compressed 3D surgical video. In: 2nd International Workshop on Service Science for e-Health, pp. 71–76. IEEE HEALTHCOM (2014)

21. Razaak, M., Martini, M.G.: Rate-distortion and rate-quality performance analysis of HEVC compression of medical ultrasound videos. Procedia Comput. Sci. **40**, 230236 (2014)

22. Hongtao, Y., et al.: Applications and improvement of H.264 in medical video compression. IEEE Trans. Circ. Syst. I Regul. Pap. **52**(12), 2707–2716 (2005)

23. Razaak, M., Martini, M.G.: Rate-distortion and rate-quality performance analysis of HEVC compression of medical ultrasound videos. Procedia Comput. Sci. **40**, 230–236 (2014)

24. ITU-R BT.500-13: Methodology for the subjective assessment of the quality of television pictures (2012)

25. Istepanaian, R.S., Zhang, Y.T.: Guest editorial introduction to the special section: 4G health - the long-term evolution of m-Health. IEEE Trans. Inf. Technol. Biomed. **16**, 1–5 (2012)

26. Yi, C., et al.: Energy analysis and QoE of wireless sensor networks. In: Adibi, S. (ed.) Mobile Health. Springer Series in Bio-/Neuroinformatics, vol. 5, pp. 947–970. Springer, Heidelberg (2015)

27. Varga, N., et al.: Network-assisted smart access point selection for pervasive real-time mHealth applications. In: The 5th International Conference on Current and Future Trends of Information and Communication Technologies in Healthcare, Procedia Computer Science, vol. 63, pp. 317–324 (2015)

28. Kirtava, Z., et al.: mHealth for cardiac patients telemonitoring and integrated care. IEEE HEALTHCOM **9**, 21–25 (2013)

29. Skorin-Kapov, L., et al.: Towards evaluating the quality of experience of remote patient monitoring services - a study considering usability aspects. IJMHCI **6**(4), 59–89 (2014)

30. Akter, S., et al.: User perceived service quality of m-Health services in developing countries. In: 18th European Conference on Information Systems, pp. 1–12 (2010)

31. Martini, M.G.: Wireless broadband multimedia health services: current status and emerging concepts. In: Personal, Indoor and Mobile Radio Communications, pp. 1–6. IEEE (2008)

32. Skorin-Kapov, L., Matijasevic, M.: Analysis of QoS requirements for e-Health services and mapping to evolved packet system QoS classes. Int. J. Telemedicine Appl. **2010**, 18 (2010)

33. Istepanian, R.S.H., et al.: Medical quality of service (m-QoS) and quality of experience (m-QoE) for 4G-health systems. In: Multimedia Networking and Coding, pp. 359–376. IGI Global (2013)

34. Lin, D., et al.: QoE-based optimal resource allocation in wireless healthcare networks: opportunities and challenges. Wirel. Netw. **21**, 2483–2500 (2015). Springer Science+Business Media, New York

35. Vidhya, K., Shenbagadevi, S.: Performance analysis of medical image compression. In: International Conference on Signal Processing Systems, pp. 979–983. IEEE Computer society (2009)

36. Kumar, B., et al.: Performance of quality metrics for compressed medical images through mean opinion score prediction. J. Med. Imaging Health Inform. **2**, 17 (2012). American Scientific Publishers

37. Dendumrongsup, T., et al.: Multi-reader multi-case studies using the area under the receiver operator characteristic curve as a measure of diagnostic accuracy: systematic review with a focus on quality of data reporting. PLoS ONE **9**(12), e116018 (2014)

38. Istepanian, R.S.H., Martini, M.G.: Subjective and objective quality assessment in wireless teleultrasonography imaging. In: 30th Annual International IEEE EMBS Conference, pp. 5346–5349 (2008)
39. Martini, M.G., et al.: A cross-layer approach for wireless medical video streaming in robotic teleultrasonography. In: Conference Proceedings of IEEE Engineering in Medicine and Biology Society, pp. 3082–3085 (2007)
40. Ojanperä, T., et al.: QoE-based management of medical video transmission in wireless networks. In: Network Operations and Management Symposium (NOMS), pp. 1–6. IEEE (2014)
41. Powell, A.C., et al.: Interrater reliability of mHealth app rating measures: analysis of top depression and smoking cessation apps. JMIR mHealth uHealth 4(1), e15 (2016)
42. Wicks, P., et al.: 'Trust but verify'-five approaches to ensure safe medical apps. BMC Medicine (2015)
43. Boudreaux, E.D., et al.: Evaluating and selecting mobile health apps: strategies for healthcare providers and healthcare organizations. Transl. Behav. Med. 4, 363–371 (2014)
44. Martnez-Prez, B., et al.: Development and Evaluation of Tools for Measuring the Quality of Experience (QoE) in mHealth Applications, pp. 9975–9982. Springer Science+Business Media, New York (2013)
45. Stoyanov, S.R., et al.: Mobile app rating scale: a new tool for assessing the quality of health mobile apps. JMIR mHealth uHealth 3(1), e27 (2015)

Monitoring of Fetal Heart Rate via iPhone

Gábor Sipka[1], Tibor Szabó[1], Ráhel Zölei-Szénási[1], Melinda Vanya[2],
Mária Jakó[2], Tamás Dániel Nagy[1], Márta Fidrich[1(✉)], Vilmos Bilicki[1],
János Borbás[2], Tamás Bitó[2], and György Bártfai[2]

[1] Department of Informatics, University of Szeged,
Dugonics squr. 13, Szeged, 6725, Hungary
fidrich@inf.u-szeged.hu
[2] Albert Szent-Györgyi Clinical Centre, University of Szeged,
Semmelweis str. 1, Szeged, 6725, Hungary

Abstract. Recording of fetal heart rate can be reassuring for the mother about the fetus' wellbeing. Our smart phone application can detect, record and evaluate fetal heart rate at any time. This method is based on sound wave thus free from the effects of ultrasound, and can be used all day without harming the fetus. It does not require medical assistance and easy to use at home. It reduces the queue at outpatient care units, helps pregnant women to relieve stress by listening to their unborn baby's heartbeat. It improves mother-child relationship yet sends an alarming message if further examinations are needed to prevent the consequences of hypoxia.

Keywords: Fetal heart rate · Mobile application · Home monitoring · Phonocardiography

1 Introduction

There are several solutions for the acoustic detection of fetal heart rate (FHR) that can help obstetricians determine whether the fetus is at risk or not [1, 3–5]. From the 38th week (or incase of any complications from the 24th week) cardiotocograph (CTG) is used to monitor the changes and characteristics of fetal pulse and movements. Two transducers are placed on the maternal abdomen; one to detect fetal heart actions (cardio-), the other registers the uterine activity (tocogram). This way the FHR is detected by Doppler ultrasound, while the uterine contractions via a pressure-sensitive contraction transducer, called tocodynamometer. Phonocardiography (PCG) is also proper way to detect fetal heartbeat. The device can record the rhythmic contractions due to the resonance made by the valves.

Brown and Patrick (1981) showed that apart from fetal activity and normal basic FHR the alteration of higher and lower heart rates is also important factor to evaluate the fetal state [2]. They have set up some alternatives for ultrasonographic non-invasive FHR monitoring such as fetal electrocardiography (fECG), fetal magnetocardiography (fMCG), fetal phonocardiography (fPCG). While the fECG requires several electrodes and the form of the recorded waves highly depends on their positions, the fMCG is too

© ICST Institute for Computer Sciences, Social Informatics and Telecommunications Engineering 2017
K. Giokas et al. (Eds.): eHealth 2016, LNICST 181, pp. 492–496, 2017.
DOI: 10.1007/978-3-319-49655-9_60

big and expensive for long time home-monitoring, therefore the fPCG has unquestionable advantages for a safe long lasting use at home environment.

2   Materials and Methods

There are numerous electric stethoscopes available (Welch-Allyn, 3 M Littmann, Thinklabs, Cardionics) but the prices go from 200 to 600 EUROs [4]. Our aim was to develop a small, inexpensive, non-invasive device that can easily be used at home to record FHR constantly. The developed measurement device has three main components:

1. Acoustic sensor, which in our case is a modified stethoscope, with a built-in microphone. The sensor transforms the acoustic signal into electric signal and it is sensitive enough in the target frequency range. The acoustic signal can be conveniently captured by placing the stethoscope on mother's abdomen without usage of gel as in CTG monitor. Furthermore, this stethoscope sensor offers a totally passive means, which promises its potential of long term and safe use.
2. A small-sized amplifier and filtering unit, whose main components are pre-amplifier, band filter, amplifier. To separate fetal heart signal from mother's heartbeat and noise, spectral separation method was used, the acceleration sensor or the piezo sensor was not successful [1, 3, 5]. We note that fetal heart signal is lower, by orders of magnitude, than mother's heartbeat and noises (breathing or bowel sound). The filtered signal is transferred to the signal processing and storage medium by frequency modulator. We included the possibility to listen to the filtered fetal heart signal.
3. Signal processing and storage medium, which in our case is an iPhone or iPad, and its software. The software records the fetal heart signal and after the demodulation finds the position of the fetal heartbeats (real-time) with an automatic process, then shows the number of beats per minute and its variability. It plays an alarming sound in case of unsatisfying (badly recorded) signal. Also, it can evaluate the FHR. A healthy FHR is between 120 and 160 beats per minute, a low (bradycardia) or high (tachycardia) FHR indicates the necessity of other examinations or a closer check up by specialists. The indication of fetal movement is also possible.

Figure 1 presents an example of measured signal vs. background noise after filtering, while Fig. 2 shows screenshots of the running application.

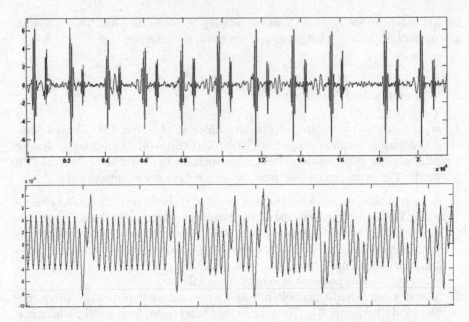

Fig. 1. Measured signal is shown in the top row, where the detected heartbeats S1 and S2 can be clearly seen. Background noise is shown in the bottom row. Signal to noise ratio is 750.

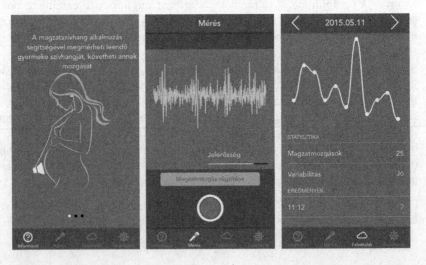

Fig. 2. Menu of the application: Information, Record, Recordings, Settings. the first screen shot is about the information panel. The second screenshot shows the application in work; the recording, the signal, and the fetal movement button. The third screenshot is the statistic evaluation of fetal movements; date, recording, fetal movements (25), evaluation (good), start of the recording.

We compared several stethoscope heads and different recording methods while detecting FHR. Our standard points of auscultation were 3 cm left to the navel and one cm up and down and same points on the right side.

The least accurate method was using the membrane face of stethoscopes used in present clinical practice. This approach is not ideal for FHR detection because stethoscopes are made to detect the maternal heart rate frequency and bowel noises. To get a clarified, noise-free voice file, there are other possible methods. The second best choice is the cone face of a stethoscope. In that case the skin serves as membrane and it reproduces the vibration of fetal heart sound better. The recordings are free from the outer noises (speaking, coughing, traffic). The best approach, however, is to rely on the waveform of the searched sound. We performed several measurements with a 70 mm long and 12 mm wide plastic tube sealed with 5 mm of thread layer. It seems to be optimal for detecting FHR.

We did 60 measurements with 7 patients. The separation of maternal and fetal heart sound was successful in all cases, while the calculation of fetal heart rate and heart rate variability was possible in most of the cases (nearly 70%).

3 Discussion

This PCG recording does not require healthcare assistance and still can provide signals of excellent quality. Although the usability of the FHR recording depends on the relative position of the stethoscope head to the fetal heart, it is sensitive enough to let pregnant women listen to their baby's heart. The method is completely passive, it does not radiates or harms the fetus. Thus it may be used even permanently or only for a shorter time at a family event. It helps women make sure their fetus is healthy, e.g. prevents dysfunctions caused by oxygen deficit. The saved recordings may be sent to doctors, who can immediately provide a diagnosis, hence it is not needed to queue in front of the outpatient care unit. It helps relieve stress, it improves mother-baby relationship, and helps the whole family to prepare to welcome the new member.

To summarize, with this device and application future child's heartbeat & movements may be listened & registered, and medical evaluation may be asked to make sure that the fetus is healthy.

Acknowledgments. This study was supported by "Telemedicine focused Researches on the Fields of Medicine, Mathematics and Informatics" TÁMOP- 4.2.2.A-11/1/KONV-2012-0073 project. The research was financed by the European Union and the European Social Fund.

References

1. Zukerwar, A., Pretlow, R., Stoughton, J., Baker, D.: Development of a piezo-polymer pressure sensor for a portable fetal heart rate monitor. IEEE Trans. Biomed. Eng. **40**(9), 963–969 (1993)
2. Brown, R., Patrick, J.: The nonstress test: How long is enough? Am. J. Obstet. Gyn. **151**, 646–651 (1981)

3. Talbert, D.G., Davies, W.L., Johnson, F., Abraham, N., Colley, N., Southall, D.P.: Wide band with fetal phonography using a sensor matched to the compliance of the mother's abdominal wall. IEEE Trans. Biomed. Eng. **33**, 175–181 (1986)
4. Andrés, E., Hajjam, A., Brandt, C.: Advances and innovations in the field of auscultation, with a special focus on the development of new intelligent communicating stethoscope systems. Health Technol. **2**, 5–16 (2012)
5. Goovaerts, H.G., Rompelman, O., van Geijn, H.P.: A transducer for detection of fetal breathing movements. IEEE Trans. Biomed. Eng. **36**, 471–478 (1989)
6. Nagel, J.: New diagnostic and technical aspects of fetal phonocardiography. Euro. J. Obstet. Gynecol. Reprod. Biol. **23**, 295–303 (1986)

Use of Infertility Handling Among Women of Reproductive Age

Melinda Vanya[1], Mária Jakó[1], Győző Füle[2], Márta Fidrich[2(✉)], Andrea Surányi[1], Tamás Bitó[1], and György Bártfai[1]

[1] Albert Szent-Györgyi Clinical Centre, University of Szeged,
Semmelweis str. 1, Szeged 6725, Hungary
[2] Department of Informatics, University of Szeged,
13 Dugonics square, Szeged 6725, Hungary
fidrich@inf.u-szeged.hu

Abstract. Our primary objective was to develop a mobile application for monitoring the changes of menstrual cycle for clinical treatment planning. Participating woman can use the application called "Infertility Handling", which will be soon available from Google Play Store for general public. This Android-based application provides basic biological and physiological information to women using the application at different stages of the cycle. They will receive useful help and advice concerning their health. The application provides also quick and convenient information gathering for short and long-term management of patient's treatment and excellent tool for the personal medical monitoring. In this paper we present a short summary of the developed application.

Keywords: Menstrual cycle · Monitoring · Android · Basal body temperature

1 Introduction

Telemedicine programs offer potential low-cost and quick solutions for management of several diseases, but infertility. The diagnosis is settled when a couple fail to achieve a successful pregnancy after 6–12 months of regular unprotected sexual intercourse [1]. However fertility can be reduced in both men and women, the diagnosis is usually valid for a couple, and sometimes for a person. The incidence is approximately 15% [2].

The female reproductive system is far more complicated than that in males. Focusing on female infertility, one of the most common causes is ovulatory dysfunction. It might be identified in approximately 15% of all infertile couples and accounts for up to 40% of infertility in women. The most common causes of ovulatory dysfunction include polycystic ovary syndrome, obesity, weight gain or loss, thyroid dysfunction, and hyperprolactinemia. However, the exact cause of ovulatory dysfunction often remains unclear. Basal body temperature (BBT) measurements provide a simple and low cost method for evaluating ovulatory function. If the menstrual cycle is monitored with BBT, it is clear that the period of highest fertility span is the mid-cycle rise in BBT. Healthy ovulatory cycles generally are associated with clearly biphasic BBT recordings and anovulatory cycles typically result in monophasic patterns [3, 4].

© ICST Institute for Computer Sciences, Social Informatics and Telecommunications Engineering 2017
K. Giokas et al. (Eds.): eHealth 2016, LNICST 181, pp. 497–501, 2017.
DOI: 10.1007/978-3-319-49655-9_61

498   M. Vanya et al.

The aim of our study was to monitor and document biphasic BBT and menstrual pattern with mobile phone application among women, in particular among women having irregular cycles and infertility problems. We intend to use this information for successful infertility treatment planning.

2 Materials and Methods

A mobile application was developed to monitor the menstrual cycle of reproductive aged women. It relies on the smartphone's own calendar. After registration, women participating in our study can download the "Infertility handling" mobile phone application from Google Play Store. For each day patients may assign body weight, basal body temperature, medication, complaints, examinations and comments. They can also record the date and duration of menstrual bleeding. On the basis of the recorded information (beginning of menstrual cycle, basal body temperature) the application will predict the potentially best time for a successful fertilization. It may also calculate the first day of the next bleeding, of course (Figs. 1, 2 and 3).

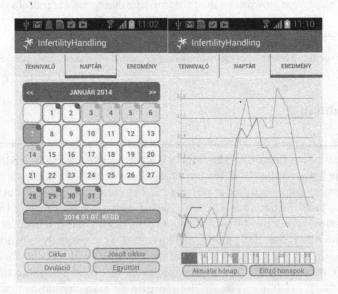

Fig. 1. Design of the "Infertility Handling" application

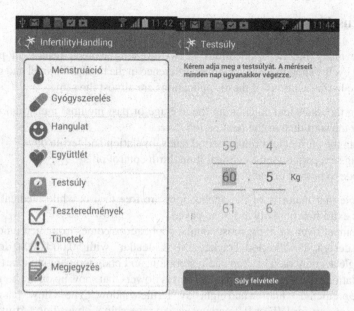

Fig. 2. Management of the events related to BBT measurements

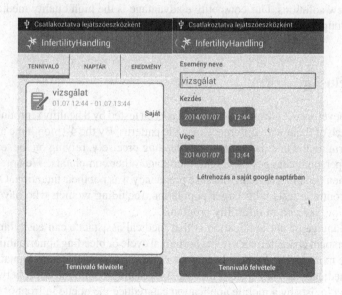

Fig. 3. Usage of the diary function to ask for appointment

3   Discussion

There are many mobile applications (50+) targeting women health, in particular menstrual cycle. Though there are subtle difference in the business model and graphical design, the basic functions of these applications are almost the same:

- logging the dates and calculating the average of past months' menstrual cycles to predict the start date of the next period
- showing the current and future period dates, ovulation and fertile days
- tracking sex, pain, moods, cervical fluid, birth control pills
- passcode to protect privacy

We note that majority of the applications are free to use, while medical services offered as extra functionality are to be payed.

The competitiveness of the most popular applications comes from their unique functions and design. The "Period Tracker - My Calendar" with 50.000.000+ downloads uses Google account data backup and restoration, and body temperature chart to determine ovulation date. The "Period Tracker" uses flowers that show up on the home screen during the predicted ovulation and eight day "fertile window." The "Glow" has a fertility treatment support for IVF or IUI patients, and partnership with leading fertility clinics. The "WomanLog" helps the user to self-exam breast and carry out ovulation test.

Assisting communication between users and gynaecologists still offers opportunity to create new solutions. Our competitive advantage is the high quality medical and IT support through telemedicine services.

4   Conclusion

So far the developed Android application has been tested by 8 healthy reproductive aged women, each of them with difference in cycle patterns. By the 4th month the application could determine the first day of the next bleeding precisely, relying on the temperature curve and personal changes in weight, mood and other complaints. We note that none of the women became pregnant, because pregnancy was not their intention. Our present aim is to continue tests with larger population, including women who have irregular cycles and/or take part in infertility programs.

An advantage of our application is that medical assistance can easily and quickly identify personal characteristics of the hormonal cycle or bleeding abnormalities. Therapies can be more patient-centered and doctors may assign pause or continuation of one or more medications via e.g. text messages. Assisting communication between users and gynaecologists by a mobile application can reduce the queue in front of the outpatient care unit and make the therapy more comfortable. For researchers this programme may provide a huge database to find out new trends in the background of reducing fertility and establish new medications and policy for women.

Acknowledgements. This study was supported by "Telemedicine focused Researches on the Fields of Medicine, Mathematics and Informatics" TÁMOP- 4.2.2.A-11/1/KONV-2012-0073 project. The research was financed by the European Union and the European Social Fund. Special thanks to Péter Seffer, who helped us to compare our application with others in the market.

References

1. Practice Committee of American Society for Reproductive Medicine: Definitions of infertility and recurrent pregnancy loss. Fertil. Steril. **90**, S60 (2008)
2. Mosher, W.D., Pratt, W.F.: Fecundity and infertility in the United States: incidence and trends. Fertil. Steril. **56**, 192 (1991)
3. Luciano, A.A., Peluso, J., Koch, E.I., Maier, D., Kuslis, S., Davison, E.: Temporal relationship and reliability of the clinical, hormonal, and ultrasonographic indices of ovulation in infertile women. Obstet. Gynecol. **75**, 412 (1990)
4. Ecochard, R., Duterque, O., Leiva, R., Bouchard, T., Vigil, P.: Self-identification of the clinical fertile window and the ovulation period. Fertil. Steril. **103**(5), 1319–1325 (2015)
5. Berglund Scherwitzl, E., Lindén Hirschberg, A., Scherwitzl, R.: Identification and prediction of the fertile window using Natural Cycles. Eur. J. Contracept. Reprod. Health Care **16**, 1–6 (2015)
6. Freundl, G., Frank-Herrmann, P., Brown, S., Blackwell, L.: A new method to detect significant basal body temperature changes during a woman's menstrual cycle. Eur. J. Contracept. Reprod. Health Care **19**(5), 392–400 (2014)

Author Index

Printed in the United States
By Bookmasters